Surgical Anatomy of the Sacral Plexus and Its Branches

Surgical Anatomy of the Sacral Plexus and Its Branches

Edited by

R. SHANE TUBBS, MS, PA-C, PHD

JOE IWANAGA, DDS, PHD

MARIOS LOUKAS, MD, PHD

AARON S. DUMONT, MD, MBA, FACS, FAHA, FAANS

MIGUEL ANGEL REINA, MD, PHD

ELSEVIER

Notices

Practitioners and researchers must always rely on their own experience and knowledge in evaluating and using any information, methods, compounds or experiments described herein. Because of rapid advances in the medical sciences, in particular, independent verification of diagnoses and drug dosages should be made. To the fullest extent of the law, no responsibility is assumed by Elsevier, authors, editors or contributors for any injury and/or damage to persons or property as a matter of products liability, negligence or otherwise, or from any use or operation of any methods, products, instructions, or ideas contained in the material herein.

Publisher: Cathleen Sether
Acquisitions Editor: Humayra Rahman
Editorial Project Manager: Megan Ashdown
Production Project Manager: Kiruthika Govindaraju
Cover Designer: Alan Studholme

3251 Riverport Lane
St. Louis, Missouri 63043

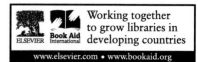

Working together to grow libraries in developing countries

www.elsevier.com • www.bookaid.org

To Maegan Tubbs who is tenacious and David Fisher without whom,
this book would not be possible.

List of Contributors

Nihail Apaydin, MD, PhD
Department of Anatomy
Ankara University School of Medicine
Ankara, Turkey

Department of Neuroscience
Brain Research Center
Ankara University
Ankara, Turkey

André P. Boezaart, MD, PhD
Professor
Department of Anesthesiology and
Department of Orthopaedic Surgery
University of Florida College of Medicine
Gainesville, Florida, United States

The Alon P. Winnie Research Institute
Gainesville, FL, United States

The Alon P. Winnie Research Institute
Still Bay, South Africa

Stephen J. Bordes, Jr., MD
Department of Anatomical Sciences
School of Medicine
St. George's University
St. George's, Grenada

Halle E.K. Burley, MD
Western University of Health Sciences
College of Osteopathic Medicine of the
    Pacific — Northwest
Lebanon, OR, United States

Amarilis Camacho, MD
University of Puerto Rico School of Medicine
San Juan, Puerto Rico

Anna Carrera, MD, PhD
Professor
Department of Medical Sciences (Human Anatomy
    and Embryology Unit)
School of Medicine
University of Girona
Girona, Spain

Claudia Cejas, MD
Head, Radiology Department
Head, MRI Division
Fundación para la Lucha de Enfermedades
    Neurológicas (Fleni)
Buenos Aires, Argentina

Marielle Esteves Coelho, MVD, PhD
Experimental Surgery Unit
Vall d'Hebron Research Institute (VHIR)
Universitat Autònoma de Barcelona
Barcelona, Spain

Graham C. Dupont, BS
Department of Neurosurgery
Tulane University School of Medicine
New Orleans, LA, United States

Paloma Fernández, BS, PhD
Histology Unit
Institute of Applied Molecular Medicine
School of Medicine
CEU San Pablo University
Madrid, Spain

Virginia García-García, TCH
Histology Unit
Institute of Applied Molecular Medicine
School of Medicine
CEU San Pablo University
Madrid, Spain

Santiago Gutierrez, MD
Pontificia Universidad Javeriana
Bogotá, Colombia

Dia R. Halalmeh, MD
Neurological Surgery
Detroit Medical Center
Detroit, MI, United States

Amgad S. Hanna, MD
Associate Professor
Department of Neurological Surgery
University of Wisconsin School of Medicine and
    Public Health
Madison, WI, United States

Joe Iwanaga, DDS, PhD
Associate Professor
Department of Neurosurgery
Clinical Neuroscience Research Center (CNRC)
Tulane University School of Medicine
New Orleans, LA, United States

Division of Gross and Clinical Anatomy
Department of Anatomy
Kurume University School of Medicine
Kurume, Fukuoka, Japan

Skyler Jenkins, MD
Department of Anatomical Sciences
School of Medicine
St. George's University
St. George's, Grenada

Marios Loukas, MD, PhD
Professor and Dean
St. George's University School of Medicine
St. George's, Grenada

Department of Anatomy
University of Warmia and Mazury
Olsztyn, Poland

Malcon Andrei Martinez-Pereira, SR., PhD
Veterinary Doctor, Professor, Animal Anatomy
    and Histology
Embryology and Neurology
Center of Rural Sciences
Federal University of Santa Catarina
Curitibanos, Santa Catarina, Brazil

Antonia Matamala-Adrover, MD, PhD
Spine Unit
Orthopaedic Surgery Department
Hospital Vall d'Hebron
Barcelona, Spain

Karishma Mehta, MD
Department of Anatomical Sciences
St. George's University
St. George's, Grenada

Marc Moisi, MD
Neurological Surgery
Detroit Medical Center
Detroit, MI, United States

Javier Moratinos-Delgado, TCH
Histology Unit
Institute of Applied Molecular Medicine
School of Medicine
CEU San Pablo University
Madrid, Spain

Paul Page, MD
Department of Neurological Surgery
University of Wisconsin School of Medicine and
    Public Health
Madison, WI, United States

Francisco Reina, MD, PhD
Professor
Department of Medical Sciences (Human Anatomy
    and Embryology Unit)
School of Medicine
University of Girona
Girona, Spain

Miguel A. Reina, MD, PhD
Professor, Anesthesiology
Department of Clinical Medical Sciences and
    Institute of Applied Molecular Medicine
School of Medicine
University of CEU San Pablo
Madrid, Spain

Department of Anesthesiology
Madrid-Montepríncipe University Hospital
Madrid, Spain

Félix D. Rodríguez, MD
University of Puerto Rico School of Medicine
San Juan, Puerto Rico

Xavier Sala-Blanch, MD
Associate Professor
Human Anatomy and Embryology Unit
Faculty of Medicine
Department of Anesthesiology
Hospital Clinic
Universitat de Barcelona
Barcelona, Spain

Mercedes Serra, MD
MRI Division
Fundación para la Lucha de Enfermedades
    Neurológicas (Fleni)
Buenos Aires, Argentina

Anna Server, MD, PhD
Department of Anesthesiology
Hospital Universitari Vall d'Hebron
School of Medicine
Universitat de Barcelona
Barcelona, Spain

R. Shane Tubbs, MS, PA-C, PhD
Professor
Department of Neurosurgery
Clinical Neuroscience Research Center (CNRC)
Tulane University School of Medicine
New Orleans, LA, United States
Department of Neurosurgery and Ochsner
    Neuroscience Institute
Ochsner Health System
New Orleans, LA, United States

Tyler Warner, MD
Department of Anatomical Sciences
St. George's University
St. George's, Grenada

Ashley K. Yearwood, MD
Department of Anatomical Sciences
St George's University
St Georges, Grenada

Preface

The anatomy of the sacral plexus (Figs. 1–3) is complex and unlike other plexuses of the body has been less studied and taught in medical curricula. However, with improved technology and newer surgical approaches, e.g., minimally invasive, an increased knowledge of this anatomy and its variations are important in order to minimize complications from invasive procedures and surgery. Therefore, the goal of this book is to provide a detailed look at the human sacral plexus both in regard to detailed anatomy and its importance in clinical medicine and surgery. Examples of recent advances that necessitate an improved knowledge of the sacral plexus and its branches include sacral plexus stimulation (e.g., ventral ramus of S3 for fecal incontinence and pain following cauda equina syndrome), pudendal nerve stimulation (for both urinary and fecal incontinence), new neurotization procedures for restoring function to structures supplied by branches of the sacral plexus, minimally invasive approaches to the lumbosacral spine, and new techniques for anesthetic blockade of branches of the sacral plexus.

The sacral plexus is formed from the upper four sacral ventral rami and forms a large flattened mass lying on the piriformis muscle. Quain summed up (an over-simplification) this anatomy as follows:

…that the several nerves entering into it unite into one broad flat cord…from which the subsidiary branches arise; and which, finally, in the region of the buttock, becomes the great sciatic nerve.

The first two of these ventral rami are large in size and then progressively become smaller as one moves caudally. Visceral efferent rami leave the second to fourth sacral rami as the pelvic splanchnic nerves, containing parasympathetic fibers to minute ganglia in the walls of the pelvic viscera. As with other spinal levels, each sacral nerve communicates with the sympathetic trunk, and the sympathetic ganglia here lie near the medial margin of the anterior sacral foramina. In addition, once the

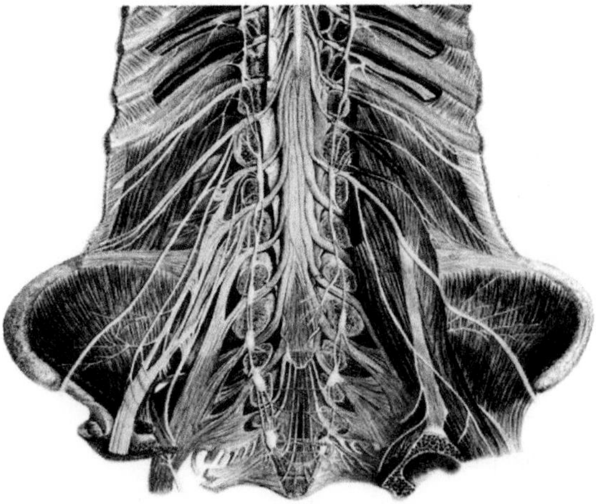

FIGURE 1 Drawing of the sacral plexus. *After Bock.*

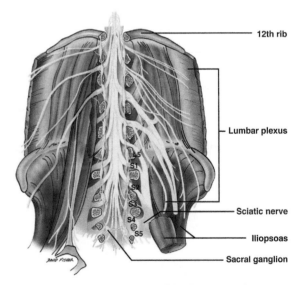

FIGURE 2 Schematic drawing of the abdominopelvic region with the vertebral bodies removed and the vertebral canal and cauda equina exposed. The lumbar plexus and its branches are seen superiorly and the L5 to S4 fibers inferiorly forming the sacral plexus. Note that the psoas major has been mostly removed on the left side.

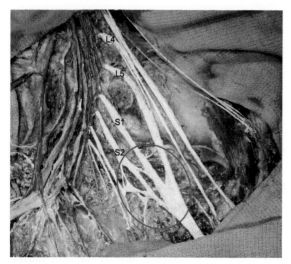

FIGURE 3 Cadaveric dissection focusing on the left sacral plexus. Sacral fibers are colored yellow and lumbar fibers blue. For reference, the ventral rami of L5-S2 are labeled. The blue oval shows the primary parts of the sacral plexus with its main outflow, the sciatic nerve, seen extending distal to the blue oval.

lumbosacral trunk, formed from some of the L4 ventral ramus and all of the L5 ventral ramus, joins with the first sacral ventral ramus, the lumbosacral plexus is formed. Teasing these two plexuses apart from one another is semantic. However, the focus of this book is to detail the clinical and surgical anatomy of the sacral component of the conjoined lumbosacral plexus.

Typically, the sacral plexus is said to have approximately 12 branches. About one half of these travel to the pelvis and the other half to the gluteal region and lower limb. Obviously, some branches of this plexus have received much more attention in the literature and are more clinically significant. However, a comprehensive knowledge of all of these branches is necessary for the physician or surgeon who diagnoses, treats, or operates patients with lesions of the plexus as a whole or its individual branches.

Herein, the reader will find dedicated chapters on each of the branches of the sacral plexus (Figs. 4 and 5) as well as chapters on comparative anatomy, imaging, histology, variations, pathology, and surgery. Additionally, nearby neural structures such as the superior and inferior hypogastric plexuses are detailed. As texts

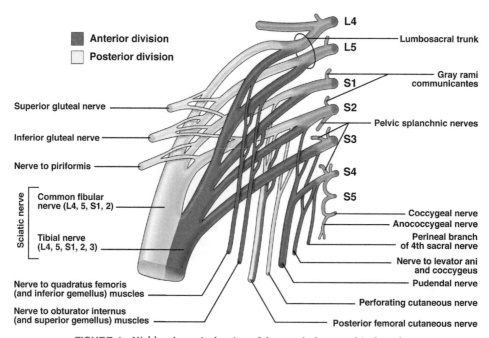

FIGURE 4 Highly schematic drawing of the sacral plexus and its branches.

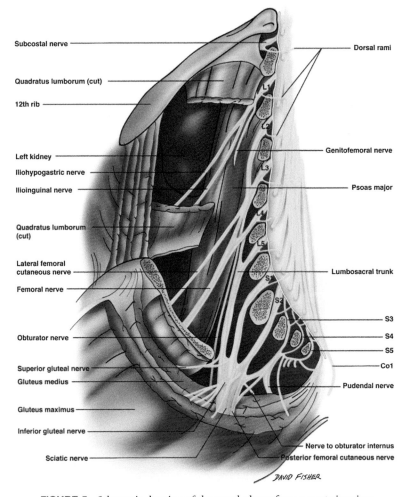

Subcostal nerve

Quadratus lumborum (cut)

12th rib

Left kidney

Iliohypogastric nerve

Ilioinguinal nerve

Quadratus lumborum
(cut)

Lateral femoral
cutaneous nerve

Femoral nerve

Obturator nerve

Superior gluteal nerve

Gluteus medius

Gluteus maximus

Inferior gluteal nerve

Sciatic nerve

Dorsal rami

Genitofemoral nerve

Psoas major

Lumbosacral trunk

S3

S4

S5

Co1

Pudendal nerve

Nerve to obturator internus

Posterior femoral cutaneous nerve

L1 L2 L3 L4 L5 S1 S2

DAVID FISHER

FIGURE 5 Schematic drawing of the sacral plexus from a posterior view.

dedicated to the clinical anatomy of the sacral plexus are lacking in the literature, this book should serve as an important resource and hopefully, decrease iatrogenic injury and improve patient outcomes.

R. Shane Tubbs
Joe Iwanaga
Marios Loukas
Aaron S. Dumont
Miguel Angel Reina

ADDITIONAL READING

Carbone, A., Palleschi, G., Pastore, A.L., Messas, A. (Eds.), 2016. Functional Urologic Surgery in Neurogenic and Oncologic Diseases. https://doi.org/10.1007/978-3-319-29191-8.

Franco, C.D., 2008. Applied anatomy of the lower extremity. Tech. Reg. Anesth. Pain Manag. 12 (3), 140–145. https://doi.org/10.1053/j.trap.2008.02.003.

Jueneman, K.P., Lue, T.F., Schmidt, R.A., Tanagho, E.A., 1988. Clinical significance of sacral and pudendal nerve anatomy. J. Urol. 139, 74–80.

Kinder, M.V., Bastiaanssen, E.H.C., Janknegt, R.A., Marani, E., 1999. The neuronal control of the lower urinary tract: a model of architecture and control mechanisms. Arch. Physiol. Biochem. 107 (3), 203–222.

Marani, E., Koch, W.F.R.M., 2014. Innervation of the mature human pelvis. In: The Pelvis, pp. 337–359. https://doi.org/10.1007/978-3-642-40006-3_14.

Marani, E., Fiji, M.E.J., Kraan, M.C., Lycklama à Nijeholt, G.A.B., Videleer, A.C., 1993. Interconnections of the upper ventral rami of the human sacral plexus: a reappraisal for dorsal rhizotomy in neurostimulation operations. Neurourol. Urodyn. 12 (6), 585–598. https://doi.org/10.1002/nau.1930120611.

Tubbs, R.S., Shoja, M., Loukas, M., 2015. Bergman's Comprehensive Encyclopedia of Human Anatomic Variation. Wiley, Hoboken.

Standring, S., 2016. Gray's Anatomy. Elsevier, Philadelphia.

Wohlgemuth, W.A., Rottach, K.G., Stoehr, M., 1999. Intermittent claudication due to ischaemia of the lumbosacral plexus — ProQuest Medical Library — ProQuest. J. Neurol. Neurosurg. Psychiatry 793–795.

Contents

CHAPTER 1

The Lumbosacral Trunk

JOE IWANAGA • R. SHANE TUBBS

After exiting the intervertebral foramen, the L4 ventral ramus trifurcates into an anterior division (forming part of the obturator nerve), a posterior division (forming part of the femoral nerve), and a caudal division, which fuses with the L5 ventral ramus to form the lumbosacral trunk (Figs. 1.1 and 1.2). As it traverses inferiorly along the sacrum, the L5 ventral ramus travels through the lumbosacral tunnel. The lumbosacral ligament, which forms the wall of the tunnel, attaches medially at the L5 vertebral body and/or transverse process and laterally at the sacral ala.

The lumbosacral trunk passes caudally over the sacral ala, crossing the sacroiliac joint about 2 cm below the pelvic brim. For the most part, the lumbosacral trunk is anchored to the sacral ala by fibrous connective tissue. It eventually joins the sacral plexus, forming the lumbosacral plexus. Most of the motor and sensory innervation to the fibular division of the sciatic nerve is provided by the lumbosacral trunk.

Injury to the lumbosacral trunk manifests as foot drop (of the same clinical spectrum as a fibular nerve palsy) along with more proximal weakness such as the tibialis posterior muscle innervated by the tibial nerve, and the gluteal muscles innervated by the superior and inferior gluteal nerves. Although the clinical presentation is similar, lumbosacral trunk injury can be differentiated from L5 nerve root radiculopathy through electrical testing and examining the paraspinal muscles for wasting, which occurs in L5 radiculopathy but not lumbosacral trunk injury. Prior diagnosis of lumbosacral trunk injury occurs mainly in obstetric patients, the newborn's head pressing against and injuring neural structures against the hip, or after hip fractures or hip surgeries.

Variants of nerve root contributions to the lumbar and lumbosacral plexuses are also well documented in the literature. In the prefixed, high form of the plexus, the lumbosacral trunk may draw fibers from the L3 level. Should the patient possess this particular variant, it would be reasonable to find L3-pattern deficits after lumbosacral trunk injury.

In some cases, the lumbosacral trunk may present as two ununited parallel trunks. It has also been found more superiorly than typical, medial to the psoas. Lastly, if the L4 ventral ramus fails to communicate with the L5 ventral ramus, a lumbosacral trunk will not be formed and no L4 fibers will enter the lumbosacral plexus.

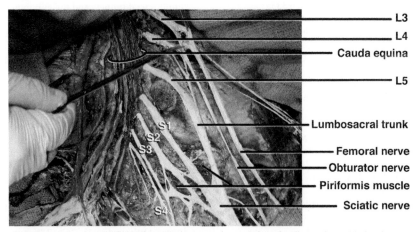

L3
L4
Cauda equina
L5
Lumbosacral trunk
Femoral nerve
Obturator nerve
Piriformis muscle
Sciatic nerve

S1
S2
S3
S4

FIG. 1.1 Anterior view of the left lumbosacral plexus in a cadaveric dissection with lumbar components colored blue and sacral components colored yellow. Note the lumbosacral trunk.

Surgical Anatomy of the Sacral Plexus and Its Branches. https://doi.org/10.1016/B978-0-323-77602-8.00001-5

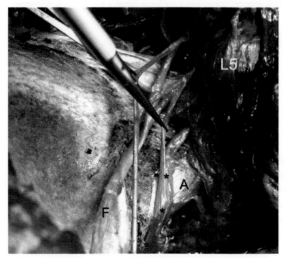

FIG. 1.2 Right-sided lumbosacral trunk (asterisks) in a cadaver, anterior view. The fifth lumbar vertebra's body (L5) is seen at midline. Also note the femoral nerve (F) and ala of the sacrum (A). The obturator nerve (unlabeled) is seen coursing between the lumbosacral trunk medially and the femoral nerve laterally. The forceps are holding the L4 contribution to the lumbosacral trunk and joining the L5 ventral ramus (not labeled).

ADDITIONAL READING

Ahmadian, A., Deukmedjian, A.R., Abel, N., Dakwar, E., Uribe, J.S., 2013. Analysis of lumbar plexopathies and nerve injury after lateral retroperitoneal transpsoas approach: diagnostic standardization. J. Neurosurg. Spine 18, 289–297.

Bartynski, W.S., Kang, M.D., Rothfus, W.E., 2010. Adjacent double–nerve root contributions in unilateral lumbar radiculopathy. Am. J. Neuroradiol. 31, 327–333.

Bina, R.W., Zoccali, C., Skoch, J., Baaj, A.A., 2015. Surgical anatomy of the minimally invasive lateral lumbar approach. J. Clin. Neurosci. 22, 456–459.

Brailsford, J.F., 1929. Deformities of the lumbosacral region of the spine. Br. J. Surg. 16, 562–627.

Briggs, C.A., Chandraraj, S., 1995. Variations in the lumbosacral ligament and associated changes in the lumbosacral region resulting in compression of the fifth dorsal root ganglion and spinal nerve. Clin. Anat. 8, 339–346.

Ebraheim, N.A., Lu, J., Biyani, A., Huntoon, M., Yeasting, R.A., 1997. The relationship of lumbosacral plexus to the sacrum and the sacroiliac joint. Am. J. Orthop. 26, 105–110.

Hashavardhana, N.S., Dabke, H.V., 2014. The furcal nerve revisited. Orthop. Rev. 6, 5428.

Houten, J.K., Alexandre, L.C., Nasser, R., Wollowick, A.L., 2011. Nerve injury during the transpsoas approach for lumbar fusion. J. Neurosurg. Spine 15, 280–284.

Jones 2nd, T.L., Hisey, M.S., 2012. L5 radiculopathy caused by L5 nerve root entrapment by an L5-S1 anterior osteophyte. Internet J. Spine Surg. 6, 174–177.

Katirji, B., 2007. Electromyography in Clinical Practice, a Case Study Approach. Mosby Elsevier, Philadelphia, pp. 81–97.

Kikuchi, S., Hasue, M., Nishiyama, K., Ito, T., 1986. Anatomic features of the furcal nerve and its clinical significance. Spine 11, 1002–1007.

Louis, P.K., Narain, A.S., Hijji, F.Y., Yacob, A., Yom, K.H., Phillips, F.M., Singh, K., 2017. Radiographic analysis of psoas morphology and its association with neurovascular structures at L4-5 with reference to lateral approaches. Spine 42, E1386–E1392.

Mandelli, C., Colombo, E.V., Sicuri, G.M., Mortini, P., 2016. Lumbar plexus nervous distortion in XLIF® approach: an anatomic study. Eur. Spine J. 25, 4155–4163.

Matsumoto, M., Chiba, K., Nojiri, K., Ishikawa, M., Toyama, Y., Nishikawa, Y., 2002. Extraforaminal entrapment of the fifth lumbar spinal nerve by osteophytes of the lumbosacral spine: anatomic study and a report of four cases. Spine 27, 169–173.

Matsumoto, M., Chiba, K., Ishii, K., Watanabe, K., Nakamura, M., Toyama, Y., 2006. Microendoscopic partial resection of the sacral ala to relieve extraforaminal entrapment of the L-5 spinal nerve at the lumbosacral tunnel. J. Neurosurg. Spine 4, 342–346.

Matsumoto, M., Watanabe, K., Ishii, K., Tsuji, T., Takaishi, H., Nakamura, M., Toyama, Y., Chiba, K., 2010. Posterior decompression surgery for extraforaminal entrapment of the fifth lumbar spinal nerve at the lumbosacral junction. J. Neurosurg. Spine 12, 72–81.

Mitchell, G.A.G., 1936. The lumbosacral Junction. J. Bone Jt. Surg. 16, 233–254.

Nathan, H., 1968. Compression of the sympathetic trunk by osteophytes of the vertebral column in the abdomen: an anatomical study with pathological and clinical consideration. Surgery 63, 609–625.

Nathan, H., Weizenbluth, M., Halperin, N., 1982. The lumbosacral ligament (LSL), with special emphasis on the "lumbosacral tunnel" and the entrapment of the 5th lumbar nerve. Int. Orthop. 6, 197–202.

Olsewski, J.M., Simmons, E.H., Kallen, F.C., Mendel, F.C., 1991. Evidence from cadavers suggestive of entrapment of fifth lumbar spinal nerves by lumbosacral ligaments. Spine 16, 336–347.

Pawar, A., Hughes, A., Girardi, F., Sama, A., Lebl, D., Cammisa, F., 2015. Lateral lumbar interbody fusion. Asian Spine J. 9, 978–983.

Pecina, M.M., Krmpotic-Nemanic, J., Markiewitz, A.D., 2001. Tunnel Syndromes: Peripheral Nerve Compression Syndromes, third ed. CRC Press, Boca Raton, pp. 199–200.

Protas, M., Edwards, B., Loukas, M., Oskouian, R.J., Tubbs, R.S., 2017. The lumbosacral tunnel: Cadaveric study and review of the literature. Spine Scholar 1, 99–102.

Silber, J.S., Anderson, D.G., Hayes, V.M., Vaccaro, A.R., 2002. Advances in surgical management of lumbar degenerative disease. Orthopedics 25, 767–771 quiz 72-3.

Skovrlj, B., Gilligan, J., Cutler, H.S., Qureshi, S.A., 2015. Minimally invasive procedures on the lumbar spine. World J. Clin. Cases 3, 1–9.

Transfeldt, E.E., Robertson, D., Bradford, D.S., 1993. Ligaments of the lumbosacral spine and their role in possible extraforaminal spinal nerve entrapment and tethering. J. Spinal Disord. 6, 507–512.

Tubbs, R.S., Shoja, M.M., Loukas, M., 2016. Bergman's Comprehensive Encyclopedia of Human Anatomic Variation. John Wiley & Sons, Inc., Hoboken, pp. 1113–1127.

Tubbs, R.I., Gabel, B., Jeyamohan, S., Moisi, M., Chapman, J.R., Hanscom, R.D., Loukas, M., Oskouian, R.J., Tubbs, R.S., 2017. Relationship of the lumbar plexus branches to the lumbar spine: anatomical study with application to lateral approaches. Spine J. 17, 1012–1016.

Yuan, P.S., Rowshan, K., Verma, R.B., Miller, L.E., Block, J.E., 2014. Minimally invasive lateral lumbar interbody fusion with direct psoas visualization. J. Orthop. Surg. Res. 9, 20.

CHAPTER 2

The Superior Gluteal Nerve

STEPHEN J. BORDES, JR. • R. SHANE TUBBS

EMBRYOLOGY

The lower limb buds appear during week 4 of fetal development, about 2 days after the upper limb buds form. The preaxial (cranial) and postaxial (caudal) borders of the limbs form by week 7. As the limbs rotate, the ventral and dorsal surfaces appear. In adults, the preaxial border of the lower limb can be defined as the area extending from the medial foot to the groin in line with the saphenous vein (Paterson, 1893). The postaxial border extends from the lateral foot to the lower border of the gluteus maximus and finally the coccyx (Paterson, 1893). Muscles and nerves can then be classified as preaxial, postaxial, ventral, and dorsal. The superior gluteal nerve (Figs. 2.1 and 2.2) is a nerve of the dorsal surface and primarily innervates the dorsal musculature (Paterson, 1893).

ANATOMY

The superior gluteal nerve arises from the posterior, or dorsal, divisions of the L4, L5, and S1 ventral rami (Figs. 2.3 and 2.4) (Lung and Lui, 2018; Ray et al., 2013; Akita et al., 1994a; Piersol, 1916; Tubbs et al., 2018; Bozkurt et al., 2012). Within the sacral plexus, the superior gluteal nerve is more proximal and dorsal than its counterpart, the inferior gluteal nerve (Akita et al., 1992). It is unique in that it is the only structure to descend inferiorly from the lumbosacral plexus and pass superiorly to the piriformis muscle in the suprapiriform foramen (Fig. 2.5) (Lung and Lui, 2018; Ray et al., 2013; Pecina et al., 1997). It tends to run on the ventral surface of the piriformis; however, cases have been reported in which branches penetrate this muscle's belly (Akita et al., 1994b).

Following emergence from the greater sciatic foramen, the superior gluteal nerve branches into superior and inferior divisions (Akita et al., 1994a). The inferior division is derived from a thick cranial portion (L4, L5) of the nerve, while the superior division comes from a thin, caudal portion (L5 and S1) (Akita et al., 1992). These segments cross prior to the gluteal muscles. The superior division typically innervates the gluteus medius and, on occasion, the gluteus minimus (Lung and Lui, 2018; Ray et al., 2013). The inferior division more commonly innervates the gluteus minimus and terminates in the tensor fasciae latae (Lung and Lui, 2018; Akita et al., 1994a). It is the major division of the superior gluteal nerve, and insult to this branch entails more devastating consequences for gait (Bos et al., 1994).

The superior gluteal nerve travels together with the superior gluteal artery and vein (Lung and Lui, 2018). Deep branches of both the artery and the nerve supply the hip joint, gluteus medius, gluteus minimus, tensor fasciae latae, and superior portion of the femoral neck (Williams and Stranding, 2005; Trescot, 2016). The most inferior, caudal roots of the superior gluteal nerve also contribute to innervating the piriformis along with the inferior, caudal roots of the inferior gluteal and common peroneal nerves (Akita et al., 1992). This was noted by Iwanaga et al., who showed the piriformis to have primary superior gluteal nerve innervation (70%) in addition to innervation from the inferior gluteal nerve and the L5-S2 ventral rami (Tubbs et al., 2018). Consequently, transection of one branch of these nerves to the piriformis would probably leave the muscle partially innervated (Tubbs et al., 2018). Some branches of the superior gluteal nerve penetrating the tensor fasciae latae also innervate the cutaneous surface, a role originally attributed solely to branches of the lateral femoral cutaneous, iliohypogastric, posterior femoral cutaneous, and dorsal rami of the lumbar nerves (Medical, 1992). In the past, the L4 and L5 nerve roots were thought not to be involved in the cutaneous innervation of the gluteal region; however, it can be concluded that such innervation is truly segmentally arranged (Medical, 1992).

IMAGING

Owing to the small dimensions of the superior gluteal nerve and its course, ultrasound and MR imaging are difficult (Martinoli et al., 2013). MR imaging remains

Surgical Anatomy of the Sacral Plexus and Its Branches. https://doi.org/10.1016/B978-0-323-77602-8.00002-7

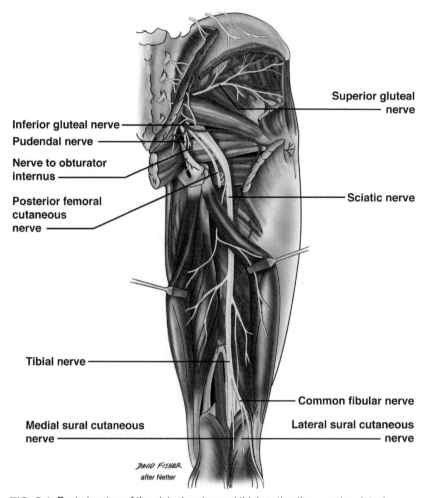

Inferior gluteal nerve

Pudendal nerve

Nerve to obturator
internus

Posterior femoral
cutaneous
nerve

Superior gluteal
nerve

Sciatic nerve

Tibial nerve

Common fibular nerve

Medial sural cutaneous
nerve

Lateral sural cutaneous
nerve

DAVID FISHER
after Netter

FIG. 2.1 Posterior view of the gluteal region and thigh noting the superior gluteal nerve.

the gold standard for visualization of this nerve (Garwood et al., 2018). The main landmark used to identify image pathology is the fatty area between the gluteus minimus and gluteus medius (Martinoli et al., 2013). The superior gluteal nerve enters this fatty space and runs between the gluteal muscles upon its exit from the greater sciatic foramen. Entrapment of the nerve can be best diagnosed through recognition of denervation of the gluteus maximus, gluteus minimus, or tensor fasciae latae (Prost et al., 2013). Indirect detection is most common and includes signs of muscle atrophy, edema, and effacement of the suprapiriformis fat plane (Prost et al., 2013). Direct detection, while less common, includes differences in MR signal intensity, morphological changes, location, and size (Prost et al., 2013).

VARIATIONS

Variants of the superior gluteal nerve are not common; however, when there is a variation, it often involves the nerve's inferior branch course in proximity to the greater trochanter or the superior branch point of termination (Lung and Lui, 2018). In the latter case, the superior branch of the nerve descends beneath the inferior branch and inserts directly into the tensor fasciae latae inferolaterally (Lung and Lui, 2018; Ray et al., 2013). In most cases, the superior branch does not travel to this muscle as the tensor fasciae latae is primarily innervated by the inferior branch of the superior gluteal nerve.

Nearly 90% of cases show the superior gluteal nerve branching into two divisions, superior and

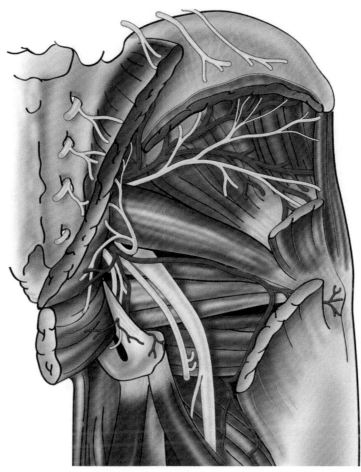

FIG. 2.2 Zoomed-in view of the superior gluteal nerve and its exit above the piriformis muscle.

inferior; however, in the remaining cases, there are typically three branch divisions (Miguel-Perez et al., 2010).

A double-bellied piriformis muscle is occasionally seen entrapping the superior gluteal nerve (Rask, 1980). While piriformis syndrome typically involves entrapment of the sciatic nerve, this rare occurrence can present with nonspecific deep gluteal pain, weakness upon abduction, and tenderness; this was dubbed the "triad of superior gluteal nerve entrapment" by Rask (Rask, 1980; Hernando et al., 2015).

A 1994 case report described a presentation in which an inferior division of the superior gluteal nerve innervated the rectus femoris and vastus lateralis on the right lower limb of a Japanese male (Akita et al., 1994c). Previous investigations have revealed communications between the superior gluteal and femoral nerves (Akita et al., 1994c). Such cases have demonstrated anastomoses among the rectus femoris, vastus lateralis, and tensor fasciae latae, probably because the nerves to those muscles are dorsal, cranial, lumbosacral derivatives (Akita et al., 1994c).

PATHOLOGY

The most common cause of injury to the superior gluteal nerve is iatrogenic, frequently a complication of hip arthroplasty (Prost et al., 2013). The nerve is extremely variable in course and branching pattern. As a result, postoperative complications are not easily predictable preoperatively. The inferior branch of the nerve is frequently injured during anterior or anterolateral dissection (Prost et al., 2013). As such, the tensor fasciae latae is commonly affected.

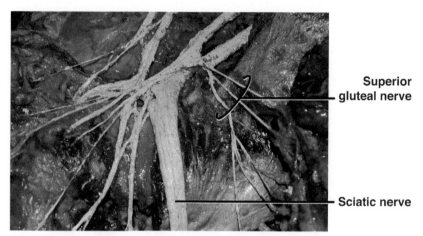

FIG. 2.3 Cadaveric dissection of the proximal sacral plexus noting the superior gluteal nerve.

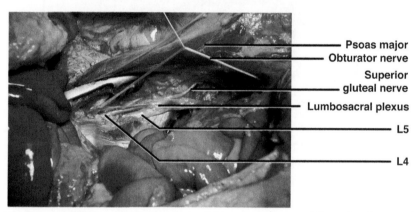

FIG. 2.4 Cadaveric dissection of the left pelvis medial to psoas major and illustrating the superior gluteal nerve at its origin. Note the nerve leaving the pelvis through the greater sciatic foramen and above the piriformis muscle (not labeled).

The gluteal region is a common site for administering drugs. Intramuscular injection into the superomedial quadrant of the buttock carries a high risk of superior gluteal nerve injury. Sciatic nerve injury can result from superomedial, inferomedial, or inferolateral quadrant injection (Small et al., 2004). Therefore, the safest area for an intramuscular buttock injection is the superolateral quadrant or anterogluteal area (von Hochstetter triangle) (Eksioglu et al., 2003).

Superior gluteal nerve entrapment is another possible pathological complication. This can be caused by various factors, including local inflammation, active infection, bone fracture, osteophytic growth, vascular or muscular compression commonly associated with external rotation of the leg, or a mass effect arising from tumor lesions (Trescot, 2016; Prost et al., 2013).

As mentioned above, piriformis syndrome, while most commonly involving the sciatic nerve, can also affect the superior gluteal nerve. Indications of entrapment include a "pseudo-sciatica" presentation in which pain can travel down the posterior thigh, leg, and foot (Tubbs et al., 2018; Trescot, 2016). From a clinical perspective, the pain improves with rest in a seated position and worsens while standing, walking, climbing stairs, lifting objects, and twisting away from the side of injury (Trescot, 2016). The pain also often worsens through the night. Isolated nerve compression, while rare, can result from muscle hypertrophy, anatomical distortion due to fracture, or stretch injuries (Pecina et al., 1997).

The gluteus medius, gluteus minimus, and tensor fasciae latae work in unison to support and stabilize

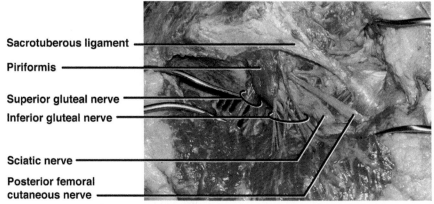

Sacrotuberous ligament

Piriformis

Superior gluteal nerve

Inferior gluteal nerve

Sciatic nerve

Posterior femoral
cutaneous nerve

FIG. 2.5 Posterior view of the left piriformis muscle with the exiting of the superior and inferior gluteal nerves.

the pelvis (Lung and Lui, 2018; Pecina et al., 1997). While the gluteus medius serves as the primary internal rotator of the hip, the gluteus minimus facilitates this action. The tensor fasciae latae externally rotates the hip. All three muscles abduct the hip. In the event of injury to the superior gluteal nerve or its branches, the hip joint can destabilize, resulting in a clinical sign known as the Trendelenburg gait (Lung and Lui, 2018). Ipsilateral nerve insult results in contralateral hip sag during tasks such as raising the contralateral leg while balancing on the ipsilateral foot. The Trendelenburg gait is considered positive when the unaffected limb, or swing leg, swings laterally and the patient leans toward the side of injury to balance their center of gravity (Pecina et al., 1997). In the event of bilateral superior gluteal injury, the opposite can occur: the hip rises on the unsupported side and the leg swings laterally on the contralateral side. This waddling gait is occasionally referred to as the Duchenne limp (Lung and Lui, 2018).

Treatments include observation, physical therapy, electrotherapy, and, in some cases, surgery to preserve range of function (Pecina et al., 1997).

SURGICAL APPROACH

The superior gluteal nerve can be injured iatrogenically during hip arthroplasty. The nerve courses between the gluteus minimus and medius after emerging from the greater sciatic foramen. It is most vulnerable within this area during surgery (Kenny et al., 2003). The incidence is mainly related to the nerve's branching course, which varies among individuals. While surgical advances have decreased the incidence of nerve injury, each procedure still carries risk and most individuals

manifest some form of nerve insult postoperatively (Beaulieu and Laurin, 1990).

Landmarks of importance include the posterior inferior iliac spine (PIIS), anterior superior iliac spine (ASIS), a line connecting the PIIS to the greater trochanter, and the iliac tubercle (Bozkurt et al., 2012; Putzer et al., 2018). The Smith-Peterson direct anterior dissection is recognized as a completely internerval and muscle-sparing approach, in contrast to the Watson-Jones anterolateral interval, as a safe zone is hard to define in the latter (Putzer et al., 2018). The accepted safe area for direct anterior dissection is within 4 cm of the tip of the greater trochanter for anterior segments and 5 cm for the middle and posterior thirds of the gluteus medius (Eksioglu et al., 2003; Kampa et al., 2007). Some studies have indicated that this safe zone tends to be smaller than typically reported (Bozkurt et al., 2012). In fact, such studies note that owing to variations in course and pattern the safe zone is only valid if a transverse neural trunk pattern is present, as branches to the tensor fasciae latae can produce a splay pattern above the greater trochanter in which distal superior gluteal nerve branches loop with upper branches (Bozkurt et al., 2012; Trescot, 2016). The safe area in the context of a neural trunk pattern lay at a mean distance of 3.8 cm from the greater trochanter (Bozkurt et al., 2012). It is crucial to determine the nerve's course and distance, which vary as a function of patient height (Bos et al., 1994). Lateral transgluteal dissection, also known as the Hardinge approach, provides the best exposure of the hip but carries the greatest risk of nerve injury, gluteal insufficiency, and fatty degeneration of the gluteus medius, minimus, and tensor fasciae latae (Bos et al., 1994; Putzer et al., 2018; Ramesh et al., 1996). Specifically, the anterior portions of the gluteus medius and tensor fasciae latae are at greatest risk (Bos et al., 1994). While posterior approaches decrease the risk of insult to the gluteus medius and maximus muscles and anterior approaches best preserve superior gluteal nerve integrity with risk of denervation of branches to the tensor fasciae latae, all approaches carry a similarly lower risk as long as the safe area is respected (Bozkurt et al., 2012; Huráček et al., 2015). Careful attention should be paid to where the terminal branch of the superior gluteal nerve inserts into the tensor fasciae latae as preservation can preclude fatty degeneration of the muscle (Putzer et al., 2018). It is important to note that while the direct anterior approach carries the lowest risk of superior gluteal nerve injury, it commonly carries risk for femoral nerve injury; however, the prognosis is better than that following insult to the sciatic nerve (Putzer et al., 2018).

Femoral nail and percutaneous iliosacral screw placements can also cause superior gluteal nerve or gluteus medius injury (Prost et al., 2013). The risks in these procedures are reduced by flexing and adducting the hip to a greater degree (Ozsoy et al., 2007). As such, lateral positioning on the operating table allows the best results to be achieved (Ozsoy et al., 2007).

REFERENCES

Akita, K., Sakamoto, H., Sato, T., 1992. Stratificational relationship among the main nerves from the dorsal division of the sacral plexus and the innervation of the piriformis. Anat. Rec. 233 (4), 633–642. https://doi.org/10.1002/ar.1092330417.

Akita, K., Sakamoto, H., Sato, T., 1994a. Origin, course and distribution of the superior gluteal nerve. Cells Tissues Organs 149 (3), 225–230. https://doi.org/10.1159/000147581.

Akita, K., Sakamoto, H., Sato, T., 1994b. Arrangement and innervation of the glutei medius and minimus and the piriformis: a morphological analysis. Anat. Rec. 238 (1), 125–130. https://doi.org/10.1002/ar.1092380114.

Akita, K., Sakamoto, H., Sato, T., 1994c. A case in which a branch from the superior gluteal nerve innervated the rectus femoris and the vastus lateralis. Ann. Anat. 176 (2), 181–183. https://doi.org/10.1016/S0940-9602(11)80449-8.

Beaulieu, M.A., Laurin, C.A., 1990. Gluteal nerve damage following total hip arthroplasty: a prospective analysis. J. Arthroplasty 5 (4), 319–322. https://doi.org/10.1016/S0883-5403(08)80090-3.

Bos, J.C., Stoeckart, R., Klooswijk, A., van Linge, B., Bahadoer, R., 1994. The surgical anatomy of the superior gluteal nerve and anatomical radiologic bases of the direct lateral approach to the hip. Surg. Radiol. Anat. 16 (3), 253–258. https://doi.org/10.1007/BF01627679.

Bozkurt, M., Apaydin, N., Tubbs, R.S., Kendir, S., Loukas, M., 2012. Surgical anatomy of the superior gluteal nerve and landmarks for its localization during minimally invasive approaches to the hip. Clin. Anat. 26 (5), 614–620. https://doi.org/10.1002/ca.22057.

Eksioglu, F., Uslu, M., Gudemez, E., Atik, O.S., Tekdemir, I., 2003. Reliability of the safe area for the superior gluteal nerve. Clin. Orthop. Relat. Res. 412, 111–116. https://doi.org/10.1097/01.blo.0000068768.86536.7e.

Garwood, E.R., Duarte, A., Bencardino, J.T., 2018. MR imaging of entrapment neuropathies of the lower extremity. Radiol. Clin. N. Am. 56 (6), 997–1012. https://doi.org/10.1016/j.rcl.2018.06.012.

Hernando, M.F., Cerezal, L., Pérez-Carro, L., Abascal, F., Canga, A., 2015. Deep gluteal syndrome: anatomy, imaging, and management of sciatic nerve entrapments in the subgluteal space. Skeletal Radiol. 44 (7), 919–934. https://doi.org/10.1007/s00256-015-2124-6.

Huráček, J., Kubeš, R., Munzinger, U., et al., 2015. Lesion of gluteal nerves and muscles in total hip arthroplasty through 3 surgical approaches. An electromyographically controlled study. HIP Int. 25 (2), 176–183. https://doi.org/10.5301/hipint.5000199.

Kampa, R.J., Prasthofer, A., Lawrence-Watt, D.J., Pattison, R.M., 2007. The internervous safe zone for incision of the capsule of the hip. J. Bone Jt. Surg. Br 89-B (7), 971–976. https://doi.org/10.1302/0301-620x.89b7.19053.

Kenny, P., O'Brien, C.P., Synnott, K., Walsh, M.G., 2003. Damage to the superior gluteal nerve after two different approaches to the hip. J. Bone Jt. Surg. 81 (6), 979–981. https://doi.org/10.1302/0301-620x.81b6.9509.

Lung, K., Lui, F., 2018. Anatomy, Abdomen and Pelvis, Superior Gluteal Nerve.

Martinoli, C., Miguel-Perez, M., Padua, L., Gandolfo, N., Zicca, A., Tagliafico, A., 2013. Imaging of neuropathies about the hip. Eur. J. Radiol. 82 (1), 17–26. https://doi.org/10.1016/j.ejrad.2011.04.034.

Medical, T., 1992. The Cutaneous Branches of the Superior Gluteal Nerve with Special Reference to the Nerve to Tensor Fascia Lata, pp. 105–108.

Miguel-Perez, M., Ortiz-Sagrista, J., Lopez, I., et al., 2010. How to avoid injuries of the superior gluteal nerve. HIP Int. 20 (7), S26–S31. https://doi.org/10.5301/HIP.2010.2761.

Ozsoy, M.H., Basarir, K., Bayramoglu, A., Erdemli, B., Tuccar, E., Eksioglu, M.F., 2007. Risk of superior gluteal nerve and gluteus medius muscle injury during femoral nail insertion. J. Bone Jt. Surg. A. 89 (4), 829–834. https://doi.org/10.2106/JBJS.F.00617.

Paterson, A.M., 1893. The origin and distribution of the nerves to the lower limb. J. Anat. Physiol. 28 (1), 84. https://www.ncbi.nlm.nih.gov/pmc/articles/PMC1328325/.

Pecina, M., Krmpotic-Nemanic, J., Markiewitz, A., 1997. In: Petralia, P. (Ed.), Tunnel Syndromes: Peripheral Nerve Compression Syndromes, second ed. CRC Press, Inc., Boca Raton.

Piersol, G., 1916. Human Anatomy, first ed. JP Lippincott Company, Philadelphia.

Prost, R., Bencardino, J.T., Rosenberg, Z.S., 2013. Superior gluteal nerve entrapment: imaging evaluation. Electron. Present. Online Syst. 1—15.

Putzer, D., Haselbacher, M., Hörmann, R., Thaler, M., Nogler, M., 2018. The distance of the gluteal nerve in relation to anatomical landmarks: an anatomic study. Arch. Orthop. Trauma Surg. 138 (3), 419—425. https://doi.org/10.1007/s00402-017-2847-z.

Ramesh, M., O'Byrne, J.M., McCarthy, N., Jarvis, A., Mahalingham, K., Cashman, W.F., 1996. Damage to the superior gluteal nerve after the Hardinge approach to the hip. J. Bone Jt. Surg. Br 78 (6), 903—906. http://www.ncbi.nlm.nih.gov/entrez/query.fcgi?cmd=Retrieve&db=PubMed&dopt=Citation&list_uids=8951004.

Rask, M.R., 1980. Superior gluteal nerve entrapment syndrome. Muscle Nerve 3 (4), 304—307. https://doi.org/10.1002/mus.880030406.

Ray, B., D'Souza, A., Saxena, A., et al., 2013. Morphology of the superior gluteal nerve: a study in adult human cadavers, 114, 409—412. https://doi.org/10.4149/BLL.

Small, S.P., Rn, M., Small, S., 2004. Integrative Literature Reviews and Meta-Analyses Preventing Sciatic Nerve Injury from Intramuscular Injections: Literature Review, pp. 287—296.

Trescot, A.M., January 2016. Peripheral Nerve Entrapments: Clinical Diagnosis and Management, pp. 1—902. https://doi.org/10.1007/978-3-319-27482-9.

Tubbs, R.S., Simonds, E., Loukas, M., Schumacher, M., Iwanaga, J., Eid, S., 2018. The majority of piriformis muscles are innervated by the superior gluteal nerve. Clin. Anat. 32 (2), 282—286. https://doi.org/10.1002/ca.23311.

Williams, A., 2005. In: Stranding, S. (Ed.), Pelvic Girdle and Lower Limb. Gray's Anatomy, thirtyninth ed. Elsevier, New York.

CHAPTER 3

The Inferior Gluteal Nerve

SKYLER JENKINS • R. SHANE TUBBS

INTRODUCTION

The inferior gluteal nerve (IGN; Figs. 3.1 and 3.2) is a component of the sacral plexus nerve roots L5-S2 and innervates the gluteus maximus muscle. Its primary role is in the extension and lateral rotation of the hip. Interventionalists and surgeons who perform procedures near this nerve or its origin need a comprehensive knowledge of its form and function. Therefore, this chapter is focused on the clinical anatomy of the IGN.

Embryology

In regard to the nervous and musculoskeletal development of the leg, it can be helpful to delineate between the "preaxial" and "postaxial," dorsal and ventral aspects. According to Paterson, the "preaxial" plane extends from the medial foot, through the medial ankle, along the tibia and medial femoral condyle, and to the pubis, whereas the "postaxial" plane runs along the lateral border of the leg to the border of the gluteus and medially to the coccyx. The IGN, since it innervates the gluteus maximus muscle, can be classified as of dorsal, "preaxial" origin (Paterson, 1894). It was also shown that the external popliteal nerve and IGN share common spinal origin and their respective muscles share similar morphology. This anatomy is also seen in ruminants where the short head of the biceps femoris and gluteus maximus form a common large muscle, homologous in its anterior portion with the gluteus maximus and in its posterior portion to the femoral part of the biceps muscle (Paterson, 1894). This was further posited by Akita et al., suggesting the nerve to the short head of the biceps femoris arises from the ventral surface of the IGN (Akita et al., 1992).

Anatomy

The IGN arise from the lumbosacral plexus with its nerve roots being in the dorsal rami of the last lumbar and rostral two sacral spinal cord levels (Figs. 3.3 and 3.4). The plexus (L4-S4) contains the sciatic nerve, the superior and IGNs, the pudendal nerve, and the posterior femoral cutaneous nerve among others (Trescot,

2016). The roots of the IGN exit the spinal column below their respective vertebra and courses, running close and medial to the sciatic nerve, inferomedially to exit the pelvis via the infrapiriformis foramen before bending retrograde around the piriformis and branching into a superior and inferior branch (Trescot, 2016; Merryman and Varacallo, 2018). These two branches then innervate the gluteus maximus muscle. Ling (Ling and Kumar, 2006) reported that the IGN entered the deep surface of the gluteus maximus over the inferior one-third of the muscle belly as one bundle approximately 5 cm from the tip of the greater trochanter (GT). Apaydin et al. (Apaydin et al., 2009) observed the origin of the IGN averaged 5.4 cm from the GT and radiated through the "danger zone" with the possibility of one of its branches running just above the GT. In a study done by Akamatsu et al. to locate myofascial trigger points for relieving pain, it was seen that branches of the IGN entered the gluteus maximus in all quadrants (Akamatsu et al., 2017).

Recently, Iwanaga et al. reported a cutaneous branch of the IGN (Figs. 3.5 and 3.6). One to two cutaneous branches were identified as arising from the IGN on nine sides (75%) (Iwanaga et al., 2018). The branches were usually located in the lower right quadrant of the gluteus maximus. These branches had a mean distance of 12.5 cm from the midline (Iwanaga et al., 2018). Their mean diameter and length was 0.7 mm and 28.6 cm, respectively (Iwanaga et al., 2018). On all sides with a cutaneous branch of the IGN, the skin over the posterior aspect of the GT was innervated by superior and inferior cluneal nerves and supplemented by cutaneous branches of the IGN (Iwanaga et al., 2018).

According to Apaydin et al. (Apaydin et al., 2009) there is an anatomical landmark to locate the IGN. This triangular-shaped anatomic area's boundaries are set by the posterior inferior iliac spine (PIIS), the GT, and the ischial tuberosity (IT). This triangle may be divided in half, connecting a line from the midpoint between the PIIS and IT with the GT, the superior portion becoming the "danger zone" with respect to iatrogenic

Surgical Anatomy of the Sacral Plexus and Its Branches. https://doi.org/10.1016/B978-0-323-77602-8.00003-9

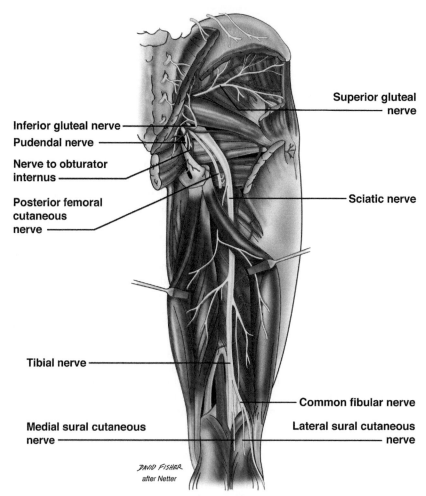

Inferior gluteal nerve

Pudendal nerve

Nerve to obturator internus

Posterior femoral cutaneous nerve

Superior gluteal nerve

Sciatic nerve

Tibial nerve

Common fibular nerve

Medial sural cutaneous nerve

Lateral sural cutaneous nerve

DAVID FISHER
after Netter

FIG. 3.1 Posterior drawing of the right lower limb with the gluteus maximus mostly dissected away to illustrate the course of the inferior gluteal nerve in the buttock.

damage of the IGN and its branches (Apaydin et al., 2009). After branching off the main trunk, the motor branches course medially and dorsally, entering the deep surface of the gluteus maximus.

In a study conducted by Skalak et al., to elucidate a minimally invasive technique to implant a nerve stimulator to prevent pressure ulcers, there was no clinically significant relationship found between the course of the IGN and artery, so vascular imaging would be challenging to locate the nerve. However, they did find an external anatomical landmark to locate the IGN apart from the sciatic nerve. This landmark targeted the region inferior to the most prominent aspect of the GT, medial to the IT, at a depth of the posterior border of the proximal femur (Skalak et al., 2008).

The IGN is the sole innervation of the gluteus maximus muscle. The gluteus maximus extends and laterally rotates the hip joint.

Variations

In a case report, Yan et al. (Yan et al., 2013) found that the IGN exited the pelvis from the upper edge of the piriformis with a frequency of 0.2%–4.26% of the time, traveling with the superior gluteal nerve. Paval and Nayak (Paval and Nayak, 2006) discovered that the nerve consisted of two branches that split superiorly and inferiorly to surround the piriformis before reuniting and coursing to innervate the gluteus maximus. The IGN may also send a branch to the posterior femoral cutaneous nerve (Petchprapa et al., 2010). In addition, the IGN was

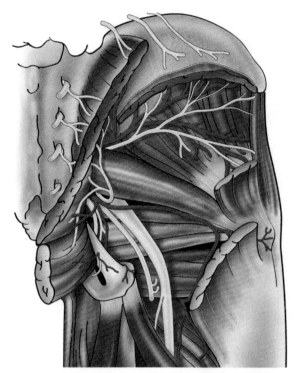

FIG. 3.2 Close-up view of the inferior gluteal nerve from Fig. 3.1.

described as one of two divisions of the "posterior cutaneous nerve of the thigh" (Sforsini and Wikinski, 2006; Martinoli et al., 2013). Finally, Tillmann (Tillmann, 1979) noted that in 15% of the cases studied, the IGN coursed through the piriformis when leaving the pelvis.

In a rare case, it was noted that an anomalous branch from the sciatic nerve innervated the gluteus maximus on one side with the IGN being absent on the corresponding side (VanithaD'Souza and Nayak, 2014). In addition, Sumalatha et al. discovered another rare variant where the IGN was absent and the gluteus maximus was supplied by a short, thin medial trunk from the common peroneal nerve (Sumalatha et al., 2014). Similarly to this finding, Jacomo et al. produced a case study showing the IGN receiving a branch originating from the lateral portion of the sciatic nerve, the common peroneal nerve (Jacomo et al., 2014).

Imaging/Studies

The basis for MR imaging of nerves is that neural enlargement, loss of normal fascicular appearance, or blurring of the perifascicular fat are morphological changes that can indicate nerve damage (Petchprapa et al., 2010). This makes MR imaging of the deep peripheral nerves of the pelvis complex due to the small size and "out-of-plane course" of the nerves (Martinoli et al., 2013). The reference point for the IGN is the deep surface of the gluteus maximus. It is often seen on coronal images, exiting the pelvis adjacent to the sciatic nerve and can also be traced on axial images in the fat plane deep to the gluteus maximus (Petchprapa et al., 2010).

As of date, there are no specific fluoroscopy-guided techniques, ultrasound-guided techniques, cryoneuroablation, or radiofrequency techniques to locate the IGN. However, using an ultrasound-guided approach to locate the sciatic nerve at the level of the piriformis should mark the IGN medial to it (Trescot, 2016).

Pathology

IGN entrapment neuropathy can take place due to increased stresses on the piriformis muscle. Since the IGN most often courses inferiorly to the piriformis with the sciatic, lumbar lordosis and internal rotation of the hip add stresses to the piriformis and may cause the IGN to become entrapped between the piriformis, gluteus minimus, and dorsal rim of the greater sciatic notch (Trescot, 2016).

In a patient with hypoesthesia of the inferior lateral buttocks with a concomitant history of colorectal carcinoma, considerations should be given to the possibility of a compression of the IGN. LeBan et al. (LaBan et al., 1982) showed that the IGN may become entrapped due to its medial, intrapelvic fixation at the origin of the sciatic nerve and from the crowding effect of the piriformis muscle superiorly, the dorsal rim of the sciatic notch posteriorly, and the inferior gluteal vessels and nodes inferiorly.

Isolated compression injury of the IGN is a rare occurrence; however, it has been noted by Stohr and should be taken into consideration for patients who are comatose or undergoing anesthesia. In the same study, it was found that lumbosacral injuries may also affect the IGN (Stohr, 1978).

Intramuscular injection–related injury to the IGN is relatively uncommon, but is usually combined with injury to the sciatic nerve. In a study of 137 patients with infrapiriformis foramen syndrome, performed by Obach et al. (Obach et al., 1983), only two had damage to the IGN.

There was an isolated case that described a patient with substantial lordosis from wearing high heels that led to piriformis entrapment of the superior gluteal nerve. Even though it was not elicited how the IGN was involved, it was posited that an aberrant variation of the IGN running above or through the piriformis was the cause of entrapment and weakness of the

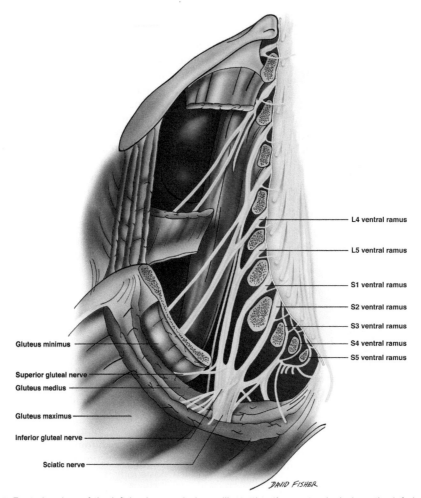

FIG. 3.3 Posterior view of the left lumbosacral plexus illustrating the anatomical plane the inferior gluteal nerve courses in after leaving the pelvis.

gluteus maximus. The entrapment of these two nerves leads to a lack of gluteal muscle function and ultimately hip fracture (De Jong and van Weerden, 1983).

Finally, pelvic fractures can distort the anatomy, potentially leading to stretch injuries of the IGN if the stretch is more than 4 cm (Hersche et al., 1993; Dhillon and Nagi, 1992).

Clinical/Surgical Considerations

Clinical presentation of patients with IGN entrapment may include pain, weakness, and numbness of the buttocks, as well as a gluteus maximus "lurch," where the trunk hyperextends the heel strike to compensate for weak hip extension (Trescot, 2016). Because the IGN runs with the sciatic and posterior femoral cutaneous nerve, the patient may also complain of pain that

radiates down the leg. As the IGN is the only innervation to the gluteus maximus, the patient may also have weakness rising from a seated position or climbing stairs (Trescot, 2016).

The two primary surgical approaches to the hip are the posterior and posterolateral, with the posterior approach being the most commonly used. The IGN, however, is more vulnerable to injury when utilizing this approach. The posterior approach allows for optimal visualization of the femoral shaft, making it ideal for surgical procedures of the hip. Because of its deep location and limited visibility, the IGN can be easily damaged when the gluteus maximus is divided by handheld or self-retaining retractors from stretching or direct damage (Apaydin et al., 2009; Martinoli et al., 2013). In a study comparing preop and postop

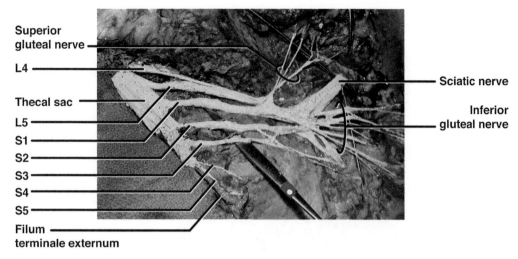

Superior
gluteal nerve

L4

Thecal sac

L5

S1

S2

S3

S4

S5

Filum
terminale externum

Sciatic nerve

Inferior
gluteal nerve

FIG. 3.4 Right posterior cadaveric dissection with the exposed thecal (dural) sac and fibers contributing to the right-sided sacral plexus and noting the origin of the inferior gluteal nerve.

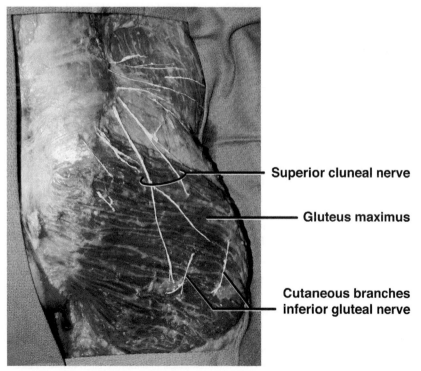

Superior cluneal nerve

Gluteus maximus

Cutaneous branches
inferior gluteal nerve

FIG. 3.5 Dissection of the right gluteal region noting cutaneous branches of the inferior gluteal nerve piercing the gluteus maximus to supply the overlying skin.

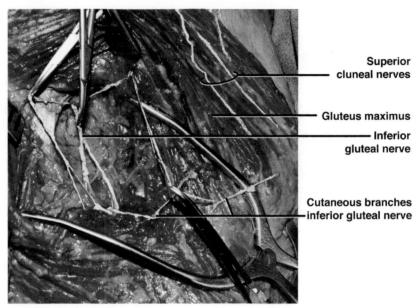

FIG. 3.6 Deeper dissection of Fig. 3.5 noting the proximal inferior gluteal nerve and the two terminal cutaneous branches illustrated in Fig. 3.5.

electromyographies, 88% of hips had abnormal EMG findings of the gluteus maximus (Abitbol et al., 1990). In an effort to understand the course of the IGN through the gluteus maximus, Hwang et al. (Hwang et al., 2009) used gross dissection to elicit that most branches of the IGN run "deeper than 60% of muscle thickness" above the GT coccyx line. Therefore, for minimally invasive posterior approaches to the hip, it is recommended that one use the inferior aspect of the triangle to avoid damaging the IGN.

It had been posited that the surgical fixation of the sacrospinous ligament could potentially lead to IGN damage. In a cadaveric study conducted by Florian-Rodriguez et al. it was shown that the median distance from either attachment point of the sacrospinous ligament would make the damage to the IGN an unlikely source of postoperative gluteal pain (Florian-Rodriguez et al., 2016).

REFERENCES

Abitbol, J., Gendron, D., Laurin, C., Beaulieu, M., 1990. Gluteal nerve damage following total hip arthroplasty. A prospective analysis. J. Arthroplasty 5 (4), 319–322.

Akamatsu, F.E., Yendo, T.M., Rhode, C., Itezerote, A.M., Hojaij, F., Andrade, M., Hsing, W.T., Jacomo, A.L., 2017. Anatomical basis of the myofascial trigger points of the gluteus maximus muscle. BioMed Res. Int. 4821968.

Akita, K., Sakamoto, H., Sato, T., 1992. Innervation of an aberrant digastric muscle in the posterior thigh: stratified relationships between branches of the inferior gluteal nerve. J. Anat. 181, 503–506.

Apaydin, N., Bozkurt, M., Loukas, M., Tubbs, R.S., Esmer, A., 2009. The course of the inferior gluteal nerve and surgical landmarks for its localization during posterior approaches to hip. Surg. Radiol. Anat. 31, 415–418.

De Jong, P., van Weerden, T., 1983. Inferior and superior gluteal nerve paresis and femur neck fracture after spondylolisthesis and lysis. A case report. J. Neurol. 230 (4), 267–270.

Dhillon, M.S., Nagi, O.N., 1992. Sciatic nerve palsy associated with total hip arthroplasty. Ital. J. Orthop. Traumatol. 18 (4), 521–526.

Florian-Rodriguez, M.E., Hare, A., Chin, K., Phelan, J.N., Ripperda, C.M., Corton, M.M., 2016. Inferior gluteal and other nerves associated with sacrospinous ligament: a cadaver study. Am. J. Obstet. Gynecol. 251 (5), 646.

Hersche, O., Isler, B., Aebi, M., 1993. Follow-up and prognosis of neurologic sequelae of pelvic ring fractures with involvement of the sacrum and/or the iliosacral joint (German). Unfallchiring 96 (6), 311–318.

Hwang, K., Seok, N., Seung Ho, H., Won, H., 2009. The intramuscular course of the inferior gluteal nerve in the gluteus maximus muscle and augmentation gluteoplasty. Ann. Plast. Surg. 63 (4), 361–365.

Iwanaga, J., Simonds, E., Vetter, M., Patel, M., Oskouian, R.J., Tubbs, R.S., 2018. The inferior gluteal nerve often has a cutaneous branch: a discovery with application to hip surgery and targeting gluteal pain syndromes. Clin. Anat. 31 (6), 937–941.

Jacomo, A.L., Martinez, C., Saleh, S., Andrade, M., Akamatsu, F., 2014. Unusual relationship between the piriform muscle and sciatic, inferior gluteal and posterior femoral cutaneous nerve. Int. J. Morphol. 32 (2), 432–434.

LaBan, M.M., Meerschaert, J.R., Taylor, R.S., 1982. Electromyographic evidence of inferior gluteal nerve compromise: an early representation of recurrent colorectal carcinoma. Arch. Phys. Med. Rehabil. 63 (1), 33–35.

Ling, Z., Kumar, V., 2006. The course of the inferior gluteal nerve in the posterior approach to the hip. J. Bone Jt. Surg. 88-B, 1580–1583.

Martinoli, C., Miguel-Perez, M., Padua, L., Gandolfo, N., Zicca, A., Tagliafico, A., 2013. Imaging of neruopathies about the hip. Eur. J. Radiol. 82, 17–26.

Merryman, J., Varacallo, M., January 2018. Anatomy, Abdomen and Pelvis, Inferior Gluteal Nerve. StatPearls Publishing, Treasure Island (FL). Available from: https://www.ncbi.nlm.nih.gov/books/NBK532884/.

Obach, J., Aragones, J., Ruano, D., 1983. The infrapiriformis foramen syndrome resulting from intragluteal injection. J. Neurol. Sci. 58 (1), 135–142.

Paterson, A., 1894. The origin and distribution of the nerves to the lower limb. J. Anat. Physiol. 28 (2), 169–193.

Paval, J., Nayak, S., 2006. A case of bilateral high division of sciatic nerve with a variant inferior gluteal nerve. Neuroanatomy 5, 33–34.

Petchprapa, C., Rosenberg, Z., Sconfienza, L., Cavalcanti, C., Vieira, R., Zember, J., 2010. MR imaging of entrapment neuropathies of the lower extremity. Part 1. The pelvis and hip. Radiographics 30 (4), 983–1000.

Sforsini, C., Wikinski, J., 2006. Anatomical review of the lumbosacral plexus and nerves of the lower extremity. Tech. Reg. Anesth. Pain Manag. 10, 138–144.

Skalak, A.F., McGee, M.F., Wu, G., Bogie, K., 2008. Relationship of the inferior gluteal nerves and vessels: target for application of stimulation devices for the prevention of pressure ulcers in spinal cord injury. Surg. Radiol. Anat. 30 (1), 41–45.

Stohr, M., 1978. Traumatic and postoperative lesions of the lumbosacral plexus. Arch. Neurol. 35, 757–760.

Sumalatha, S., D'Souza, A.S., Yadav, J.S., Mittal, S.K., Singh, A., Kotian, S.R., 2014. An unorthodox innervation of the gluteus maximus muscle and other associated variations: a case report. Australas. Med. J. 7 (10), 419–422.

Tillmann, B., 1979. Variations in the pathway of the inferior gluteal nerve. Anat. Anzeiger 145 (3), 293–302.

Trescot, A., 2016. Inferior gluteal nerve entrapment. In: Peripheral Nerve Entrapments: Clinical Diagnosis and Management., pp. 581–587. https://doi.org/10.1007/978-3-319-27482-9_54.

Vanitha D'Souza, A., Nayak, V., 2014. Variations in the innervations to the gluteus maximus muscle: a case report. Int. J. Med. Res. Health Sci. 3 (3), 721–722.

Yan, J., Takechi, M., Hitomi, J., 2013. Variations in the course of the inferior gluteal nerve and artery: a case report and literature review. Surg. Sci. 4, 429–432.

CHAPTER 4

The Nerve to Piriformis

JOE IWANAGA • R. SHANE TUBBS

INTRODUCTION

The piriformis muscle is an important anatomical landmark in the pelvis that is closely associated with the sciatic nerve. Multiple anatomical variations exist regarding the position of the sciatic nerve in relation to the piriformis muscle. However, variant innervation to the piriformis muscles has also been reported in the literature. The piriformis muscle can lead to buttock and lower limb pain due to a condition referred to as the piriformis syndrome. This chapter highlights the anatomy of the variant innervation of the piriformis muscle.

ANATOMY

The piriformis muscle originates from the anterior surface of the second to fourth sacral vertebrae near the sacral foramina, the gluteal surface of the ilium, sacroiliac joint capsule, and sometimes, the sacrotuberous ligament. The piriformis tendon inserts into the medial aspect of the greater trochanter of the femur, together with the tendons of the obturator internus muscle and the superior and inferior gemellus muscles (Standring, 2016). The greater sciatic foramen is divided into two parts by the piriformis muscle, the supra- and infrapiriform foramina. Anterior to the piriformis are the sacral plexus, internal iliac vessels, and the rectum, while the sacrum lies on the posterior side of the piriformis. The piriformis muscle is one of the lateral rotators of the thigh and functions as an abductor of the flexed thigh (Standring, 2016). The sciatic nerve runs in close proximity to the piriformis muscle and exhibits different variations with the most common being the undivided sciatic nerve traveling under the piriformis to go outside the pelvis through infrapiriform foramen (Beaton and Anson, 1937). Beaton et al. described six different variations to the sciatic nerve with some branches of the sciatic nerve piercing through or above the piriformis muscle (Beaton and Anson, 1937). Another similar study was conducted and also revealed that the most common morphology is the sciatic nerve passing undivided under the piriformis muscle (Natsis et al., 2013). Smoll et al. conducted an extensive review of the literature, which revealed that an anomaly between the piriformis muscle and the sciatic nerve was present in about 16% of both cadaveric and surgical cases (Smoll, 2010). This may lead to entrapment and irritation of the nerve, which results in neural pain. Innervation to the piriformis is provided by the nerve to piriformis, which has been reported to have multiple origins from the sacral plexus (Standring, 2016; Akita et al., 1992, 1994; Kirschner et al., 2009; Tubbs et al., 2015).

The literature contains variant reports regarding the direct innervation of the piriformis muscle, which are listed in Table 4.1. Akita et al. performed detailed dissections on human cadavers to observe the origin of the nerve to the piriformis from the sacral plexus (Akita et al., 1992). The majority of the nerves to the piriformis arose from the caudal branch of the superior gluteal nerve (SGN) (Fig. 4.1), which the authors described as S1–S2 with only one specimen arising from solely S2 (Akita et al., 1992). The second most common origin found was the inferior gluteal nerve (IGN), as well as nerves originating from the common fibular nerve and S2 ventral ramus (Akita et al., 1992). These authors performed a similar study and found consistent results of the origin of the nerves to the piriformis, in which the majority of the piriformis innervation was the SGN (Akita et al., 1994). These anatomical studies have consistently revealed that all specimens contained multiple branches from different nerves instead of just one nerve to the piriformis (Akita et al., 1992, 1994). The latest edition of *Gray's Anatomy* states that the nerve to piriformis arises from L5 and S1, and reports that it sometimes arises only from S2 (Standring, 2016). Another source reported that the nerve to piriformis was derived from the posterior divisions of the S1 and S2 ventral rami (Tubbs et al., 2015). Based on a comparative study of the pelvic muscles between humans and animals, some have suggested that the piriformis should be regarded as a compound muscle (Akita, 1997).

Surgical Anatomy of the Sacral Plexus and Its Branches. https://doi.org/10.1016/B978-0-323-77602-8.00004-0

TABLE 4.1
Variations Reported Regarding the Innervation of the Piriformis Muscle.

Author	Source	Nerves to Piriformis

Akita et al. (1992)	Cadaveric	6 pelvic halves (2 male and 1 female)
		• Right female: −3 branches of caudal SGN
		  −1 branch of caudal IGN
		• Left female: −3 branches of SGN
		• Right male 1: −4 branches of caudal SGN nerve
		  −2 branches of CPN
		• Left male 1: −1 caudal SGN,
		  −1 cranial IGN and 1 caudal IGN
		• Right male 2: −5 branches of SGN, IGN, and S1−S2 trunks
		• Left male 2: −2 branches of caudal SGN
		  −2 branches from S2 trunk

Akita et al. (1994)	Cadaveric	5 branches found: −3 branches of caudal SGN
		  −1 branch of IGN
		  −1 branch of CPN

Standring (2016)	Textbook	L5, S1, and S2 (sometimes only S2)
Kirschner et al. (2009)	Article	S1 and S2
Tubbs et al. (2015)	Textbook	S1 and S2
Iwanaga et al. (2019)	Cadaveric	20 hemipelves. **SGN in 70%**, IFN in 5%, L5 in 5%, **S1 in 85%**, and **S2 in 70%**. Note that most muscles receive more than a single nerve branch.

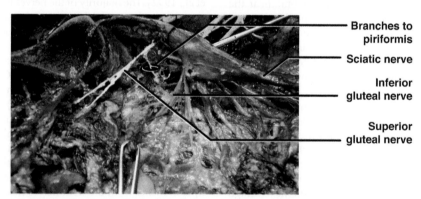

FIG. 4.1 Cadaveric example of the piriformis muscle being innervated by the superior gluteal nerve.

CLINICAL SIGNIFICANCE

Many reports exist in the literature regarding the diagnosis and management of the piriformis syndrome (Cassidy et al., 2012; Jankovic et al., 2013). In a retrospective study of patients suffering from piriformis syndrome, the main symptoms were gluteal pain and sciatica, as well as low back pain, dyspareunia, and difficulty in sitting and walking (Durrani and Winnie, 1991). In addition, these authors revealed that 92% patients reported trauma as the main factor for the pain (Durrani and Winnie, 1991). Reports in the literature have shown pain relief with local anesthetic and steroid injection into the piriformis (Benzon et al., 2003; Fishman et al., 2002).

Iatrogenic injury to the piriformis can also lead to neural damage and pain, such as in the posterior approach to total hip arthroplasty and needle insertion into the piriformis. The posterior approach for total hip arthroplasty involves detachment of the piriformis and obturator internus and externus and is associated with a higher risk of dislocation after surgery than other approaches (Ritter et al., 2001; Vicar and Coleman, 1984). This higher rate has led surgeons to develop different muscle sparing techniques, such as preservation of the piriformis and the obturator internus (Hanly et al., 2017).

CONCLUSION

This chapter provides insights into the innervation of the piriformis and its clinical implications. This innervation is variable. In fact, a recent cadaveric study by us found that the majority of piriformis muscles are innervated by the SGN (Fig. 4.1), S1 or S2 with most muscles being innervated by multiple branches (Iwanaga et al., 2019).

REFERENCES

Akita, K., 1997. A comparative anatomical study of muscles of the pelvic outlet and the piriformis with special reference to their innervation. Acta. Anat. Nippon. 72, 9−12.

Akita, K., Sakamoto, H., Sato, T., 1992. Stratificational relationship among the main nerves from the dorsal division of the sacral plexus and the innervation of the piriformis. Anat. Rec. 233, 633−642. https://doi.org/10.1002/ar.1092330417.

Akita, K., Sakamoto, H., Sato, T., 1994. Arrangement and innervation of the glutei medius and minimus and the piriformis: a morphological analysis. Anat. Rec. 238, 125−130. https://doi.org/10.1002/ar.1092380114.

Beaton, L.E., Anson, B.J., 1937. The relation of the sciatic nerve and of its subdivisions to the piriformis muscle. Anat. Rec. 70, 1−5. https://doi.org/10.1002/ar.1090700102.

Benzon, H.T., Katz, J.A., Benzon, H.A., Iqbal, M.S., 2003. Piriformis syndrome: anatomic considerations, a new technique, and a review of the literature. Anesthesiology 98, 1442−1448. https://doi.org/10.1097/00000542-200306000-00022.

Cassidy, L., Walters, A., Bubb, K., Shoja, M.M., Tubbs, R.S., Loukas, M., 2012. Piriformis syndrome: implications of anatomical variations, diagnostic techniques, and treatment options. Surg. Radiol. Anat. 34, 479−486. https://doi.org/10.1007/s00276-012-0940-0.

Durrani, Z., Winnie, A.P., 1991. Piriformis muscle syndrome: an underdiagnosed cause of sciatica. J. Pain. Symptom. Mange 6, 374−379. https://doi.org/10.1016/0885-3924(91)90029-4.

Fishman, L.M., Anderson, C., Rosner, B., 2002. BOTOX and physical therapy in the treatment of piriformis syndrome. Am. J. Phys. Med. Rehabil. 81, 936−942. https://doi.org/10.1097/00002060-200212000-00009.

Hanly, R.J., Sokolowski, S., Timperley, A.J., 2017. The SPAIRE technique allows sparing of the piriformis and obturator internus in a modified posterior approach to the hip. Hip. Int. 27, 205−209. https://doi.org/10.5301/hipint.5000490.

Iwanaga, J., Eid, S., Simonds, E., Schumacher, M., Loukas, M., Tubbs, R.S., 2019. The majority of piriformis muscles are innervated by the superior gluteal nerve. Clin. Anat. 32, 282−286.

Jankovic, D., Peng, P., van Zundert, A., 2013. Brief review: piriformis syndrome: etiology, diagnosis, and management. Can. J. Anaesth. 60, 1003−1012. https://doi.org/10.1007/s12630-013-0009-5.

Kirschner, J.S., Foye, P.M., Cole, J.L., 2009. Piriformis syndrome, diagnosis and treatment. Muscle Nerve 40, 10−18. https://doi.org/10.1002/mus.21318.

Natsis, K., Totlis, T., Konstantinidis, G.A., Paraskevas, G., Piagkou, M., Koebke, J., 2013. Anatomical variations between the sciatic nerve and the piriformis muscle: a contribution to surgical anatomy in piriformis syndrome. Surg. Radiol. Anat. 36, 273−280. https://doi.org/10.1007/s00276-013-1180-7.

Ritter, M.A., Harty, L.D., Keating, M.E., Faris, P.M., Meding, J.B., 2001. A clinical comparison of the anterolateral and posterolateral approaches to the hip. Clin. Orthop. Relat. Res. 385, 95−99. https://doi.org/10.1097/00003086-200104000-00016.

Smoll, N.R., 2010. Variations of the piriformis and sciatic nerve with clinical consequence: a review. Clin. Anat. 23, 8−17. https://doi.org/10.1002/ca.20893.

Standring, S., 2016. Gray's Anatomy: The Anatomical Basis of Clinical Practice, 41st ed. Elsevier Limited, Philadelphia.

Tubbs, R.S., Rizk, E., Shoja, M.M., Loukas, M., Barbaro, N.M., Spinner, R.J., 2015. Nerves and Nerve Injuries: History, Embryology, Imaging and Diagnostics, vol. 1. Academic Press, London, UK.

Vicar, A.J., Coleman, C., 1984. A comparison of the anterolateral, transtrochanteric, and posterior surgical approaches in primary total hip arthroplasty. Clin. Orthop. Relat. Res. 188, 152−159. https://doi.org/10.1097/00003086-198409000-00019.

CHAPTER 5

The Nerve to Levator Ani

GRAHAM C. DUPONT • R. SHANE TUBBS

INTRODUCTION

The pelvic floor is a musculofascial funnel consisting of the levator ani and ischiococcygeus muscles, and the superior and inferior diaphragmatic fasciae covering both muscles. The pelvic floor acts as a concave barrier separating the pelvic viscera and the perineum. These muscles intermingle with the pelvic contents and provide structural and functional support for the prostate, urethra, vagina, and anorectal junction. The levator ani consists of three parts: pubococcygeus, puborectalis, and iliococcygeus.

Major medical texts provide little description to the nerve to levator ani (nLA); however, its relevance warrants description. For example, the nLA, if injured during invasive procedures or childbirth, may result in various pelvic floor pathologies such as urinary and fecal incontinence, pelvic organ prolapse, and sexual dysfunction. Variations of this nerve are common and will be discussed herein.

Surgical approaches to the anorectal region must be skillfully performed as the relationships of the various interposing fascial folds and peritoneal reflections may obfuscate the urogenital or colorectal specialist.

ANATOMY

The nLA may be observed through various approaches. It may be accessed transabdominally by reflecting the pelvic viscera laterally and exposing the sacral plexus and pudendal nerve roots. After tracing the sacral and pudendal branches, the contributions to the levator ani are all considered nLA (Loukas et al., 2015). The nerve may be approached directly via the perineum and ischiorectal fossae and the anal canal and lower rectum may be incised and bisected, and the pelvic viscera reflected to expose the nLA and its course to innervate the levator ani muscles. The nLA may be seen traveling into the pelvis above or piercing through the ischiococcygeus muscle. The nerve courses along the ventral surface of the ischiococcygeus and pubococcygeus while also sending fibers to puborectalis (Standring, 2016).

Alternatively, the nerve may be accessed parasacrally by reflecting the gluteus maximus and sacrotuberous ligament. A musculoligamentous flap can then be created by transecting the sacrospinous ligament, coccygeus, and posterior portion of the levator ani to expose the pelvic section of the nLA (Roberts et al., 1988) (Fig. 5.1).

The nLA is most commonly formed from the ventral rami of S4–S5 and is supported by the most current human cadaveric study of the nLA by Loukas et al. (2015). Out of the 200 specimens used in the Loukas et al. study, 50% ($n = 100$) of the nLA were contributions from S4–S5. Of 12 human cadavers, Barber et al. (2002) found 40% of nLA to emerge from S3–S4, yet the number of specimens may present as a limitation to this study. It has been mentioned that the pudendal nerve may also convey branches to the levator ani thorough its inferior rectal and perineal nerve branches (Sato, 1980; Sato and Sato, 1981; Shafik et al., 1995), yet Loukas et al. (2015) found no such contribution in their specimens. Early descriptions insist the pudendal nerve is the essential nerve for the levator ani with the direct branches of S3–S4 serving as minor contributions to the peripheral parts. Percy et al. (1981) described three cases in which the pudendal nerve exclusively provided innervation to the external anal sphincter muscle. Major medical texts incorporate contributions from S2, as well as branches of the pudendal nerve (Standring, 2016). Barber et al. (2002) witnessed no pudendal nerve contributions in all 12 cadaveric specimens, only branches from S3–S5. One possible limitation to this study is that it utilized only human female specimens. Wallner et al. (2006) observed the nLA conveying fibers intramuscularly to puborectalis.Wallner et al. (2007) described the nLA running on the superior surface of the pelvic floor, but under the pelvic diaphragmatic fascia. The study concluded the pudendal nerve's contribution to the levator ani was minimal. The contradictions regarding the S2 and pudendal nerve contributions, as well as the variations of the nerve supply to the nLA, may contribute to iatrogenic injury in pelvic reconstructive surgeries.

Surgical Anatomy of the Sacral Plexus and Its Branches. https://doi.org/10.1016/B978-0-323-77602-8.00005-2

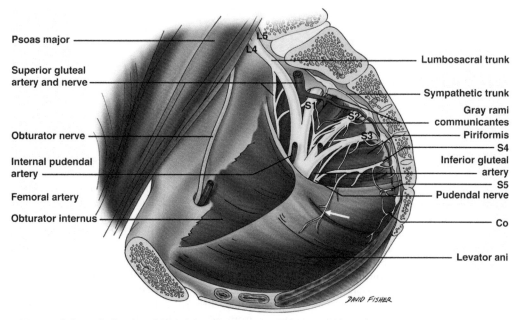

FIG. 5.1 Schematic drawing of the pelvis noting the nerve to levator ani (arrow) arising from S4 and S5 ventral rami.

Electrophysiological study of the levator ani (Percy et al., 1981) was performed in order to determine the involvement of the pudendal and S3–S4 direct branches in pelvic floor contraction. Surgical stimulating electrodes were inserted into each pelvic floor muscle. During pudendal nerve stimulation, EMG activity was only detected in the ipsilateral external anal sphincter muscle. Again, the results may be conflicting, as sources have reported the pudendal nerve supplying pubococcygeus, and deeper, puborectalis. Waller et al. (2008) found 50%–60% of specimen ($n = 9$) to have communicating nerve branches between the pudendal and nLA from the inferior surface of the pelvic floor. Grigorescu et al. (2007) found the levator ani to be innervated by pudendal, perineal, and inferior rectal nerves, and S3 and/or S4.

ORIGINS IN THE SPINAL CORD

In 1899, Bronislaw Onufrowicz observed a unique collection of neural cells in the sacral segments of the spinal cord and named them group X, now termed Onuf's nucleus. Onuf's nucleus, having been determined to be comprised of motoneurons in the ventral sacral horn, is suggested to be the origin point for the innervation of the external anal sphincter and urethral muscles. This nucleus is thus responsible for micturition and defecation; serves as the origin of the pudendal

nerve; and contributes to motor control of the pelvic sphincter muscles, skin of the genitalia, perineum, and anus, as well as having varying contributions to the levator ani (Schröder, 1981). Onuf's nucleus is regularly found in the S2–S3 segments; however, S1–S3 have been consistently involved. Longitudinally, Onuf's nucleus measures between 3.5 and 7.9 mm. From transverse, it is located at the ventral border of the ventral sacral horn, medial to the lateral motoneuron group, lateral to the anteromedial group, and dorsal to the anterior funiculus (Schröder, 1981). The cytoarchitecture of Onuf's nucleus is as follows: a transversely oriented cranial group; a ventrolateral division containing longitudinally arranged medium-sized neurons and small fusiform neurons; a dorsomedial division containing medium-sized clusters with no predictable orientation.

VARIATION

Shafik et al. (1995) reported the presence of an "accessory rectal nerve" arising from the pudendal nerve. Shafik et al. (1995) described the trajectory of the nerve as arising from the medial side of the pudendal nerve behind the sacrospinous ligament. The nerve then dove inferolaterally and split into cutaneous and motor branches, supplying the perineal skin, as well as the levator ani muscle. Loukas et al. (2015) reported five variations of the nLA: (1) contributions from S4–S5 (50%), (2) contributions only from S5 (19%), (3) contributions only from S4 (16%), (4) contributions from S3–S4 (11%), and (5) contributions from S3–S5 (4%). Two patterns of nerve termination are observed in the nLA: first, the nerve may penetrate the coccygeus and then course externally along the surface of the levator ani. Second, the nerve may cross the coccygeus superiorly, course along the superior surface of the iliococcygeus, and then give rise to various penetrating branches that continue to the pubococcygeus, and puborectalis. Loukas et al. (2015) also observed contributions from the inferior rectal nerve to the levator ani.

BLOOD SUPPLY

Day (1964) cites the lateral sacral, median sacral, gluteal, and pudendal arteries as supplying the lumbar and sacral plexuses, along with other nearest accessible vessels from the abdominal aorta. Branches of the deep iliac circumflex artery have also been observed to supply these structures (Wohlgemuth et al., 1999). The blood supply for the sacral plexus is segmental. As determined by Day (1964), the sacral roots are supplied by the lateral sacral artery (left 60%, right 60%); superior gluteal artery (22% left, 16% right); inferior gluteal artery (7% left, 5% right); iliolumbar artery (7% left, 5% right); medial sacral artery (2% left, 11% right); and internal iliac arteries (4% left, 5% right). The superior gluteal artery is distributed segmentally over the roots and ganglia of L5–S3 segments and the inferior gluteal artery from S2–S4 segments.

From the intervertebral foramina, the ventral rami of sacral nerves receive their blood supply. Arterial branching occurs at the interface of the lumbar and sacral plexuses. Day (1964) mentions that it was difficult to assign distinct arteries to nerve trunks. In the sacral region, the largest proportion of blood to the sacral ventral rami was from the lateral sacral arteries.

SURGERY

The anorectum and perineum both have complicated surgical anatomy due to the various intervening fasciae, rich blood supply from the rectal arteries (median sacral, superior rectal, middle rectal, and inferior rectal arteries), and rectal venous plexus. The rectal venous plexus is constituted by the external and internal rectal plexuses, as well as a perimuscular plexus (Godlewski and Prudhomme, 2000). The pelvic splanchnic nerves derived from S3–S4 provide parasympathetic innervation to the rectum and upper half of the anal canal.

Damage to these nerves during invasive approaches to the anorectum or genitourinary regions, such as in rectal tumor resection, genital or pelvic floor reconstructive surgery, may damage the parasympathetics resulting in dyssynergic defecation. The correction of pelvic organ prolapse, when approached posteriorly, may also result in damage to the pelvic splanchnics and nLA if they are not properly located (Takeyama et al., 2007). Damage to the nLA may result in loss of sexual function in men and women. The contraction of the levator ani muscle results in urination and defecation, therefore injury to this nerve may result in urinary incontinence.

Although small and infrequently described in the literature, the nLA should be remembered as a branch of the sacral plexus. Its exact innervation patterns still require study and consensus.

REFERENCES

Barber, M.D., Bremer, R.E., Thor, K.B., Dolber, P.C., Kuehl, T.J., Coates, K.W., 2002. Innervation of the female levator ani muscles. Am. J. Obstet. Gynecol. 187 (1), 64–71. https://doi.org/10.1067/mob.2002.124844.

Day, M.H., 1964. The blood supply of the lumbar and sacral plexuses in the human foetus. J. Anat. 98 (Pt 1), 105.

Godlewski, G., Prudhomme, M., 2000. Embryology and anatomy of the anorectum. Surg. Clin. 80 (1), 319–343. https://doi.org/10.1016/s0039-6109(05)70408-4.

Grigorescu, B.A., Lazarou, G., Olson, T.R., Downie, S.A., Powers, K., Greston, W.M., Mikhail, M.S., 2007. Innervation of the levator ani muscles: description of the nerve branches to the pubococcygeus, iliococcygeus, and puborectalis muscles. Int. Urogynecol. J 19 (1), 107–116. https://doi.org/10.1007/s00192-007-0395-8.

Loukas, M., Joseph, S., Etienne, D., Linganna, S., Hallner, B., Tubbs, R.S., 2015. Topography and landmarks for the nerve supply to the levator ani and its relevance to pelvic floor pathologies. Clin. Anat. 29 (4), 516–523. https://doi.org/10.1002/ca.22668.

Percy, J.P., Swash, M., Neill, M.E., Parks, A.G., 1981. Electrophysiological study of motor nerve supply of pelvic floor. Lancet 317 (8210), 16–17. https://doi.org/10.1016/s0140-6736(81)90117-3.

Roberts, W.H., Harrison, C.W., Mitchell Jr., D.A., Fischer, F., 1988. The levator ani muscle and the nerve supply of its puborectalis component. Clin. Anat. 1, 267–283.

Sato, K., 1980. A morphological analysis of the nerve supply of the sphincter ani externus, levator ani and coccygeus. Acta. Anat. Nippon. 55, 187–223.

Sato, K., Sato, T., 1981. Composition and distribution of the pudendal and pelvic plexuses. Jpn. J. Coloproctol. SOC 34, 515–529.

Schrøder, H.D., 1981. Onuf's nucleus X: a morphological study of a human spinal nucleus. Anat. Embryol. 162 (4), 443–453. https://doi.org/10.1007/bf00301870.

Shafik, A., El-Sherif, M., Youssef, A., Olfat, E.-S., 1995. Surgical anatomy of the pudendal nerve and its clinical implications. Clin. Anat. 8 (2), 110–115. https://doi.org/10.1002/ca.980080205.

Standring, S., 2016. Gray's Anatomy: Anatomical Basis for Clinical Practice, 41st ed. Elsevier.

Takeyama, M., Koyama, M., Murakami, G., Nagata, I., Tomoe, H., Furuya, K., 2007. Nerve preservation in tension-free vaginal mesh procedures for pelvic organ prolapse: a cadaveric study using fresh and fixed cadavers. Int. Urogynecol. J. 19 (4), 559–566. https://doi.org/10.1007/s00192-007-0467-9.

Wallner, C., Maas, C.P., Dabhoiwala, N.F., Lamers, W.H., DeRuiter, M.C., 2006. Evidence for the innervation of the puborectalis muscle by the levator ani nerve. Neuro. Gastroenterol. Motil. 18 (12), 1121–1122. https://doi.org/10.1111/j.1365-2982.2006.00846.x.

Wallner, C., Maas, C.P., Dabhoiwala, N.F., Lamers, W.H., DeRuiter, M.C., 2007. MP-13.07: the levator ani nerve and its clinical implications. Urology 70 (3), 107–108. https://doi.org/10.1016/j.urology.2007.06.430.

Wallner, C., van Wissen, J., Maas, C.P., Dabhoiwala, N.F., DeRuiter, M.C., Lamers, W.H., 2008. The contribution of the levator ani nerve and the pudendal nerve to the innervation of the levator ani muscles; a study in human fetuses. Eur. Urol. 54 (5), 1136–1144. https://doi.org/10.1016/j.eururo.2007.11.015.

Wohlgemuth, W.A., Rottach, K.G., Stoehr, M., 1999. Intermittent claudication due to ischaemia of the lumbosacral plexus. J. Neurol. Neurosurg. Psychiatry 67 (6), 793–795.

CHAPTER 6

The Perforating Cutaneous Nerve

AMARILIS CAMACHO • FÉLIX D. RODRÍGUEZ • R. SHANE TUBBS

ANATOMY

The perforating cutaneous nerve (n. perforans ligament tuberoso-sacri, n. cutaneous clunium inferior medialis) (Fig. 6.1) arises from the posterior rami of the second and third sacral nerves, pierces the sacrotuberous ligament not far from the coccyx, and curves around the inferior border of the gluteus maximus to then supply the skin of its respective area. The perforating cutaneous nerve is the only nerve in the gluteal region that does not enter the area through the greater sciatic foramen. Its distribution has been variably described as innervating the skin on the inferior and medial parts of the buttocks, the skin of the posteroinferior area of the gluteal region, to the skin over the inner and lower parts of the gluteus maximus or only the medial aspect of the gluteus maximus or gluteal fold.

VARIATIONS

The perforating cutaneous nerve may also arise from the same origin as the pudendal nerve or from the pudendal nerve itself, follow the same course, and then reach its normal innervated area. When absent as a separate nerve, its place is taken by gluteal branches of the posterior cutaneous nerve of the thigh or a branch from the pudendal nerve or a small nerve (n. perforans coccygeus major, Eisler), arising separately from the posterior part of the third and fourth sacral nerves and piercing the coccygeus muscle. Its territory can be supplied by the greater coccygeal perforating nerve of Eisler that arises from the third and fourth or the fourth and fifth sacral nerves. A perforating cutaneous nerve arising as above was found by Eisler 22 times in 34 plexuses: in three of these it arose at its origin with the pudendal nerve. Instead of piercing the sacrotuberous ligament, it may run with the pudendal nerve between the sacrotuberous and sacrospinous ligaments, or it may pass between the sacrotuberous ligament and gluteus maximus muscle.

Florian-Rodriguez et al., in 14 female cadavers, found that in 85% of specimens, between one and three branches from S3 and/or S4 pierced or coursed between the sacrotuberous and sacrospinous ligaments and perforated the lower medial part of the gluteus maximus or subcutaneous tissues just medial to the ischial tuberosity. These authors suggested these nerve branches might represent a variant origin/course of the perforating branch of the sacral plexus, but such nerves might also be the greater coccygeal perforating nerve as described by Eisler.

Surgical Anatomy of the Sacral Plexus and Its Branches. https://doi.org/10.1016/B978-0-323-77602-8.00006-4

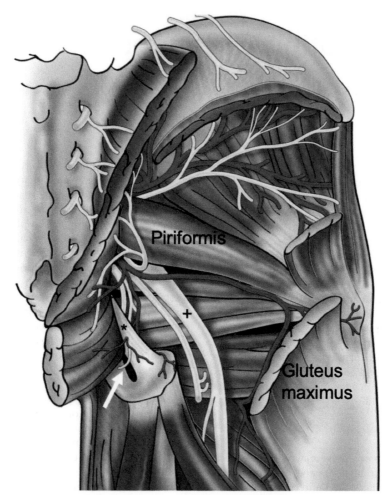

FIG. 6.1 Posterior view of the gluteal region. The perforating cutaneous nerve (arrow) is seen emanating from the sacrotuberous ligament (asterisk). For reference, note the laterally placed sciatic nerve (+).

ADDITIONAL READING

Eisler, P., 1892. Der Plexus lumbo-sacralis des Menschen, Abhandlg. D. Naturforsch.Gesellsch. zu Halle.

Florian-Rodriguez, M.E., Hare, A., Chin, K., et al., 2016. Inferior gluteal and other nerves associated with the sacrospinous ligament: a cadaver study. Am. J. Obstet. Gynecol. 215, 646.

Schafer, E.A., Thane, G.D., 1895. Quain's Elements of Anatomy, tenth ed. Longmans, Green, and Co., London.

Schaffer, J.P., 1953. Morris' Human Anatomy, eleventh ed. McGraw-Hill, New York.

CHAPTER 7

The Nerve to Obturator Internus

TYLER WARNER • R. SHANE TUBBS

ANATOMY

The nerve to the obturator internus (Figs. 7.1 and 7.2) is a branch of the lumbosacral plexus derived from the ventral rami of nerve roots L5, S1, and S2. The nerve roots aggregate inside the pelvis and exit through the greater sciatic foramen, below the piriformis muscle and posterior to the sacrospinous ligament. The nerve travels distally to innervate the obturator internus and superior gemellus. Specifically, the nerve innervates the obturator internus on its medial surface. As it continues to move anteriorly, the nerve branches off laterally and posteriorly within the obturator internus. The nerve innervates the superior gemellus on its posterior aspect and will vary in both its intramuscular path and its interaction with the nerve to the quadratus femoris. Studies have shown various intramuscular and extramuscular communication patterns between the two nerves (Aung et al., 2001). The obturator internus contributes to lateral rotation of the thigh, abduction at the hip, and stabilization of the hip joint when walking (Miniato and Varacallo, 2019).

Because of the structure, function, and variant nerve supply of the muscles, anatomists have inquired as to how the superior gemellus, inferior gemellus, and obturator internus muscles should be classified. The obturator internus muscle enters the gemellus pocket—made up of the superior and inferior gemellus muscles—giving rise to a single tendon from these three muscles. Although the nerve patterns differ among these muscles, the nerves innervating them share spinal roots, which raises the question of whether the muscles truly work independently of each other and should instead be classified as an individual muscle with three heads (Shinohara, 1995).

FUNCTION

The nerve to the obturator internus primarily innervates the obturator internus and superior gemellus muscles, which assists in lateral rotation of the hip (Miniato and Varacallo, 2019). As the former muscle is much larger, it describes much of the function that the nerve to the obturator internus is responsible for. This muscle lies on the anterolateral wall of the pelvis and exits through the lesser sciatic foramen to insert on the greater trochanter of the humerus. Until recently, it has been difficult to definitively identify the actions of the muscle because superficial electromyography recordings do not allow for information to be read from the obturator internus muscle exclusively (Hodges et al., 2014).

Recent studies have been able to effectively isolate electromyography readings to the obturator internus, which show its primary role in external rotation of and abduction at the hip. The readings revealed the greatest activation coming from extension at the hip, but most muscles in the gluteal region—including larger muscles—were highly activated during this movement, which may indicate a lower proportion of function to that particular movement coming from the obturator internus muscle. The study was able to confirm that joint stability was only proven to be evident when the muscle is activated and torque is applied to the joint. Some speculate that the obturator internus muscle even plays a role in bowel continence because the muscles of levator ani attach to the obturator internus (Hodges et al., 2014).

VARIATIONS

There is a large degree of variation for both the origin of the nerve and its muscular innervations (Hollinshead, 1967). The lumbosacral plexus usually forms from the combined nerve roots of the ventral rami but will vary if the plexus is prefixed or postfixed (Tubbs et al., 2019). Hollinshead reported variations of the nerve to the obturator internus that included L4 to S1, L4 to S2, L4 to S3, L5 to S3, S1 to S2, S1 to S3, and S2 but showed the common composition of this nerve was from L5 to S2. This nerve also shows consistency in receiving more caudally located nerve roots than the nerve to the quadratus femoris (Hollinshead, 1967).

Surgical Anatomy of the Sacral Plexus and Its Branches. https://doi.org/10.1016/B978-0-323-77602-8.00007-6

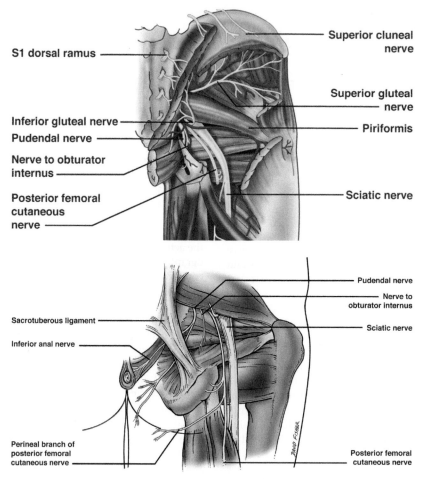

S1 dorsal ramus

Inferior gluteal nerve

Pudendal nerve

Nerve to obturator internus

Posterior femoral cutaneous nerve

Superior cluneal nerve

Superior gluteal nerve

Piriformis

Sciatic nerve

Sacrotuberous ligament

Inferior anal nerve

Perineal branch of posterior femoral cutaneous nerve

Pudendal nerve

Nerve to obturator internus

Sciatic nerve

Posterior femoral cutaneous nerve

FIGS. 7.1 AND 7.2 Schematic drawing illustrating the nerve to obturator internus and surrounding anatomy.

To thoroughly review the variants of the nerve to the obturator internus, it is necessary to compare it to the nerve to the quadratus femoris due to its similarity in course, proximity, and related functionality. There are varying degrees of communication between the nerve to the obturator internus and the nerve to the quadratus femoris because the superior gemellus can receive innervation from both nerves. One study using human specimens showed that seven specimens received innervation from the nerve to the obturator internus exclusively, four received innervation from the nerve to the quadratus femoris exclusively, and three received innervation from both nerves. This is exemplary of the great variation in the nerves that innervate the superior gemellus (Honma et al., 1998).

Studies have shown that there is consistency in the positional relationship of the two nerves but variant innervation patterns for the target muscles and the intramuscular pathway of the nerves. The nerve to the obturator internus travels dorsally, whereas the nerve to the quadratus femoris runs along the ventral aspect of the muscle. The nerve to the obturator internus will innervate the posterior and lateral aspects of the superior gemellus, but its communicating branches with the nerve to the quadratus femoris will differ as they innervate the posterior, superior, and anterior aspects of the muscle. Although there are variant pathways for the superior gemellus, the nerve to the obturator internus travels along the same intramuscular pathway through the obturator internus muscle (Aung et al., 2001).

CLINICAL

Piriformis syndrome can also involve the nerve to the obturator internus. Compression of the sciatic nerve is usually responsible for the pain associated with this complication, but the sciatic nerve is not the only nerve running through the greater sciatic foramen. Like the sciatic nerve, the nerve to the obturator internus passes under the piriformis muscle and may be compressed in piriformis syndrome or other sciatic notch syndromes (Kirschner et al., 2009; Filler, 2008). Endoscopic sciatic nerve neurolysis has been used as an effective tool in temporarily relieving symptoms of piriformis syndrome. Although proven useful, the risk of damage to the nerve to the obturator internus has been noted. The procedure is image guided, but clinicians consider the proximity of the nerve to the obturator internus because it lies just medial to the sciatic nerve (Knudsen et al., 2015).

Calcifications may also compress the nerve to the obturator internus. Although rare, ossification of the sacrotuberous ligament can present with symptoms like perineal pain and muscle weakness. The pain is not directly related to a compression of the nerve to the obturator internus, but it may indicate a problem in the deep gluteal region. If the nerve to the obturator internus were compressed, muscle weakness from the obturator internus and superior gemellus muscles would result (Arora et al., 2009). The compression of this nerve could present as spasms of the obturator internus muscle. After passing through the greater sciatic foramen, the sciatic nerve crosses over the tendon of the obturator internus muscle, which may lead to sciatic nerve impingement if the tendon is taut. The pudendal nerve—which is located medial to the nerve to the obturator internus as it courses over the sacrospinous ligament—may also be susceptible to impingement in Alcock's canal, which could cause pain in the perineum and dysfunction of the muscles; this nerve is responsible for innervating (Youmans and Winn, 2011).

COMPARATIVE ANATOMY

Although the nerves to the obturator internus and quadratus femoris are named separately, there is a large degree of overlap at the nerve root origins that make up these nerves and the muscles they are responsible for innervating. Rhesus monkeys have been used to observe the relationships between the nerves coming from the lumbosacral plexus because its anatomy has many morphological similarities to humans. Like humans, the nerve to the quadratus femoris tends to receive innervation from nerve roots more cranially located, while the nerve to the obturator internus tends to receive innervation from those more caudally located. However, in two of the eight specimens in one study (Aung et al., 2001), the nerve to the obturator internus branched from the nerve to the quadratus femoris, showing some level of variation in this species.

These specimens also showed a great deal of similarity in the target muscles and the intramuscular path through the muscle. Like humans, the nerve to the obturator internus innervates the obturator internus muscle on its medial aspect in Rhesus monkeys. It then proceeds through the muscle anteriorly with branches moving superficially and posteriorly along the muscle. The gemelli muscles received some branches from the nerve to the obturator internus, but the innervation is shared with the nerve to the quadratus femoris. The degree to which they share their innervation to the gemelli muscles varied and the differences in the muscle development may have accounted for this. Ultimately, the Rhesus monkey showed a large number of similarities, and the specimens proved useful when observing the anatomical relationships between the nerve to the obturator internus and its surrounding tissues (Aung et al., 2001).

REFERENCES

Arora, J., Mehta, V., Suri, R., Rath, G., 2009. Rom. J. Morphol. Embryol. 50 (3), 505—508.

Aung, H., Sakamoto, H., Akita, K., Sato, T., 2001. Anatomical study of the obturator internus, gemelli and quadratus femoris muscles with special reference to their innervation. Anat. Rec. 263 (1), 41—52.

Filler, A., 2008. Piriformis and related entrapment syndromes: diagnosis & management. Neurosurg. Clin. 19 (4), 609—622.

Hodges, P., McLean, L., Hodder, J., 2014. Insight into the function of the obturator internus muscle in humans: observations with development and validation of an electromyography recording technique. J. Electromyogr. Kinesiol. 24 (4), 489—496.

Hollinshead, W., 1967. Textbook of Anatomy, second. Harper & Row, New York, pp. 722—724.

Honma, S., Jun, Y., Horiguchi, M., 1998. The human gemelli muscles and their nerve supplies. Kaibogaku Zasshi 73 (4), 329—335.

Kirschner, J., Foye, P., Cole, J., 2009. Piriformis syndrome, diagnosis and treatment. Muscle Nerve 40 (1), 10—18.

Knudsen, J., McConkey, M., Brick, M., 2015. Endoscopic sciatic neurolysis. . 4 (4), e353—e358. www.ncbi.nlm.nih.gov/pmc/articles/PMC4680922/.

Miniato, M.A., Varacallo, M., January 2019. Anatomy, back, lumbosacral trunk [Updated 2019 Mar 9]. In: StatPearls. StatPearls Publishing, Treasure Island (FL). Available from: https://www.ncbi.nlm.nih.gov/books/NBK539878/.

Shinohara, H., 1995. Gemelli and obturator internus muscles: different heads of one muscle? Anat. Rec. 243 (1), 145–150.

Tubbs, et al., 2019. Bergman's Comprehensive Encyclopedia of Human Anatomic Variation. John Wiley & Sons, Inc., pp. 1113–1114

Youmans, J., Winn, H., 2011. Youmans Neurological Surgery. Saunders/Elsevier, Philadelphia, pp. 2447–2456.

CHAPTER 8

The Nerve to Quadratus Femoris

KARISHMA MEHTA • R. SHANE TUBBS

The nerve to quadratus femoris is a branch of the sacral plexus arising from ventral rami L4, L5, and S1. It provides innervation to the quadratus femoris and inferior gemellus muscles, which function to laterally rotate and abduct the hip.

EMBRYOLOGY

Before discussing the embryology of the nerve to quadratus femoris, it is useful to first understand the "preaxial" and "postaxial" borders of the limbs. Paterson (Paterson, 1894) describes the preaxial border as running in line with the great saphenous vein (i.e., originating at the medial border of the foot, to the medial border of the tibia and sartorius muscle, and ending at the groin). The postaxial border starts at the outer edge of the foot, to the lateral border of the thigh, and then runs posteriorly to the gluteus maximus and coccyx. Each border is then subdivided into the conventional definitions of ventral and dorsal muscles. The dorsal surface is defined as the anterior plane of the lower limb, while the ventral surface pertains to the upper medial thigh and the posterior plane of the lower limb. The nerve to quadratus femoris and its associated muscles are located ventrally along the preaxial border.

The nerve to quadratus femoris has been found to be in close association with the nerve to obturator internus. Paterson (Paterson, 1894) states that as a general rule, muscles located near the preaxial border are innervated by more proximal nerves, while those near the postaxial border by more distal nerves, with a few exceptions. For example, according to this rule, a nerve more distal to that of which supplies the obturator internus should innervate the quadratus femoris and inferior gemellus muscles (e.g., the obturator internus should be innervated by more proximal ventral rami). Instead, the obturator internus muscle is innervated by the nerve to obturator internus derived from the ventral rami of S1-3 and the nerve to quadratus femoris is supplied by ventral rami of L4-S1. This suggests a

rotation of the lower limb during embryological development in which the ventral quadratus femoris and inferior gemellus muscles likely began more distal to the obturator internus (Paterson, 1894).

ANATOMY

The nerve to quadratus femoris originates from the lumbosacral plexus via the fourth and fifth lumbar ventral rami and the first sacral ventral rami. The nerve exits the pelvis and enters the gluteal region through the greater sciatic foramen (Fig. 8.1). It passes below the piriformis muscle and anterior to the sciatic nerve, anterior to the plane of the gluteal muscles. It then courses toward the ischial tuberosity, deep to the obturator internus tendon (Figs. 8.2–8.4), finally supplying branches to the deep surfaces of quadratus femoris and inferior gemellus muscles. The nerve also has numerous smaller branches, including a periosteal branch supplying the ischial tuberosity and an articular branch supplying the hip joint (Walji and Tsui, 2016; Drake et al., 2009; Cruveilhier, 1853).

Kampa et al. studied this articular nerve in 20 cadaveric hips and determined that the average number of capsular branches was 1.65, ranging from one to four. The majority of the branches innervated the medial aspect of the hip joint (Kampa et al., 2007). The innervation of this articular branch to the hip joint can explain the basis behind quadratus femoris nerve blockade as an alternative to obturator nerve blockade in alleviation of hip pain (James and Little, 1976).

Kikuchi (1987) studied the anatomy of the nerve to quadratus femoris in different mammals, including dogs, cats, rabbits, guinea pigs, and rats. He noted that among these animals, guinea pigs have a common trunk between the obturator internus nerve and the quadratus femoris nerve that joins the sciatic nerve. Cats do not have this bigeminal nerve, but rather the nerve to quadratus femoris arises from the pudendal nerve or its ventral rami (Kikuchi, 1987).

Surgical Anatomy of the Sacral Plexus and Its Branches. https://doi.org/10.1016/B978-0-323-77602-8.00008-8

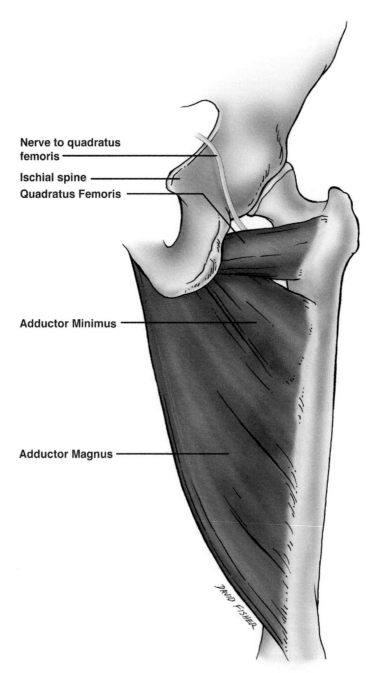

Nerve to quadratus femoris

Ischial spine

Quadratus Femoris

Adductor Minimus

Adductor Magnus

DAVID FISHER

FIG. 8.1 Schematic drawing of the posterior hip and thigh and noting the exit of the nerve to quadratus femoris out of the greater sciatic foramen. Note the nerve's proximity to the hip joint and ischial spine.

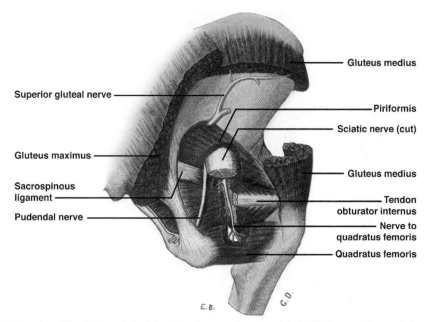

Gluteus medius

Superior gluteal nerve

Piriformis

Sciatic nerve (cut)

Gluteus maximus

Gluteus medius

Sacrospinous ligament

Tendon obturator internus

Pudendal nerve

Nerve to quadratus femoris

Quadratus femoris

E.B.

C.D.

FIG. 8.2 Drawing of the right posterior hip noting the muscles associated with the nerve to quadratus femoris. (After Testut.)

VARIATIONS

Numerous variations have been noted when studying the anatomy of the nerve to quadratus femoris. Wilson et al. noted an enlarged right-sided nerve to quadratus femoris in a cadaver. This specimen's nerve descended distally and also innervated the adductor magnus muscle (Wilson, 1889; Aung et al., 2001). Aung et al. observed variations in the supply and branching patterns of this nerve. Although most commonly observed with contributions from ventral rami L4-S1, the nerve to quadratus femoris may originate from L5-S1 (Aung et al., 2001; Campbell, 2012). Furthermore, in 84.6% of their specimens, there was a common nerve root shared between the nerve to quadratus femoris and the nerve to obturator internus. They also found a communicating branch between these two nerves in several of their cadavers. Lastly, innervation to the superior gemellus muscle was noted in 60.4% of their dissections (Aung et al., 2001).

Petchprapa et al. noted that different planes of view are optimal when viewing the lumbosacral plexus at various points along its trajectory. Normally, the lumbar plexus forms posterior to the psoas major muscle. And while most nerves of the plexus travel lateral to

the psoas major, the obturator nerve and nerve roots of the lumbosacral plexus exit medial to the psoas major muscle. They then coalesce with the rest of the sacral plexus anterior to the piriformis muscle (Soldatos et al., 2013). The lumbosacral plexus can best be seen using axial images at this point. However, as the sacral ventral rami continue distally, the use of a coronal oblique, axial oblique, or sagittal plane is optimal (Petchprapa et al., 2010).

There are also certain landmarks to keep in mind when viewing MR imaging of the lumbosacral plexus. The common iliac vessels are located anteromedial to the plexus at the S1 ventral ramus level. Also, the superior gluteal vessels pass between the lumbosacral plexus and the S1 nerve, while the inferior gluteal vessels pass between the S1 and S2 nerves (Gierada et al., 1993).

PATHOLOGY

Little research has been conducted on a quadratus femoris nerve pathology. Instead, more studies have focused on impingement or damage to the quadratus femoris muscle itself. Muscular pathologies of the quadratus femoris include but are not limited to

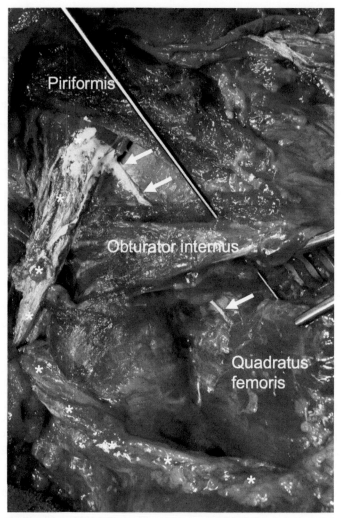

FIG. 8.3 Cadaveric dissection of the right nerve to quadratus femoris (arrows). Note that the overlying sciatic nerve (asterisks) has been retracted. The dissection probe is placed under the tendon of obturator internus in order to better visualize the superior and inferior gemelli muscles just above and just below this muscle. After traveling deep to the aforementioned muscles, the nerve is seen terminating (lowest arrows) in the quadratus femoris.

ischiofemoral impingement syndrome and muscle tear with various clinical presentations.

Ischiofemoral impingement syndrome is defined as the entrapment of the quadratus femoris muscle between the ischium and femur due to space narrowing (Lee et al., 2013; Torriani et al., 2009). This syndrome presents as hip pain exacerbated by lateral rotation, adduction, and extension of the hip. It is usually caused by trauma, surgery, or, very rarely, degenerative nerve lesions. Women are predisposed to the condition due to their broad and shallow pelvis. Diagnosis is made via T2-weighted MRI that demonstrates increased signal in the quadratus femoris muscle and possible edema, tearing, and fatty infiltration (Torriani et al., 2009).

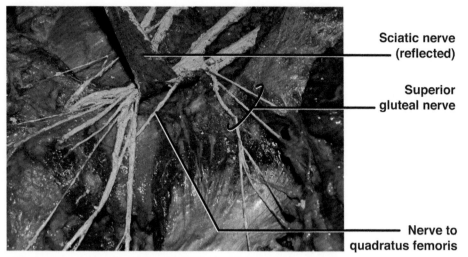

Sciatic nerve (reflected)

Superior gluteal nerve

Nerve to quadratus femoris

FIG. 8.4 Cadaveric dissection noting the nerve to quadratus femoris with the sciatic nerve lifted superiorly.

REFERENCES

Aung, H.H., Sakamoto, H., Akita, K., et al., 2001. Anatomical study of the obturator internus, gemelli and quadratus femoris muscles with special reference to their innervation. Anat. Rec. 263 (1), 41–52.

Campbell, W.W., 2012. Dejong's the Neurologic Examination, seventh ed. Lippincott's Williams & Wilkins, Philadelphia.

Cruveilhier, J., 1853. The Anatomy of the Human Body, third ed. Harper & Brothers, New York.

Drake, R., Vogl, A.W., Mitchell, A.W.M., 2009. Gray's Anatomy for Students, second ed. Churchill Livingstone Elsevier, Philadelphia, PA.

Gierada, D.S., Erickson, S.J., Haughton, V.M., Estkowski, L.D., Nowicki, B.H., 1993. MR imaging of the sacral plexus: normal findings. Am. J. Roentgenol. 160 (5), 1059–1065.

James, C.D.T., Little, T.F., 1976. Regional hip blockade: a simplified technique for the relief of intractable osteoarthritic pain. Anaesthesia 31, 1060–1067.

Kampa, R.J., Prasthofer, A., Lawrence-Watt, D.J., et al., 2007. The internervous safe zone for incision of the capsule of the hip. A cadaver study J. Bone Joint Surg. Br. 89, 971–976.

Kikuchi, T., 1987. A macroscopical observation of the nerves to the pelvic floor muscles, the obturator internus and the quadratus femoris in some mammals. Hokkaido Igaku Zasshi 62 (1), 96–107.

Lee, S., Kim, I., Lee, S.M., Lee, J., 2013. Ischiofemoral impingement syndrome. Ann. Rehabil. Med. 37, 143–146.

Paterson, A., 1894. The origin and distribution of the nerves to the lower limb. J. Anat. Physiol. 28 (2), 169–193.

Petchprapa, C., Rosenberg, Z., Sconfienza, L., Cavalcanti, C., Vieira, R., Zember, J., 2010. MR imaging of entrapment neuropathies of the lower extremity. Part 1. The pelvis and hip. Radiographics 30 (4), 983–1000.

Soldatos, T., Andreisek, G., Thawait, G.K., Guggenberger, R., Williams, E.H., Carrino, J.A., Chhabra, A., 2013. High-resolution 3-T MR neurography of the lumbosacral plexus. Radiographics 33 (4), 967–987.

Torriani, M., Souto, S.C.L., Thomas, B.J., et al., 2009. Ischiofemoral impingement syndrome: an entity with hip pain and abnormalities of the quadratus femoris muscle. Am. J. Roentgenol. 193, 186–190.

Walji, A.H., Tsui, B.C.H., 2016. Clinical anatomy of the sacral plexus. In: Tsui, B., Suresh, S. (Eds.), Pediatric Atlas of Ultrasound and Nerve Stimulation Guided Regional Anesthesia. Springer, New York.

Wilson, J.T., 1889. Abnormal distribution of the nerve to quadratus femoris in man, with remarks on its significance. J. Anat. Physiol 23, 354–357.

CHAPTER 9

The Posterior Femoral Cutaneous Nerve

HALLE E.K. BURLEY • R. SHANE TUBBS

INTRODUCTION

The posterior femoral cutaneous nerve (Fig. 9.1), also known as the small sciatic nerve, arises from the dorsal and ventral divisions of the ventral rami of S1, S2, and S3. Along its course, it splits into inferior cluneal, perineal, and femoral branches supplying skin of the inferior buttock, posterior genitalia, posterior thigh, and variable amounts of the superior posterior calf. The posterior femoral cutaneous nerve may be implicated in a number of entrapment or iatrogenic neuralgias.

ANATOMY

The posterior femoral cutaneous nerve arises from the dorsal divisions of S1 and S2 and the ventral divisions of S2 and S3. It exits the pelvis via the greater sciatic foramen, below the piriformis and just medial to the sciatic nerve. It follows the sciatic nerve medially and the inferior gluteal vessels through the subgluteal space, trending superficially. Eventually, it splits into a cutaneous or femoral branch, a gluteal branch, and a perineal branch. The femoral branch runs superficial to the long head of the biceps femoris deep to the fascia lata. It pierces the fascia lata with the short saphenous vein in the popliteal fossa, its terminal fibers joining with the sural nerve. The gluteal branch, also called the inferior cluneal nerve (Fig. 9.2), follows the inferior gluteal vessels until the inferior margin of the gluteus maximus, where the vessels pass into the muscle belly to perfuse it and the nerve curls around to supply the skin of that region. The perineal branch (Fig. 9.3) wraps medially toward the perineum, communicating with the inferior rectal and posterior scrotal or labial branches of the perineal nerve. Altogether, the three branches of the posterior femoral cutaneous nerve innervate the skin of the posterior thigh, superior posterior calf, inferior buttocks, and posterior labia majora or scrotum.

Piersol (1923) has included a sural branch for the posterior femoral nerve, which is the extension of the femoral branch. This author states, "The sural branches are usually two terminal twigs which innervate to a varying extent the integument of the back of the leg, sometimes not extending beyond the confines of the popliteal space and sometimes continuing all the way to the ankle. They inosculate with the external saphenous nerve, and when they are lacking their place is taken by the external saphenous (sural nerve)."

The posterior femoral cutaneous nerve has a close relationship to the inferior gluteal artery and usually, its descending branch. Pauchot et al. (2010) have found that the perforating branches of the deep femoral artery, popliteal and genicular arteries supply the posterior femoral cutaneous nerve along its course. The nerve has been targeted for anesthetic injection by inserting the needle into the gluteal fold at a point one quarter of the distance from the ischial tuberosity to the greater trochanter.

VARIATIONS

Many variations of the posterior femoral cutaneous nerve or one of its branches may occur. In a prefixed sacral plexus, the posterior femoral cutaneous nerve arises from the L5, S1, and S2 nerve roots. In a postfixed plexus, it arises from the S2, S3, and S4 nerve roots (Eisler, 1892). In some cases, the nerve may arise from two separate trunks, one from the common fibular nerve and one from the tibial nerve (Apaydin, 2016). In this variation, the common fibular nerve carries the dorsal trunk fibers and gives rise to the gluteal and femoral branches. The tibial nerve carries the ventral trunk fibers and gives rise to the perineal and femoral branches. A duplicated posterior femoral cutaneous has also been documented in the literature (Huban et al., 2012), especially when the common fibular and tibial nerves are separated by the piriformis muscle (Piersol, 1923). The nerve can join the sciatic nerve in the thigh via a small branch.

Tubbs et al. (2009) found that it arose directly from the posterior femoral cutaneous nerve in only about 55% of cases. In about 30% of cases, it split from the

Surgical Anatomy of the Sacral Plexus and Its Branches. https://doi.org/10.1016/B978-0-323-77602-8.00009-X

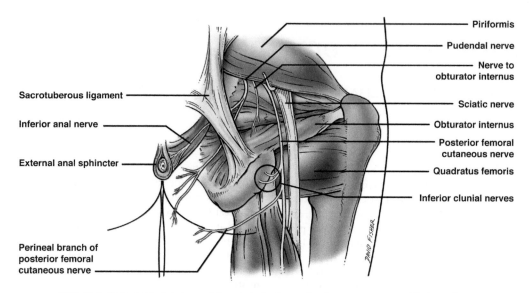

Piriformis

Pudendal nerve

Nerve to obturator internus

Sciatic nerve

Obturator internus

Posterior femoral cutaneous nerve

Quadratus femoris

Inferior clunial nerves

Sacrotuberous ligament

Inferior anal nerve

External anal sphincter

Perineal branch of posterior femoral cutaneous nerve

FIG. 9.1 Schematic drawings of the posterior femoral cutaneous nerve and its branches.

gluteal branch, and in the remaining 15% of cases, it was absent altogether. The perineal branch has also been known to pierce the sacrotuberous ligament. Given their close proximity and overlapping innervations, communications between the perineal branch of the posterior femoral cutaneous nerve and the perineal branch of the pudendal nerve are common.

The number and course of the nerves of the gluteal branch vary from person to person and even side to side. In general, there are two to three branches that separate from the main trunk of the posterior femoral cutaneous nerve, two laterally and one medially. In addition to its typical origin from the main trunk of posterior femoral cutaneous nerve, the medial branch has been known to arise directly from the nerve roots of S2, before the trunk of the posterior femoral cutaneous nerve has formed, or to split from one of the lateral branches and cross medially over the trunk of the posterior femoral cutaneous. The lateral branches may split from the posterior femoral cutaneous nerve individually or from a common trunk (Darnis et al., 2008).

The descending femoral branch may terminate in the popliteal fossa without innervating the calf. Usually in these cases, the sural nerve takes over the innervation of the skin of the superior posterior calf.

Occasionally, small communicating branches will connect the posterior femoral cutaneous and sciatic nerves. Tunali et al. (2011) reported a case where the bridging nerve was located 11 cm below the infrapiriform foramen and measured 3 cm in length. There

were no other variations of the surrounding neural or muscular structures. In cases where fibers from the sciatic join the posterior femoral cutaneous nerve, they may supply the innervation of the biceps femoris (Aasar, 1947).

COMPARATIVE ANATOMY

The origin and course of the posterior femoral cutaneous nerve were observed macroscopically in 38 Japanese adult cadavers, and the results obtained were compared with those from some other mammals (rat, rabbit, dog, and cat) and a number of bibliographical findings on the other animals (Nakanishi et al., 1976). On the basis of the archetype of the pudendal plexus, the site of origin of the posterior femoral cutaneous nerve was divided into seven portions as follows: the sciatic nerve or inferior gluteal nerve (I) and its originating roots (RI), the bigeminal nerve (L6 and boundary between pudendal and sacral plexuses) (B) and its originating roots (RB), the part of junction of I and B (CIB), the pudendal nerve (P) and its originating roots (RP). According to the origin, the posterior femoral cutaneous nerve was classified into six types: Type A (the sciatic nerve type)—the nerve arises from I and RI (horse, rat, bird, frog, and salamander); Type B (the sciatic transitional type)—the nerve arises from I, RI, CIB, RB, and B (man and monkey); Type C (the bigeminal nerve type)—the nerve arises from CIB, RB, and B (gorilla, chimpanzee, orangutan, cat, and sphenodon (*Tuatara*)); Type D (the pudendal transitional type)—

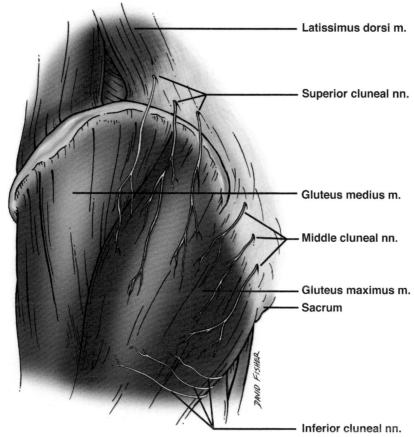

Latissimus dorsi m.

Superior cluneal nn.

Gluteus medius m.

Middle cluneal nn.

Gluteus maximus m.

Sacrum

Inferior cluneal nn.

FIG. 9.2 Schematic drawing of the inferior cluneal branch of the posterior femoral cutaneous nerve.

the nerve arises from CIB, RB, B, RP, and P (dog); Type E (the pudendal nerve type)—the nerve arises from RP and P (pig, cow, and rabbit); Type F (the mixed type)—a mixture of A to E types. From these descriptions it is reasonable to presume that the main trunk of the posterior femoral cutaneous nerve of the tetrapod below the Aves arises from the sciatic nerve and is analogous to the gluteal branches of mammals, with its main stem still retained in the pudendal nerve. If the area supplied by the posterior femoral cutaneous nerve expands to the lateral border of the buttock in company with the medial rotation of the lower limb, the part between this area and that supplied by the pudendal nerve is enlarged. At first, these expanded areas are probably supplied by the branches of the pudendal nerve, which gradually become independent to become the main stem of the posterior femoral cutaneous nerve in mammals. This nerve seems, therefore, to be primarily a division of the pudendal nerve, and so in man has various types of origin in accordance with the scheme in the phylogeny.

PATHOLOGY

Along the course of the posterior femoral cutaneous nerve, there are two areas of potential pathology. One is where the nerve passes the piriformis and ischial spine. Here, the piriformis may compress the nerve or its roots against the ischial spine. The second possible pathologic region is where the perineal branch crosses under the ischium. At this point the nerve is encased in a fatty, fibrous slip, but removal of the fat or development of mechanical or traumatic fibrosis could lead to lesions of the perineal branch. In this scenario, sitting would compress the nerve between the ischium and hamstring muscles, and internal rotation of the thigh would stretch the perineal branch.

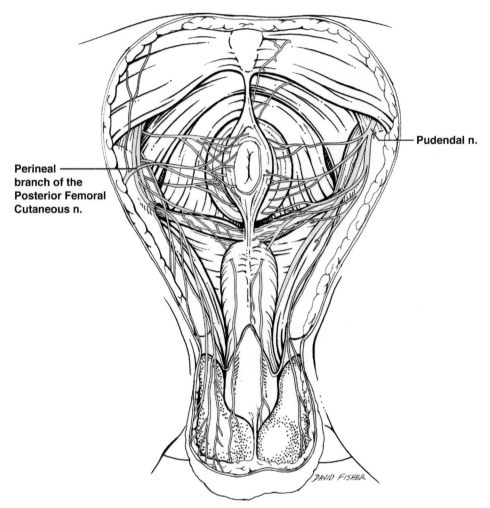

FIG. 9.3 The perineal branch of the posterior femoral cutaneous nerve and its relationship to the pudendal nerve.

Pathology of the posterior femoral cutaneous nerve often presents as pain of the skin of the inferior buttocks, posterior thigh, popliteal area, and superior posterior calf. Clunealgia, specifically, has been described as a burning sensation in the distribution of the inferior cluneal nerve and perineal branch. This distribution encompasses the inferior and medial buttock, proximal posterior thigh, lateral anal margin, and the labia majora or scrotum. Symptoms of clunealgia are aggravated by sitting in a hard chair, which compresses the nerves against the ischium and hamstring muscles. This presentation is in contrast to pudendal neuralgia, where symptoms are confined to the perineum and aggravated by sitting in a soft chair, which compresses the soft tissue of the perineum.

Vascular and neoplastic entrapment pathologies of the posterior femoral cutaneous nerve have also been documented. Chutkow (1988) recorded a case of posterior femoral cutaneous neuralgia caused by a plexus of congenitally dilated, tortuous veins that surrounded the posterior femoral cutaneous nerve and overlaid the posterior surface of the sciatic nerve in the subgluteal space. Harrer et al. (2001) documented a nonmobile lipoblastomatosis of the gluteus maximus, vastus lateralis, and subgluteal space that wrapped around both the posterior femoral cutaneous and sciatic nerves of a newborn.

Because it travels so close to the larger sciatic nerve, isolated traumatic injuries to the posterior femoral cutaneous nerve without concomitant damage to the sciatic nerve are rare. There are a few case reports of posterior femoral cutaneous nerve mononeuropathy in the literature, mostly related to intramuscular gluteal injections (Iyer and Shields, 1989; Kim et al., 2009; Tong and Haig, 2000). There was also one case that occurred in a 73-year-old male who had recently undergone a coronary angiography on his right femoral artery with a subsequent hematoma and hematoma evacuation (Gomceli et al., 2005).

Surgical injuries to the posterior femoral cutaneous nerve have been documented following total hip replacements, proximal hamstring operations, and flap surgeries. Damage incurred during hip replacements is uncommon, and likely related to overstretching (Schumm et al., 1975). In one study, approximately 19% of patients who underwent proximal hamstring avulsion repair had postoperative numbness in the distribution of the posterior femoral cutaneous nerve, especially if the gluteal crease incision was used (Wilson et al., 2019). Another study by Orava et al. (2015), corroborated this incidence range, reporting that 18% of patients developed posterior femoral cutaneous distribution numbness following resection of posttraumatic ossifications and repair of the proximal hamstrings. Fortunately, most patients report that this numbness does not significantly impact their daily lives and it is rarely accompanied by pain. Posterior femoral cutaneous nerve injuries related to gluteal and thigh flap surgeries are relatively common due to the proximity of the nerve and the inferior gluteal artery and their variable arrangement in relation to each other.

IMAGING AND TREATMENT

Should posterior femoral cutaneous neuropathies prove painful, conservative treatment options include physical therapy and oral pain therapy. Nerve blockades, perineural injections, and cryoablation have also proven effective in reducing pain. A number of imaging modalities are available for localization before and during these procedures, including ultrasound, high-resolution MRI, and CT. On the most invasive end of the spectrum, surgical neurectomy may provide long-lasting relief if the diagnosis of posterior femoral cutaneous neuropathy has been confirmed with a nerve block.

REFERENCES

Aasar, Y.H., 1947. Anatomical Abnormalities. Fouad I University Press, Cairo, pp. 92–101.

Apaydin, N., 2016. Lumbosacral plexus. In: Tubbs, R.S., Shoja, M.M., Loukas, M. (Eds.), Bergman's Comprehensive Encyclopedia of Human Anatomic Variation, vol. 1. John Wiley & Sons, Inc, Hoboken, pp. 335–368.

Chutkow, J.G., 1988. Posterior femoral cutaneous neuralgia. Muscle Nerve 11, 1146–1148.

Darnis, B., Robert, R., Labat, J.J., Riant, T., Gaudin, C., Hamel, A., Hamel, O., 2008. Perineal pain and inferior cluneal nerves: anatomy and surgery. Surg. Radiol. Anat. 30 (3), 177–183.

Eisler, P., 1892. Der Plexus lumbosacralis des Menschen (Berlin: Halle).

Gomceli, Y.B., Kapukiran, A., Kutlu, G., Kurt, S., Baysal, A.I., 2005. A case report of an uncommon neuropathy: posterior femoral cutaneous neuropathy. Acta Neurol. Belg. 105, 43–45.

Harrer, J., Hammon, G., Wagner, T., Bolkenius, M., 2001. Lipoblastoma and lipoblastomatosis: a report of two cases and review of the literature. Eur. J. Pediatr. Surg. 11 (5), 342–349.

Huban, T.R., Nayak, V.S., D'Souza, A.S., 2012. A rare variation in the innervation of the gluteus maximus muscle. A case report. Proceed. Anat. Assoc. Thai. 1, 12.

Iyer, V.G., Shields, C.B., 1989. Isolated injection injury to the posterior femoral cutaneous nerve. Neurosurgery 25, 835–838.

Kim, J.E., Kang, J.H., Choi, J.C., Lee, J.S., Kang, S.Y., 2009. Isolated posterior femoral cutaneous neuropathy following intragluteal injection. Muscle Nerve 40, 864–866.

Nakanishi, T., Kanno, Y., Kaneshige, Y., 1976. Comparative morphological remarks on the origin of the posterior femoral cutaneous nerve. Anat. Anzeiger 139, 8–23.

Orava, S., Hetsroni, I., Marom, N., Mann, G., Sarimo, J., Ben-Zvi, O., Lempainen, L., 2015. Surgical excision of posttraumatic ossifications at the proximal hamstrings in young athletes: technique and outcomes. Am. J. Sports Med. 43, 1331–1336.

Pauchot, J., Lepage, D., Fyad, J.P., Braun, M., 2010. Anatomy of the artery of the cutaneous posterior nerve of the thigh. Ann. Chir. Plast. Esthet. 55, 297–301.

Piersol, G.A., 1923. Human Anatomy. Including Structure and Developmental and Practical Considerations. J.B. Lippincott Company, Philadelphia.

Schumm, F., Stohr, M., Bauer, H.L., Eck, T., 1975. Peripheral nerve injury due to total replacement of the hip-joint. Z. Orthop. Ihre Grenzgeb. 113, 1065–1069.

Tong, H.C., Haig, A., 2000. Posterior femoral cutaneous nerve mononeuropathy: a case report. Arch. Phys. Med. Rehabil. 81, 1117–1118.

Tubbs, R.S., Miller, J., Loukas, M., Shoja, M.M., Shokouhi, G., Cohen-Gadol, A.A., 2009. Surgical and anatomical landmarks for the perineal branch of the posterior femoral cutaneous nerve: implications in perineal pain syndromes. Laboratory investigation. J. Neurosurg. 111, 332–335.

Tunali, S., Cankara, N., Albay, S., 2011. A rare case of communicating branch between the posterior femoral cutaneous and the sciatic nerves. Rom. J. Morphol. Embryol. 52 (1), 203–205.

Wilson, T.J., Spinner, R.J., Krych, A.J., 2019. Surgical approach impacts posterior femoral cutaneous nerve outcomes after proximal hamstring repair. Clin. J. Sport. Med. 29 (4), 281–284.

CHAPTER 10

The Pudendal Nerve

ASHLEY K. YEARWOOD • R. SHANE TUBBS

ANATOMY

The pudendal nerve (PN) (Figs. 10.1−10.3) is a paired nerve formed from the sacral plexus, which is a network of nerve fibers located in the posterior pelvic wall. It carries sensory, motor, and autonomic fibers, innervating the skin and muscles of the perineum.

It commonly originates from the ventral rami (anterior divisions) of the spinal nerve roots S2, S3, S4. The first root derived from S2, passes through the second anterior sacral foramen and passes laterally and downwards over the sacrum to form the first (upper) cord, while the second and third roots formed by S3 and S4 pass through the third and fourth anterior sacral foramina and fuse to form the second (lower) cord. After, the upper and lower cords unite just proximal to the sacrospinous ligament or ischial spine, medially and caudally to the sciatic nerve to form the PN.

The course of this nerve is complex in that it initially travels in the pelvis, then leaves for a short extrapelvic course in the gluteal area (Fig. 10.2), then reenters the pelvis and where it courses into the pudendal canal (Alcock's canal), to innervate the perineal area.

In more detail, once the distinct PN is formed, it travels laterally and inferiorly along the anterior surface of the piriformis, coursing between this muscle and posterior surface of the coccygeus (ischiococcygeus) muscles. Sometimes branches for the levator ani and coccygeus leave the nerve at the inferior margin of the piriformis.

The PN then leaves the pelvis to enter the gluteal region via the infrapiriformis notch of the greater sciatic foramen, ventral to the sciatic nerve. In this region, it accompanies the pudendal vessels medially, and runs inferiorly and laterally to the interligamentous space (the area between the sacrospinous ligament, found posterior to the nerve, and sacrotuberous ligament, which is anterior). After this, it winds posterior-laterally around the inferior margin of the sacrospinous ligament in close proximity to the ischial spine (here it

is posterior to the sacrotuberous ligament due to the way these ligaments intersect).

It is common to find the PN attached to the dorsal surface of the sacrospinous ligament by connective tissue. The PN then reenters the pelvis via the lesser sciatic foramen. While in the perineal region, it courses with the internal pudendal artery and vein along the lateral wall of the ischiorectal fossa within the pudendal canal above the obturator internus muscle, below the levator ani. This canal is made of the split sheath of the obturator internus muscle and internally contains a connective tissue that surrounds the nerves and vessels. The canal follows the superior edge of the ischiopubic ramus toward the base of the urogenital diaphragm, where it terminates.

Normally, three nerves arise from the PN (Fig. 10.3). The inferior rectal nerve is the first and usually branches either just before or just after entering the canal. The bifurcation of the PN into its terminal two branches, the dorsal nerve to the penis/clitoris and the perineal nerve, occurs within the canal. The perineal nerve pierces the sheath of the obturator internus medially to leave the canal, while the dorsal nerve to the penis/clitoris continues toward the exit. It is difficult to describe the typical path of the PN, as a hallmark of this nerve appears to be variability.

VARIATIONS

While the above describes the universally accepted classic PN, cadaveric studies suggests that there are many variations that occur at many different locations, and that a person is just as likely to have the classic PN as he/she is to have a variation.

VENTRAL RAMI

The number of axons and the nerve roots that dominate in the PN may differ depending on whether the lumbosacral plexus is prefixed or postfixed.

Surgical Anatomy of the Sacral Plexus and Its Branches. https://doi.org/10.1016/B978-0-323-77602-8.00010-6

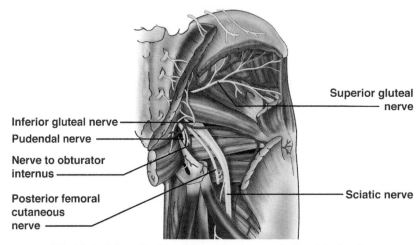

FIG. 10.1 Schematic view of the pudendal nerve in the gluteal region.

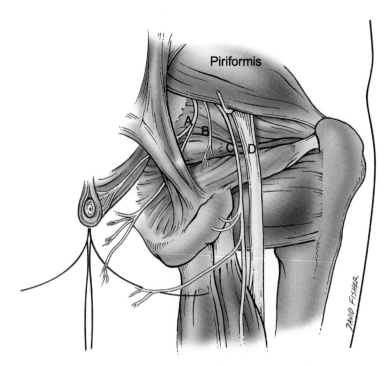

FIG. 10.2 Drawing of the pudendal nerve **(A)**, nerve to obturator internus **(B)**, posterior femoral cutaneous nerve **(C)**, and the sciatic nerve **(D)** in the gluteal region. Note the course of the pudendal nerve deep to the sacrospinous ligament (not labeled) traveling toward the perineum.

As previously mentioned, the normal roots are S2, S3, S4. In people with a prefixed plexus, that is one which originates more rostrally than normal, S1 and S2 roots are the main contributions to the PN. In people with a postfixed plexus, which is one that originates more caudally than normal, S3 is the dominant root contribution most often, while S4 is dominant less often. S5 nerve root contribution was even more minimal. These roots combine to form cords, which combine to form the single trunk of the PN.

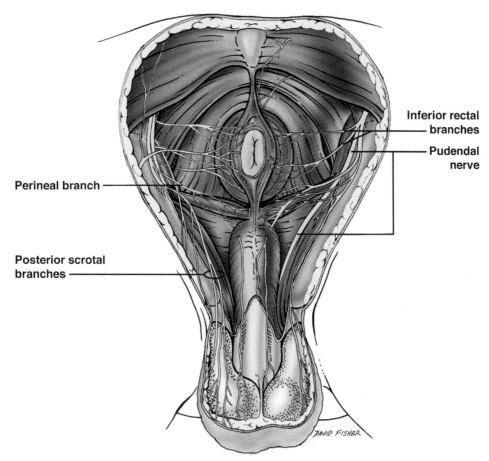

Inferior rectal
branches

Pudendal
nerve

Perineal branch

Posterior scrotal
branches

DAVID FISHER

FIG. 10.3 Perineal view in the male. The branches of the pudendal nerve are shown with the exception of the dorsal nerve of the penis.

TRUNKS

Despite the classic description of the PN and its course, studies have found that there are often multiple PN trunks, most often two but up to three have been reported, as it leaves the pelvis.

Rather than a distinct single PN, it is possible to have a common trunk for the dorsal and perineal nerves with either the inferior rectal nerve arising separately from the sacral plexus or arising from a rectal-perineal trunk.

It is also possible to have a common trunk for the rectal and perineal nerve with the dorsal nerve arising from any of the following: a unique rectal-dorsal trunk, from a classic PN, as a separate nerve branch from the pelvis or from the aforementioned perineal-dorsal trunk.

An example of a classification system based on a cadaveric study was devised, describing five PN sub-

types as follows: Type I is defined as one-trunked, Type II is two-trunked, Type III is two-trunked with one trunk as an inferior rectal nerve piercing through the sacrospinous ligament, Type IV is two-trunked with one as an inferior rectal nerve not piercing through the sacrospinous ligament, and Type V is three-trunked. This shows an example of the variability.

These trunks travel slightly apart posterolaterally toward the area of the sacrospinous ligament. Once the PN is formed, it can either descend posterior or medial to the ischial spine. When medial, it descends past the sacrospinous ligament. It is noteworthy that in studies of people with the postfixed type, the PN was not found to course near the ischial spine in any case. This has implications for using the ischial spine as a landmark for procedures such as the PN block.

BRANCHES

The inferior rectal nerve shows different branching patterns of the PN, and less commonly, a separate nerve from the sacral plexus. The typical branching description is that it branches in the posterior part of the ischiorectal fossa, just before the pudendal canal. However, cases have been described where the inferior rectal nerve entered the canal with the PN branching shortly after this.

In some cadaveric specimens, it was noted to branch at the superior border of the sacrospinous ligament and then proceed to descend, crossing the sacrospinous ligament. In others, it branched from the PN at the inferior border of the sacrospinous ligament; so these crossed the ligament as one structure. When the inferior rectal nerve branches superior to the ligament, it can also be found descending either posterior or medial to the ischial spine. There have also been reports that after branching from PN at the superior border, the inferior rectal nerve pierced the sacrospinous ligament. A study revealed that the PN and inferior rectal nerve were found further from the ischial spine, closer to the midline in African Americans compared with people of European decent.

Other variations include fusion of the PN and inferior rectal nerve after crossing the ischial spine or sacrospinous ligament, followed by an accessory inferior rectal nerve branching from the fused nerve 15 mm after fusion.

When there is an inferior rectal nerve, that is, a separate nerve from the sacral plexus, it is possible for the inferior rectal nerve from the PN to fuse with this separate inferior rectal nerve after the inferior border of the sacrospinous ligament before proceeding to the structures that it innervates.

After crossing sacrospinous ligament, the PN makes its way into the pudendal canal as described in the anatomy section to divide into its terminal branches. The perineal nerve is relatively consistent with the location of the branches that arise but may vary in the number of branches. It is possible for the perineal nerve to originate separately from the sacral plexus.

The dorsal nerve to the penis/clitoris normally arises within the pudendal canal. However, it has been observed branching before the pudendal canal, arising from the S1 root as a separate nerve.

IMAGING

Ultrasound can be used to detect the PN directly or to visualize the pudendal artery and the ischial spine, which are considered reliable landmarks. Thus, the use of ultrasound may improve therapeutic access when anesthetizing the PN.

Previously, radiologists have reported that it is difficult to use CT and MRI to accurately diagnose PN entrapment, since the PN and its branches show variation in their course, as well as in the number of trunks and branches. However, with the development of MRN, an MRI specifically dedicated to assessing peripheral nerves by providing images of superior resolution, it is possible to obtain more details of the PN anatomy and pathology.

The PNs are best seen on axial images along the distal edge of piriformis muscle entering the interligamentous space at the ischial spine. At this point, the nerve shows intermediate signal intensity with a fascicular appearance. This helps differentiate it from the surrounding artery and vein in the pudendal neurovascular bundle.

While 3D imaging is useful for large nerves of the lumbosacral plexus, its use for the PN is limited by its small size and incomplete suppression of the surrounding venous signals.

In summary, new advances in MRN that display the nerve as intermediate in signal intensity with a fascicular appearance help differentiate the PN from the hyperintense vessels. When abnormal, you may see alterations in signal or contour of the nerve, prominence of fascicles, or scarring of the nerve. Visualizing surrounding structures may also suggest pathology such as a thick obturator internus sheath, or thick sacrotuberous or sacrospinous ligaments. These suggest that there may have been previous injury or procedure done.

Imaging-guided nerve block injections are useful for the therapeutic intervention of pudendal neuralgia. Imaging offers a way to directly view the nerve at different locations: in the interligamentous space, in the level of the ischial spine, or in the pudendal canal. However, this is again limited by the variability in PN anatomy and by the difficulty associated with identifying the smaller terminal branches.

PATHOLOGY/INJURY OF THE PUDENDAL NERVE

In the clinical setting, a thorough knowledge of PN variation is necessary for a good understanding of the causes of injury and potential methods of treatment. PN injury may present clinically as anal, perineal, vaginal or scrotal, clitoral or penile pain/hyperesthesia; erectile/orgasmic dysfunction; vulvodynia; and fecal or stress urinary incontinence.

Injury to the PN may result from a variety of mechanisms. These include, but are not limited to, nerve compression or entrapment, stretch injury, and direct injury, some of which are iatrogenic due to surgery.

PN entrapment or compression can occur at many places along its course. It has been implicated as the cause of several clinical syndromes. Examples of symptoms thought to be caused by entrapment of the PN and the resulting pudendal neuropathy are pain or loss of sensation to the penis, scrotum, labia, perineum, or rectum (anorectal anesthesia). It has been implicated in rectal incontinence and erectile dysfunction. The consequences of misdiagnoses include prolongation of nerve constriction leading to chronic perineal pain, or even inappropriate surgical treatment.

While the PN could be compressed anywhere along its course, common sites of compression are as follows: between the sacrotuberous and sacrospinous ligament; in the pudendal canal, inferior surface of the pubic ramus; and by the falciform process of the sacrotuberous ligament. The PN within Alcock's canal passes behind the insertion of the sacrotuberous ligament into the ischial tuberosity. For this reason, it is a possible site for entrapment.

Entrapment of the PN may occur during pelvic surgery. Richter's procedure is a transvaginal sacrospinous colpopexy for the treatment of vaginal vault prolapse. Entrapment of the PN and injury of the neurovascular pudendal bundle are among the main issues involved in this surgical procedure. During this procedure, a stitch is placed through the wall into the sacrospinous ligament, and since the PN frequently passes near here it may become entrapped.

Pudendal neuralgia is a painful neuropathic condition in the distribution of the PN. Neuromas are a known cause of pudendal neuralgia. The PN may be compressed by neuromas caused by previous surgical interventions. Pudendal neuralgia may also stem from several other etiologies including vaginal delivery, pelvic surgery, intraoperative patient positioning, trauma, chronic compression caused by pelvic tumors. Chronic compression injuries may also occur through repetitive motion such as biking.

The relationships between the PN and inferior rectal nerve are important in evaluating anorectal symptoms of pudendal neuralgia, and as previously discussed, there is a huge potential for variations in this relationship. Moreover, the inferior rectal nerve innervates the external anal sphincter, so injury to this structure may cause fecal incontinence.

During vaginal delivery, the nerve is thought to be at risk of both compression and stretch injury during downward displacement of the pelvic floor and perineal structures because of the close relation to structures in the pelvic floor and perineal area. It is fixed the dorsal surface of the sacrospinous ligament and the pudendal canal, so moves in unison with these during childbirth. If the perineal nerve branch gets damaged, the woman may develop urinary stress incontinence as the perineal nerve innervates the urogenital sphincter.

During labor, potential compression of the inferior rectal nerve is avoided in cases where the nerve branches before the pudendal canal. Thus, the person is spared the anorectal symptoms of pudendal canal syndrome. On the other hand, in this situation where branching of the PN occurred before the canal, the inferior rectal nerve courses deeper in the ischioanal fossa close to the pelvic floor muscles, so is now more at risk for a traction injury.

Direct injury may occur when draining fistulas and ischioanal abscesses due to the location of these pathologies in relation to the PN and its branches. In cases where the branches of the inferior rectal nerve run superficially, drainage of fistulas and ischioanal abscesses put the nerves at risk. The risk of rectal incontinence following drainage of perineal abscesses has been reported to be 10%–12%, even when the anal sphincters have not been damaged. The terminal branches of the PN may also be damaged during drainage of an ischiorectal abscess, during surgery for a complex perianal fistula, or during excessive posterolateral mobilization of the sphincters during a sphincter repair.

In addition, disruption of the "pudendal plexus" in the ischiorectal fossa, might cause denervation of the anal sphincters, leading to complications that result in an increased risk of fecal incontinence. This nerve is at risk for either compression or direct injury with neuroma formation from obstetrical, urogynecologic, and rectal surgery as well as pelvic fracture and blunt trauma.

SURGICAL APPROACH

It is important to have detailed knowledge of the course and branching pattern of the PN for perineal and pelvic surgery, as well as for urogenital and rectal pain syndromes such as vulvodynia, rectal pain, perineal pain, and PN neuropathy, which may require surgical interventions.

This knowledge helps determine the appropriate surgical approach to access, expose, and safely execute various procedures on the nerve and helps avoid intraoperative complications. The PN has been accessed by many surgical approaches, but the following four are most common: transperineal, transischiorectal, trans-gluteal, or laparoscopic.

1. The transperineal approach is the technique of cutting though the region between the anus and the scrotum or vulva to access the PN.
2. The transischiorectal approach in woman is one whereby the surgeon makes a vertical incision through the vagina into the pararectal space. To access the entrance to the pararectal space in men, the surgeon must go via a paramedian transverse perineal incision.
3. The transgluteal approach involves a path across the gluteus maximus and the ischial tuberosity.

A limitation of approaches via the abdominal laparoscopic, transperineal, transischiorectal is that the surgeon is not able to visualize the complete course of the nerve and so cannot explore all the sites of possible entrapment simultaneously. The transgluteal approach, however, is minimally invasive and allows visualization of the entire nerve and surrounding structures in the gluteal region. It is proposed that this is the best approach.

Decompression surgery has been discussed as a treatment option for patients with refractory pudendal neuralgia. One way to perform this is through a vertical para-anal incision with the patient in the lithotomy position. This frees the nerve within the pudendal canal. However, the use of decompression is still controversial.

Understanding the course of the PN is critical to avoid nerve injury and allows for accurate placement of the needle for local anesthetics. Landmarks such as the tip of the ischial spine are useful for PN block injections and surgical procedures. This is palpable through the rectum or vagina. The PN can also be reached posteriorly using the sacrotuberous ligament as a landmark for the application of local anesthetics. Information about the patient's branching pattern is also crucial. During reconstructive surgery of the penis, vagina, or rectum, plastic surgeons may encounter the PN, since its course takes it through areas involved in this surgery, and puts it at risk for accidental injury.

The branching pattern is also important when approaching the nerve between the sacrotuberous and sacrospinous ligament. It is crucial for the surgeons to identify the branching pattern of the PN for effective neurolysis when treating entrapment syndrome. If the PN has branched, neurolysis of one twig of the nerve may not be sufficient to stop the symptoms, or it may not represent the branch of interest.

To perform the Richter's procedure, surgeons suggest that the medial and inferior part of the sacrospinous ligament near to the sacrum is a safe site for suture placement for the suspension of the vaginal vault posthysterectomy. This is because the PN group does not course here.

Surgeries that reconstruct the sphincter using the gluteus maximus or gracilis muscle also involve the PN. Anastomoses of the PN with the muscles are used to innervate the neosphincter.

ADDITIONAL READING

Furtmüller, G.J., Mckenna, C.A., Ebmer, J., Dellon, A.L., 2014. Pudendal nerve 3-dimensional illustration gives insight into surgical approaches. Ann. Plast. Surg. 73 (6), 670–678. https://doi.org/10.1097/sap.0000000000000169.

Hruby, S., Ebmer, J., Dellon, A.L., Aszmann, O.C., 2005. Anatomy of pudendal nerve at urogenital diaphragm—new critical site for nerve entrapment. Urology 66 (5), 949–952. https://doi.org/10.1016/j.urology.2005.05.032.

Loukas, M., Louis, R.G., Hallner, B., Gupta, A.A., White, D., 2006. Anatomical and surgical considerations of the sacrotuberous ligament and its relevance in pudendal nerve entrapment syndrome. Surg. Radiol. Anat. 28 (2), 163–169. https://doi.org/10.1007/s00276-006-0082-3.

Mahakkanukrauh, P., Surin, P., Vaidhayakarn, P., 2005. Anatomical study of the pudendal nerve adjacent to the sacrospinous ligament. Clin. Anat. 18 (3), 200–205. https://doi.org/10.1002/ca.20084.

Maldonado, P.A., Chin, K., Garcia, A.A., Corton, M.M., 2015. Anatomic variations of pudendal nerve within pelvis and pudendal canal: clinical applications. Am. J. Obstet. Gynecol. 213 (5) https://doi.org/10.1016/j.ajog.2015.06.009.

Matejčík, V., 2012. Surgical location and anatomical variations of pudendal nerve. ANZ J. Surg. 82 (12), 935–938. https://doi.org/10.1111/j.1445-2197.2012.06272.x.

Nayak, S.R., Kumar, S.M., Krishnamurthy, A., Prabhu, V.L., D'Costa, S., Jetti, R., 2006. Unusual origin of dorsal nerve of penis and abnormal formation of pudendal nerve—clinical significance. Ann.Anat. 188 (6), 565–566. https://doi.org/10.1016/j.aanat.2006.06.011.

Pirro, N., Sielezneff, I., Corroller, T.L., Ouaissi, M., Sastre, B., Champsaur, P., 2009. Surgical anatomy of the extrapelvic part of the pudendal nerve and its applications for clinical practice. Surg. Radiol. Anat. 31 (10), 769–773. https://doi.org/10.1007/s00276-009-0518-7.

Schraffordt, S.E., Tjandra, J.J., Eizenberg, N., Dwyer, P.L., 2004. Anatomy of the pudendal nerve and its terminal branches: a cadaver study. ANZ J. Surg. 74 (1–2), 23–26. https://doi.org/10.1046/j.1445-1433.2003.02885.x.

Shafik, A., El-Sherif, M., Youssef, A., Olfat, E., 1995. Surgical anatomy of the pudendal nerve and its clinical implications. Clin. Anat. 8 (2), 110–115. https://doi.org/10.1002/ca.980080205.

Wadhwa, V., Hamid, A.S., Kumar, Y., Scott, K.M., Chhabra, A., 2016. Pudendal nerve and branch neuropathy: magnetic resonance neurography evaluation. Acta. Radiol. 58 (6), 726–733. https://doi.org/10.1177/0284185116668213.

Walt, S.V., Oettlé, A.C., Patel, H.R., 2015. Surgical anatomy of the pudendal nerve and its branches in South Africans. Int. J. Impot. Res. 27 (4), 128–132. https://doi.org/10.1038/ijir.2015.10.

CHAPTER 11

The Sciatic Nerve

SKYLER JENKINS • R. SHANE TUBBS

The sciatic nerve (Fig. 11.1), a branch of the lumbosacral plexus, has the largest cross-sectional area of any nerve in the human body (15–20 mm in width) and is formed from the ventral rami of L4, L5, S1-3 (Mirjalili, 2015). Externally, the sciatic nerve divides into its component branches, the tibial and common fibular nerves (Fig. 11.2), near the popliteal fossa; however, internally, this division traces from the pelvic cavity. Previously thought to have no internal interconnections between the two parts of the sciatic nerve, it has now been shown

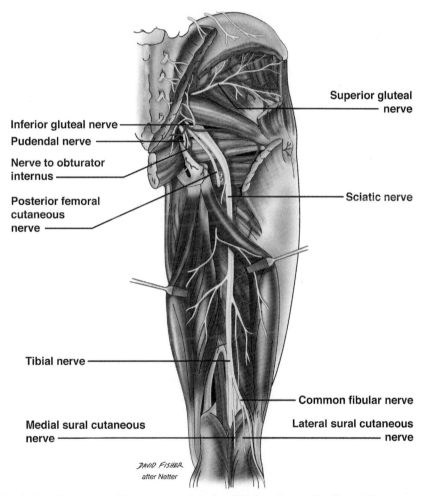

FIG. 11.1 Schematic drawing of the posterior gluteal and thigh regions noting the sciatic nerve and related neuromuscular relationships.

Surgical Anatomy of the Sacral Plexus and Its Branches. https://doi.org/10.1016/B978-0-323-77602-8.00011-8

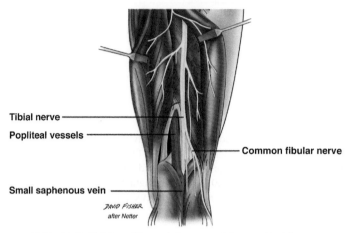

FIG. 11.2 Division of the sciatic nerve at the popliteal fossa.

that these interconnections do exist in the gluteal or proximal thigh region (Tubbs et al., 2017).

It provides motor function to both heads of the biceps femoris, semimembranosus, semitendinosus, hamstring component of the adductor magnus, as well as all muscles below the knee. This provides for knee flexion and hip adduction, dorsiflexion, plantarflexion, and inversion and eversion of the ankle. A cutaneous branch from the sciatic nerve to the perineal may be present (Gibbs, 2018), and the tibial and common fibular nerves provide sensation below the knee.

TOPOGRAPHY/MORPHOLOGY

At its origin, the sciatic nerve is large and flat but becomes smaller and more round distally. The size of the nerve is proportional to the number of funiculi. This number of funiculi decreases as the nerve progresses distally, until, at the apex of the popliteal fossa, it suddenly increases. The cross-sectional area is not an accurate predictor of the number of funiculi at a given point in the nerve, due to the amount of myelination and connective tissue present. However, it may be used as a predictor of the fiber content within the nerve at that point. Though previous literature stated that there were no intercommunications between the tibial and common fibular nerves in the gluteal and thigh region, Tubbs et al. (2017) found these intercommunications to be present (Tubbs et al., 2017). In addition, the fibers within each bundle may take an oblique course, exiting the bundle in order to anastomose with fibers of the other bundle to then innervate their target (i.e., muscle, skin).

With aging, the amount of adipose tissue between the fascicles and the amount of epineural and perineural connective tissue increases, leading to an increase in the cross-sectional area of the nerve (Sladjana, 2008). In addition, aging also led to a decrease in the myelination of the nerve fibers' area in a process called endoneural fibrosis.

The sciatic nerve has the same microarchitecture as most other peripheral nerves, meaning that there are perineurium encapsulated nerve fascicles surrounded by fat and connective tissue, all within an epineural sheath of connective tissue. These connective tissue sheaths provide protection and a structural framework for the nerve. It is a polyfascicular nerve containing anywhere between 11 and 93 fascicles with approximately 1-4 fascicles per square millimeter (Sunderland, 1978; Sladjana, 2008). In Sunderland's experiment (1948), it was found that in the smaller segments of the nerve, there were few large funiculi; however, in segments with a larger diameter, there were many smaller funiculi. The size is then attributed to the increased amount of supporting connective tissue. The sciatic nerve has its external bifurcation at the apex of the popliteal fossa; however, internally it is already divided into its branches within the pelvic cavity. These two branches are divided by the Compton-Cruveilhier septum, which lies obliquely through the nerve, not anteroposteriorly, and at no point did the fibers cross between the two bundles in the sciatic trunk (Sunderland, 1978).

The following describes the internal morphology (Fig. 11.3) of the branches of the common fibular and tibial nerve as the branches course proximally.

Common Fibular Nerve
Superficial fibular branches

a) The superficial fibular nerve (Figs. 11.4 and 11.5) consists of a bundle of 1-6 funiculi that course

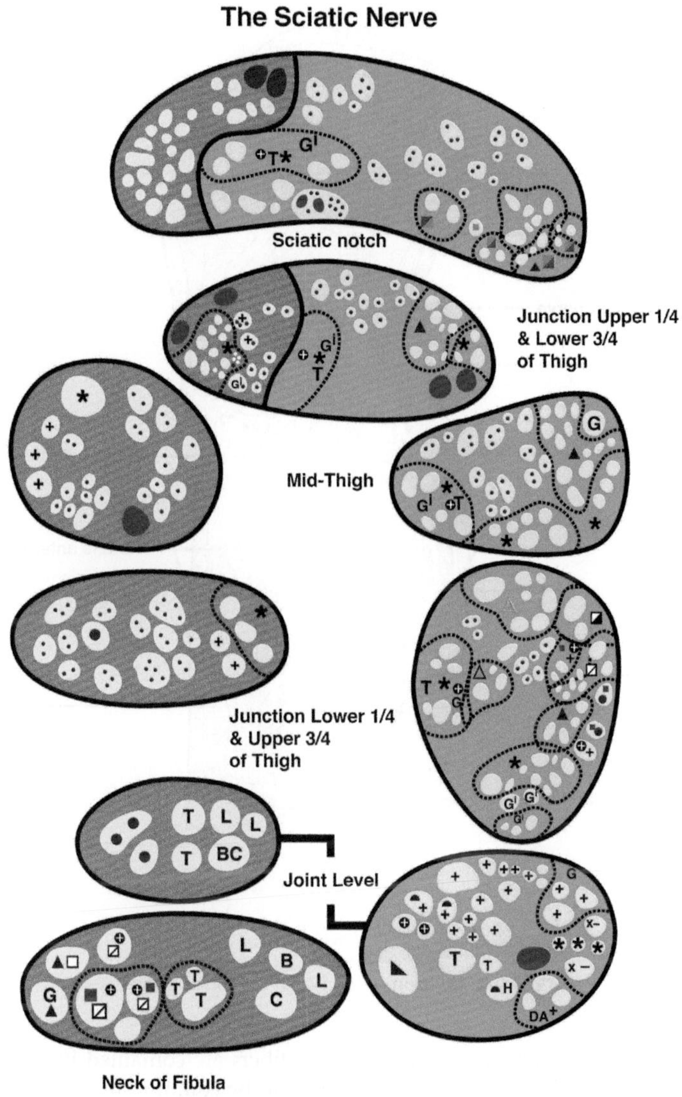

The Sciatic Nerve

FIG. 11.3 Internal topography of the sciatic nerve from proximally as it exits the greater sciatic notch (foramen) to distal with its tibial component colored blue and common fibular component colored orange. For the **common fibular nerve**, combined fibers to the biceps femoris short head (purple ovals), distal and proximal fibers to the biceps femoris short head (green ovals), combined sural communicating and lateral cutaneous branches to the calf (*), sural communicating branch (+), cutaneous fibers (C), distal genicular fibers (G), proximal genicular fibers (G¹), terminal branches of the superficial fibular nerve (T), fibularis brevis (B), terminal part of deep fibular nerve (■), fibers to TA (▲), fibers to extensor digitorum longus (□), combined superficial and deep fibular nerve fibers (..). For the **tibial nerve**, proximal articular fibers from the knee (G¹), fibers to tibialis posterior (T), medial and lateral plantar nerve fibers (+), flexor hallucis longus and plantar nerves (*), flexor digitorum longus (D), arterial fibers (A), proximal branch flexor hallucis longus (H), distal genicular fibers (G), combined branches excluding sural, flexor digitorum longus, hamstrings and arterial branches (hamstrings and arterial branches (▲), combined fibers from plantar nerves, tibialis posterior, and distal and intermediate branches to soleus (●), combined fibers from adductor magnus, semitendinosus, long head of biceps, plantar nerves, flexor hallucis longus (▨), combined fibers from popliteus and lateral head of gastrocnemius (▨), lateral plantar nerve (pink oval), flexor hallucis longus distal branch (X-), combined fibers from popliteus, medial and lateral heads of gastrocnemius, and soleus proximal branch (▨), combined fibers

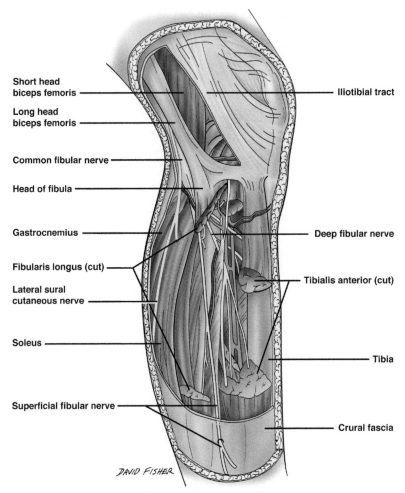

Short head
biceps femoris

Long head
biceps femoris

Common fibular nerve

Head of fibula

Gastrocnemius

Fibularis longus (cut)

Lateral sural
cutaneous nerve

Soleus

Superficial fibular nerve

Iliotibial tract

Deep fibular nerve

Tibialis anterior (cut)

Tibia

Crural fascia

DAVID FISHER

FIG. 11.4 Division of the common fibular nerve.

proximally to join at the level of the knee joint. As the funiculi extend above the knee, they comprise the middle third of the common fibular nerve, joined medially by the sural communicating and lateral cutaneous of the calf nerve bundles.

b) The nerve to the fibularis brevis and a cutaneous branch had two separate bundles that course proximally for 8 cm until fusing, forming a compound funiculus extending to the knee joint. About 1 cm above the joint, the fibers divide with one bundle joining fibers of the fibularis longus and the other with a bundle containing terminal fibers. These

fibers are contained in the anteromedial quadrant of the common fibular nerve. They then are joined medially by the sural communicating and lateral cutaneous of the calf nerve bundles until all localization is lost 6.1 cm above the knee joint.

c) The fibularis longus branch joins the superficial fibular trunk 1.5 cm below the neck of the fibula and stays a separate group until the knee joint. It ascends in the posteromedial quadrant of the common fibular until being forced centrally by the sural communicating and lateral cutaneous of the calf nerve bundles.

popliteus, medial and lateral heads of gastrocnemius, soleus proximal branch, and sural nerve (■), intermediate branches to soleus (⬭), popliteus (▲), adductor magnus and semimembranosus fibers (green ovals). Above a level 30 cm above the knee, unmarked fibers contain fibers from every branch of the nerve except genicular fibers and fibers for the short head of biceps femoris when on the common fibular side (after Sunderland).

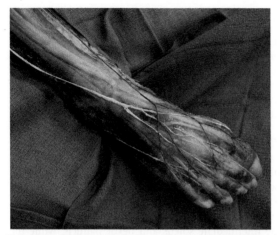

FIG. 11.5 Cadaveric dissection of the distal anterior leg and dorsum of the foot. The cutaneous nerves are highlighted in yellow, and the superficial veins in blue. Medially, on the great toe side, the dorsal venous plexus is seen culminating into the great saphenous vein. The small saphenous vein is seen on the lateral leg/foot and is traveling with the sural nerve branch to the dorsal foot. Traveling from the lateral leg to the dorsal foot, the superficial fibular nerve is observed. Note its interconnection with the terminal part of the deep fibular nerve at the first web space.

Deep fibular branches

a) The terminal deep fibular fibers from the foot ascends as an individual bundle group until approximately 1 cm below the fibular neck until it is joined by fibers from the second and third digital extensor group. In the distal leg, the nerve bundles vary from 4-6, whereas in the proximal leg there are only 1-4 bundles present.

b) Branches to tibialis anterior (TA) and knee joint have a common origin off the deep fibular nerve approximately 3 cm distal to the neck of fibula. The TA bundle group consists of three fused bundles that extend to 1 cm distal to the fibular neck. At this point, one bundle joins the first and second digital extensors. The second bundle joins the common bundle at the neck of the fibula, whereas the third bundle joins an articular bundle, consisting of one bundle, about 2 cm proximally.

c) Branches to extensor digitorum and extensor hallucis longus are supplied by three separate systems. The first system consists of three bundles and innervates the extensor digitorum longus which join the parent trunk 4.5 cm below the fibular neck. The second system, comprised of the intermediate branch to the extensor digitorum longus and proximal branch to extensor hallucis longus, fuses with the parent trunk approximately 6 cm distal to the neck of the fibula. Finally, the third system (the distal extensor digitorum and extensor hallucis longus) joins the parent trunk about 10 cm distal to the fibular head, each comprised of a single funiculus.

- 2.6 cm above the neck of the fibula, the fibers of all deep fibular branches are contained in a single bundle; however, they are in two separate bundles at the knee joint.

The deep and superficial divisions of the common fibular nerve stay separate until approximately 10 cm above the joint all bundles contain fibers from both divisions. The deep bundle comprises the lateral half of the nerve, whereas the superficial bundle occupies the medial half of the nerve until being pushed centrally by the sural cutaneous and the lateral cutaneous nerve of the calf 2.2 cm proximal to the knee joint.

Sural communicating and lateral cutaneous nerve of the calf

The fibers of these cutaneous branches kept their own identity for 3.7 cm, then joined, ascending 14.4 cm to the common stem 2.2 cm proximal to the knee joint. These nerves joined and occupied the medial aspect of the common fibular nerve for approximately 9 cm, then moved posterior for 2.2 cm, posterolateral, and finally ended on the lateral aspect of the nerve 17.6 cm above the joint. The fibers then split 2.7 cm proximally into an anterolateral and posterolateral division which ultimately became distributed over the common fibular nerve.

Genicular branch and distal branch to short head of biceps

These fibers share a common origin from the anterior surface of the sciatic nerve 15 cm above the knee joint. Each contained a single bundle of fibers that were incorporated into the common fibular nerve.

a) The genicular branch stayed in its anterior position until approximately 34 cm above the knee joint where it turned to the lateral margin. It maintained this anterolateral quadrant of the common fibular nerve to the sciatic notch.

b) The distal branch to the short head of the biceps nerve maintained the anteromedial aspect of the common fibular nerve for 19 cm until it migrated to the extreme lateral position 27.5 cm above the joint. After another 6 cm, it joined with the nerve bundle of the proximal branch to the short head of biceps femoris.

Proximal branch to the short head of biceps

This bundle joined the posterolateral quadrant of the common fibular 26 cm above the joint. It then migrated to the lateral margin where it fused with the distal branch. The branch entered the biceps femoris then migrated to a posteromedial angle 35 cm proximal to the joint where it then divided with each bundle being discretely localized.

The Tibial Nerve

The tibial nerve changed shape as it ascended from the popliteal fossa to the mid-thigh, from circular to oval. Due to this change in shape, the internal fiber systems all rotate approximately 45 degrees in a clockwise direction.

Plantar nerves

The plantar nerves are comprised of medial and lateral divisions which remain separate for 10 cm at the mid-anterior surface of the tibial nerve. Once fusing, they are located posteriorly and centrally, gradually moving to a centrolateral position over the next 7.5 cm. Three centimeters more proximally, the fibers lie in the posterolateral quadrant of the tibial nerve. As more fibers were added to the tibial nerve, they comprised the central half. They gradually intermingle until they are fully intertwined approximately 2.5 cm above the knee joint. At the sciatic notch, these fibers were represented in all funiculi.
a) The medial plantar group had some fibers branch off the main trunk 2 cm above the distal end and ascend parallel to the trunk. After 10 cm, the "offshoot" was joined by branches of the flexor hallucis longus. This whole bundle rejoined the main trunk 13.5 cm below the knee joint. These fibers were maintained in the medial or anteromedial quadrant of the tibial nerve.
b) The lateral plantar group ascends laterally within the tibial nerve for 15 cm until dividing into an anterior and posterior group. These groupings were diluted by anastomoses from medial and common plantar fibers until approximately 13.6 cm below the knee joint when only a small group of lateral plantar funiculi remained anteriorly. These remained until finally being fused with other fibers 2.4 cm above the knee joint.

Flexor hallucis longus

Innervated by two branches, the distal branch joins the medial plantar offshoot as mentioned above. The proximal branch joins the anterolateral portion of the tibial nerve 13 cm below the joint. It then migrates medially to the mid-anterior surface until joined by fibers from the intermediate branch to the soleus. More proximally, it is joined by fibers from the plantar nerves, the arterial branch, and the branch to the flexor digitorum longus. It maintained this position until 3 cm above the joint when it distributed fibers across the anterior half of the nerve. As the nerve progressed, its fibers were distributed throughout the tibial nerve.

Flexor digitorum longus

Consisting of a single bundle, this nerve joined the tibial approximately 13 cm below the knee. The arterial bundle and funiculi from both plantar nerves joined it 9 and 2 cm proximal, respectively. This common bundle divided at the knee joint; one branch joining the intermediate soleus and flexor hallucis, while the other blended with fibers from the plantar, tibialis posterior, and intermediate and distal soleus branches. The flexor digitorum fibers moved from the anterior to medial margin of the tibial nerve. After 15 cm, the bundle moved laterally until it reached the anterolateral quadrant 4 cm above the joint. From this position to the sciatic notch, the fibers were distributed over the entire tibial nerve except for the antero-medial corner and a small bundle group located laterally.

Arterial branch

A single funiculus of arterial fibers joined the anteromedial region of the tibial nerve approximately 6 cm below the joint. It then joined the flexor digitorum funiculus on the mid-anterior side of the nerve, following its course proximally.

Tibialis posterior

These fibers, comprised of three funiculi, ascended to join the tibial nerve 9 cm below the knee joint at the lateral margin. As it ascended over the next 4 cm, it migrated to the anterior margin. One of the three funiculi joined branches from the intermediate and distal branches to the soleus 1 cm above the joint. The remaining two bundles joined a bundle containing the plantar fibers, and this then fused with a bundle composed of intermediate soleus and tibialis posterior fibers. The tibialis posterior fibers then moved into the anterolateral quadrant, fanning out to fill the central and lateral portions of the tibial nerve and, furthermore, the medial portion. At the sciatic notch, there is a small bundle located laterally, but throughout the nerve, they are intermixed with all branches distal to the hamstring.

Popliteus and lateral head of gastrocnemius

The nerve to popliteus joined the tibial 3 cm below the knee joint at the extreme lateral margin. As it coursed proximally, it migrated to an anterolateral position, joined laterally by the nerve to the lateral head of the gastrocnemius near the knee joint. These two bundles fused and migrated posteriorly over their proximal course. One of these bundles fused with the fibers from the plantar nerves, flexor digitorum and hallucis, arterial, tibialis posterior, and intermediate and distal branches to soleus. As they continued to ascend, they were joined by fibers from the medial and lateral gastrocnemius, and proximal branch to soleus. Approximately 9 cm above the knee joint, these fibers were distributed across all bundles posteriorly, except for those bundles located anteriorly. At the sciatic notch, the fibers were distributed across almost all nerve bundles in the tibial nerve.

Soleus (contains a proximal, intermediate, and distal branch)

a) The distal branch joined the tibial 11 cm below the knee, coursing for 10 cm before a small bundle was joined by fibers from the intermediate branch. Ascending, they traveled in the posterolateral margin until blending with a small bundle from the intermediate soleus, just posterior to the proximal flexor hallucis bundle. The tibialis posterior bundle joined lateral to it. Then, 5 cm distal to the knee joint, the intermediate soleus group entered posterolateral to it. The soleus bundle remained at the extreme lateral margin as the flexor hallucis and tibialis posterior bundles migrated medially over the anterior surface of the tibial nerve.
b) The intermediate branch entered the lateral margin of the tibial 5 cm below the joint. These fibers proceeded to fuse with those of the distal branch.
c) One cm above the joint, the soleus bundles were joined by the plantar and tibialis posterior fibers, ascending in the posterolateral margin. This complex migrated more medially by the addition of the popliteus-lateral gastrocnemius complex. Approximately 3.5 cm proximal to the joint, the soleus fibers were distributed across all but the anteromedial quadrant. Here, it was associated with plantar fibers posteriorly; plantar and tibialis posterior fibers centrally; one or two bundles of flexor digitorum and hallucis fibers anterolaterally; proximal soleus, medial head of gastrocnemius, and sural complex posterolaterally; and popliteus-lateral head of gastrocnemius complex laterally. Approximately 5 cm above the knee, the distal and intermediate fibers are distributed in all bundles except three anterior and one posterior group.

Proximal soleus and medial head of gastrocnemius

These two branches each consisted of a single bundle that joined the posterolateral aspect of the tibial nerve 3 cm proximal to the knee joint. It quickly migrated posteriorly and within 9 cm proximal to the joint, its fibers were distributed over the posteromedial quadrant. Ascending to the sciatic notch, these fibers infiltrated all but a few antero-medially located bundles.

Sural

These fibers share a common origin with the proximal soleus and medial gastrocnemius. It entered the tibial nerve in the posteromedial quadrant 9 cm above the joint, quickly moving posteriorly just lateral to the soleus-gastrocnemius complex. It gained a branch of this complex 2 cm proximal and from there followed the course discussed in its associated complex.

Genicular branches (proximal and distal branch)

a) Distal branch: the fibers entered the tibial nerve medially about 3.5 cm below the knee joint and soon after joined bundles containing plantar fibers. Within 1 cm of the knee joint, the fibers infiltrated the posteromedial quadrant.
b) Proximal branch: containing four bundles, it entered the nerve anteriorly approximately 8.5 cm above the joint and divided into two bundles.
    a. The first bundle moved laterally, fusing with plantar, flexor hallucis, distal and intermediate soleus, and tibialis posterior fibers.
    b. The second bundle began anteriorly, migrating posteromedially over the next 20 cm above the joint when the hamstring fibers entered medially. The fibers then joined with branches except those from sural, arterial, flexor digitorum, and hamstrings. At the sciatic notch, the fibers were distributed posteromedially with some branches lateral.

Adductor Magnus

Adductor Magnus shared a common stem with semimembranosus. These fibers entered the tibial nerve 19 cm above the knee joint. All of the adductor magnus fibers fused into a common bundle after ascending 8 cm while adding fibers from plantar, flexor hallucis longus, and proximal genicular. Within the next 8 cm some of the fibers fuse with semitendinosus and long head of biceps femoris, while the other fibers travel another 1.5 cm and merge with semimembranosus. Through the whole course, the fibers are medially located.

Semimembranosus

These two bundles of fibers enter anterior to the adductor magnus fibers 19 cm above the knee joint. One bundle had a superficial mid-anterior position and the other an antero-medial position. The anteromedial bundle joined with fibers from plantar, flexor hallucis longus, proximal genicular, and adductor magnus. This bundle then split on its way to the sciatic notch with one branch fusing with plantar, flexor hallucis longus, and other hamstring fibers. The bundle in the superficial mid-anterior position ascended until, 1 cm distal to the sciatic notch, it gained fibers from all other branches except fibers from hamstring muscles.

Long head of biceps femoris and semitendinosus

These entered the tibial nerve about 7 cm distal to the sciatic notch and ascended on the medial aspect of the nerve. It gained fibers from all distal branches except the sural, arterial, and flexor digitorum longus.

Hamstring muscles

These fibers were all contained in the medial aspect of the nerve as follows and were organized at the sciatic notch. There was a varying distribution of distal fibers within the funiculi of the hamstring muscles.

ANATOMY/VARIATIONS
Sciatic Nerve
Anatomy

The sciatic nerve is the largest nerve in the body. It is almost 2 cm wide at its origin near the sacral plexus. It originates from the ventral rami of spinal nerves L4-L5, S1-S3. The greater part of S2 and S3 converge on the inferomedial aspect of the lumbosacral trunk in the greater sciatic foramen to form the sciatic nerve. The ventral and dorsal divisions of the nerve do not separate physically from each other, but their fibers remain separate within the rami. The ventral and dorsal divisions of each contributing root join within the sciatic nerve. The fibers of the dorsal divisions go on to form the common fibular nerve, and those of the ventral division form the tibial nerve.

Within the pelvic cavity, the sciatic nerve roots lie posterior to the pelvic viscera, the pelvic vasculature, and the lymph nodes. The internal iliac vessels and ureter run anteriorly, while the lateral sacral arteries are medial along the sacral plexus. In addition, the iliolumbar artery crosses anteriorly to the lumbosacral trunk, the superior gluteal artery runs posteriorly between the trunk and the first sacral nerve, and the inferior

gluteal artery courses between the second and third sacral nerve. In the gluteal region, it runs over the posterior surface of the acetabulum (with the nerve to the quadratus femoris on its deep surface) and runs downward over the obturator internus, gemelli, and quadratus femoris to enter the posterior compartment of the thigh. The posterior cutaneous nerve of the thigh and inferior gluteal artery lie on its medial side. Surface anatomy of the sciatic nerve is essential for intramuscular injections, sacral nerve block, and percutaneous drainage of deep pelvic abscesses (Small, 2004; Raj, 1975; Franco, 2007; Robards, 2009). Currin et al. (2014) showed that the sciatic nerve traversing a point approximately one-third of the way between the posterior superior iliac spine and the ischial tuberosity, curving inferolaterally to a point halfway between the greater trochanter and the ischial tuberosity (Currin, 2014).

In the thigh, the sciatic nerve runs vertically down the midline through the posterior compartment on the posterior aspect of the adductor magnus, deep to the long head of the biceps femoris. The sciatic nerve then divides into tibial and common fibular components at a variable level but usually near the apex of the popliteal fossa.

The muscular branches of the sciatic nerve supply the posterior femoral muscles which include long and short head of the biceps, the semimembranosus, semitendinosus, and hamstring component of the adductor magnus. It also innervates the hip joint.

Gibbs et al. (2018) found that the sciatic may provide a cutaneous branch to the perineal region. This branch arises approximately 0.6 cm distal to the piriformis muscle and may course posterior to the ischial tuberosity or posterior to the conjoint tendon (Gibbs, 2018).

The first branch of the sciatic arises in close proximity to the ischial tuberosity and predominantly innervates the semitendinosus and long head of biceps femoris. However, to a lesser extent, it innervates either the semitendinosus or long head of biceps femoris solely. The long head of the biceps femoris may be supplied by one, two, or three branches of the sciatic and is always innervated before the short head. The short head of the biceps femoris is either innervated by a single branch from the sciatic, or from a branch of the sciatic and a branch from the common fibular nerve. The semitendinosus is innervated by fibers that branch off the tibial division of the sciatic nerve approximately 7.5 cm below the sciatic notch. Finally, nerves to the hamstring component of the adductor magnus and semimembranosus share a common origin, 19 cm above the knee joint (Sunderland, 1978).

Variations

The sciatic nerve occasionally divides into common fibular and tibial nerves inside the pelvis. In these cases, the common fibular nerve usually runs through the piriformis. The sciatic nerve typically comes out of the pelvis through the greater sciatic foramen, entering the gluteal region anterior to the piriformis muscle. After reaching the lateral aspect of the ischial tuberosity it turns vertically downwards to run between the ischium medially and the greater trochanter laterally. For most of its trajectory in the gluteal region it runs parallel to the midline. Superiorly it lies deep to gluteus maximus, resting first on the posterior ischial surface with the nerve to the quadratus femoris between them. It then crosses posterior to the obturator internus, gemelli, and quadratus femoris, separated by the latter from the obturator externus and the hip joint. The posterior femoral cutaneous nerve and the inferior gluteal artery usually accompany it medially. The nerve then enters the thigh behind the adductor magnus and is crossed posteriorly by the long head of the biceps femoris. It corresponds to a line drawn from just medial to the midpoint between the ischial tuberosity and greater trochanter to the apex of the popliteal fossa. It gives articular branches to the posterior aspect of the hip joint. These branches are sometimes derived directly from the sacral plexus. Muscular branches are distributed to the biceps femoris, semitendinosus, semimembranosus, and the ischial part of the adductor magnus.

The sciatic nerve has two main terminal branches: the tibial nerve and the common fibular nerve. The tibial nerve arises from its medial side, being derived from the anterior divisions of the ventral rami of L4-L5, S1-S3, and the common fibular nerve arises from its lateral side, being derived from the posterior divisions of the ventral rami of L4-L5, S1-S2. However, the point of division of the sciatic nerve into its major components (tibial and common fibular) is very variable. The most common site is at the junction of the middle and lower thirds of the thigh, near the apex of the popliteal fossa, but the division can occur at any level above this point, or more rarely below it. It is also possible for these components to leave the sacral plexus separately, in which case the common fibular component usually passes through the piriformis at the greater sciatic foramen while the tibial passes below the muscle (Bergman, 1984, 1988; Williams, 2005; Mahadevan, 2008).

The tibial and common fibular components can easily be identified as two separate nerves throughout their trajectory in about 11% of cases. However, even in those cases a common sheath of connective tissue surrounds the two components. The sciatic nerve can be readily divided artificially back to the spinal nerves. Therefore, it is important not to confuse this with a true separation of the components, which generally takes place in the popliteal fossa. Upon entering the popliteal fossa, the two nerve components, fibular and tibial, finally diverge from each other, having never mixed their fibers. The tibial nerve continues to run posteriorly in the direction of the main trunk, at the center of the popliteal fossa. The common fibular component turns laterally to run just medial to the biceps tendon.

A number of variations in the course and distribution of the sciatic nerve have been reported. The main ones concern the relationship of the nerve to the piriformis. Beaton and Anson (1938) classified variations in the relationship of the sciatic nerve and its subdivisions to the piriformis muscle in 120 specimens in 1937, and in 240 specimens in 1938. Their classification is as follows:

Type 1: Undivided nerve below undivided muscle

Type 2: Divisions of nerve between and below undivided muscle

Type 3: Divisions above and below undivided muscle

Type 4: Undivided nerve between heads

Type 5: Divisions between and above heads

Type 6: Undivided nerve above undivided muscle

Patel et al. (2011) reported two other types, which were not previously defined by Beaton and Anson (Patel, 2011). These were a sciatic nerve (1) already divided in the pelvis, its two divisions traveling out below the piriformis, and (2) already divided in the pelvis, its two divisions leaving the pelvis differently—the common fibular nerve coming out after piercing the piriformis and the tibial nerve coming out below the piriformis. Additionally, Arifoglu et al. (1997) reported a case with a double superior gemellus and double piriformis associated with a high dividing sciatic nerve, which passed between the two piriformis muscles in the same lower extremity (Arifoglu, 1997). Carare and Goodwin (2008) observed the common fibular nerve and the tibial nerve to originate independently from the lumbosacral plexus in one case (Carare, 2008). Furthermore, in their case, the two roots of the common fibular nerve joined only at the inferior end of the piriformis muscle, after one of the roots pierced the muscle. The results of current studies are presented in Table 3.

The sciatic nerve can bifurcate into its two major divisions (common fibular and tibial) anywhere between the sacral plexus and the lower part of the thigh. The two terminal branches can arise directly from the sacral plexus (Santanu, 2013). The division into terminal branches has been reported to occur below the popliteal space. The nerve to the short head of the biceps femoris sometimes arises directly from the sacral plexus. In one study of 420 limbs, the sciatic nerve passed beneath the piriformis in 87.5%, through it in 12% (fibular division), and above it in 0.5%. In another study of 138 subjects, the sciatic passed beneath the piriformis in 118 cases (85.5%), the fibular division passed through it in 17 (12.3%), and the entire sciatic passed through it in 3 (2.2%) (Bergman, 1984, 1988). Babinski et al. (2003) described another anatomical variation in which the common fibular nerve passed superior, and the tibial nerve inferior, to the superior gemellus muscle (Babinski, 2003). Pokorny et al. (2006) examined 91 cadavers and found an atypical relationship in 19 cases (20.9%) (Pokorny, 2006).

Natsis et al. (2014) dissected 294 limbs and noted the typical relationship between the common fibular and tibial nerve in 275 (93.6%), demonstrating four additional variations (1.4%) not described in the Beaton and Anson classification. In one of these, the common fibular nerve passed between the superficial and the deep muscle bellies of a doubled piriformis muscle, while the tibial nerve passed below the muscle. In another, the piriformis muscle had three bellies. The common fibular nerve passed between the superficial and intermediate muscle bellies, while the tibial nerve passed through the deep muscle. The other variation presented a bilateral supernumerary muscle located just superior to the piriformis in the suprapiriform foramen. The sciatic nerve ran below the piriformis muscle. Mas et al. (2003) reported a sciatic nerve where the tibial component traveled inferior to the superior gemellus muscle, and the common fibular part left the pelvis below the piriformis muscle (Mas, 2003).

The sciatic nerve usually exits the greater sciatic foramen between the ischial tuberosity medially and the greater trochanter laterally; however, Dupont et al. (2018) presented a case in which the sciatic nerve exited the pelvis inferior to the piriformis but bifurcated around the ischial tuberosity as a type C variant as described by Kiros and Woldeyes (2015) (Dupont, 2018; Kiros, 2015).

The sciatic nerve may innervate the gluteus maximus (Huban, 2012).

Common Fibular Nerve
Anatomy
The common fibular nerve (common peroneal nerve) (Fig. 11.4) is derived from the dorsal branches of the L4, L5 and S1, S2 ventral rami. It is approximately half the size of the tibial nerve. It descends obliquely along the lateral side of the popliteal fossa to the fibular head, medial to the biceps femoris. It lies between the biceps femoris tendon and the lateral head of the gastrocnemius. It then passes into the anterolateral compartment of the leg through a tight opening in the thick fascia overlying the TA. It curves lateral to the fibular neck, deep to the fibularis longus, and divides into superficial and deep fibular nerves. The course of the common fibular nerve can be indicated by a line drawn from the apex of the popliteal fossa, passing distally, medial to the biceps tendon, to the back of the head of the fibula, where it can be rolled against the bone. In the gluteal region, Santanu et al. (2013) reported the common fibular part of the sciatic nerve as innervating the gluteus maximus muscle (Santanu, 2013).

It innervates the anterolateral part of the knee joint capsule and the proximal tibiofibular joint via three articular branches. Two of these branches accompany the superior and inferior lateral genicular arteries and can arise together. The third branch is known as the recurrent articular nerve; it arises near the termination of the common fibular nerve. It ascends with the anterior recurrent tibial artery through the TA and supplies it. Watt et al. (2014) supported the use of the term "anterior tibial recurrent nerve (ATRN)" for the branch innervating the TA and reported four major branching patterns of the common fibular nerve as follows: Type 1, neither the deep fibular nerve nor the ATRN branch before piercing the anterior intermuscular septum; Type 2, the ATRN branches before piercing the anterior intermuscular septum; Type 3, the deep fibular nerve branches before piercing the anterior intermuscular septum; Type 4, both the deep fibular nerve and the ATRN branch before piercing the anterior intermuscular septum.

The nerve usually gives off two cutaneous branches, the lateral sural and sural communicating nerves. The lateral sural nerve (lateral cutaneous nerve of the calf) supplies the skin on the anterior, posterior, and lateral surfaces of the proximal leg. The sural communicating nerve arises near the head of the fibula and joins the sural nerve crossing over the lateral head of gastrocnemius. It can descend separately as far as the heel (Bergman, 1984, 1988; Williams, 2005; Mahadevan, 2008). Occasionally the sural nerve arises purely from the tibial nerve, and even less commonly it is purely from the fibular nerve (lateral sural cutaneous nerve).

Variations
The sciatic usually divides into the common fibular and tibial nerves at the level of the lower thigh. These two

nerves usually arise separately from the sacral plexus. They can be separated in the greater sciatic foramen by the piriformis and pass into the thigh as continuous but separate structures. Huelke (1958) examined 198 adult lower extremities and reported that the fibular communicating nerve arose directly from the common fibular nerve in 54.7%, usually as a branch separate from the lateral sural cutaneous nerve (41.5%) (Huelke, 1958). The fibular communicating nerve gave rise to the lateral sural cutaneous branches in 13.2% of sides studied. The fibular communicating nerve was a terminal branch of the lateral sural cutaneous nerve in one-third of the sides, and arose from a trunk common to it and to the lateral sural cutaneous nerve in 12%. The fibular communicating nerve was absent in 19.7% of the 198 sides, so no sural nerve was formed in these cases. When this occurs, it is usually the medial sural cutaneous nerve that passes on to the dorsum of the foot as the lateral dorsal cutaneous nerve. Only 58.6% of the cadavers had the same type of origin of the fibular communicating nerve in both legs. There were no significant differences between the right and left sides, between sexes, or the place where the fibular communicating or sural nerves arose. The union between the fibular communicating and medial sural cutaneous nerves was seen on 159 sides (80.3%). This union was more often located in the lower half of the leg (75%) (Bergman, 1984, 1988).

Deep Fibular (Peroneal) Nerve

This nerve (Fig. 11.4) begins at the bifurcation of the common fibular nerve, between the fibula and the proximal part of the fibularis longus. It passes obliquely forwards deep to the extensor digitorum longus to the front of the interosseous membrane. Here, it gives muscular branches to the TA, extensor hallucis longus, extensor digitorum longus, and fibularis tertius. In the anterior compartment it accompanies the anterior tibial artery in the proximal third of the leg. It descends with this artery to the ankle, where it divides into lateral and medial terminal branches. As it descends, the nerve is first lateral to the anterior tibial artery, then anterior, and finally lateral again at the ankle. It is usually divided into medial and lateral branches. It also gives an articular branch to the ankle joint. The lateral terminal branch crosses the ankle deep to the extensor digitorum brevis and supplies that muscle. It also gives three very small interosseous branches, which supply the tarsal and metatarsophalangeal joints of the middle three toes. The medial terminal branch runs distally on the dorsum of the foot lateral to the dorsalis pedis artery and connects with the medial branch of the superficial

fibular nerve in the first web space (Figs. 11.5 and 11.6). It divides into two dorsal digital nerves, which supply adjacent sides of the great and second toes. Before dividing, it gives off an interosseous branch, which supplies the first metatarsophalangeal joint. The deep fibular nerve can end as three terminal branches instead of two. A number of variations in the digital distribution of the nerve have been reported. It can supply the medial side of the great toe, adjacent sides of the second and third toes, or the lateral three-and-one-half toes. It sometimes has no digital branches at all. Absence of the cutaneous part of the superficial fibular nerve and the deep fibular nerve and its branch to the extensor digitorum brevis has been reported. In this case the nerves were replaced by the saphenous and sural nerves (Bergman, 1984, 1988).

Superficial Fibular (Peroneal) Nerve

The superficial fibular nerve (Fig. 11.4) begins at the bifurcation of the common fibular nerve. It lies at first deep to the fibularis longus, then passes anteroinferiorly between the fibularis longus and brevis and the extensor digitorum longus, and pierces the deep fascia in the distal third of the leg. It divides into a large medial dorsal cutaneous nerve and a smaller, more laterally placed, intermediate dorsal cutaneous nerve, usually after piercing the crural fascia. But sometimes it divides while it is still deep to the fascia. Solomon et al. (2001) reported the superficial fibular nerve to branch into the medial dorsal cutaneous nerve of the foot and the intermediate dorsal cutaneous nerve of the foot before piercing the crural fascia in 24 out of 68 cases (35%). Apaydin et al. (2008a) investigated the compartmental anatomy of the superficial fibular nerve and defined three particular types in its course. In 71% of cases the SFN coursed entirely within the lateral compartment of the leg (Type I). In 23.7% it penetrated the anterior intermuscular septum, 12.7 cm inferior to the apex of the head of fibula, and coursed in the anterior compartment (Type II). In the remaining 5.3% of the specimens the SFN had branches in both the anterior and lateral compartments (Type III). Prakash et al. (2010) examined 60 specimens for the location and course of the superficial fibular nerve and found it was located in the anterior compartment of the leg in 28.3%. In 8.3% it branched before piercing between the fibularis longus and extensor digitorum longus muscles, whereas in 11.7% it branched after piercing them. In 41 out of 60 specimens the sensory division of the superficial fibular nerve branched into the medial dorsal cutaneous and the intermediate dorsal cutaneous nerve distal to its emergence from the deep fascia.

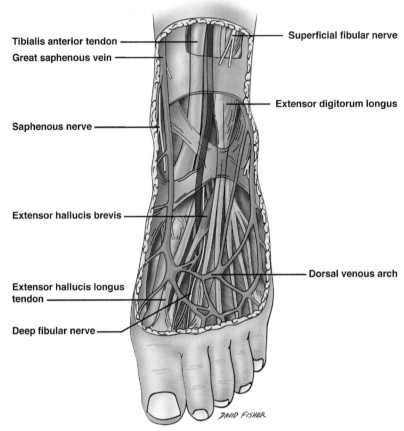

Tibialis anterior tendon

Great saphenous vein

Superficial fibular nerve

Saphenous nerve

Extensor digitorum longus

Extensor hallucis brevis

Extensor hallucis longus tendon

Dorsal venous arch

Deep fibular nerve

DAVID FISHER

FIG. 11.6 Schematic drawing of the distal anterior leg and dorsum of the foot.

As the nerve lies between the muscles of the lateral compartment of the leg, it supplies the fibularis longus, fibularis brevis, and the skin of the lower leg. The course, compartmental location, and peripheral digital distribution of the superficial fibular nerve are subject to considerable variation. For example, Browne and Morris (2007) described an adult female cadaver where the superficial fibular nerve bifurcated into two equal caliber branches 3 cm distal to the fibular head. The two branches remained in the lateral compartment of the leg and passed between the fibularis longus and brevis muscles. The anterior branch pierced the lateral intermuscular septum and then pierced the crural fascia to continue as the medial dorsal cutaneous nerve of the foot. The posterior branch pierced the crural fascia to continue as the intermediate dorsal cutaneous nerve of the foot. Variation in the distribution of the cutaneous nerves of the dorsum of the foot was reported in a series of 229 feet in 1892 by the Committee of Collective Investigation of the Anatomical Society of Great

Britain and Ireland: 12 patterns of termination of the dorsal nerves were described, which are known as Kosinski's variants (Kosinski, 1926; Solomon, 2001). Great variability was described in both the deep course (Kosinski, 1926; von Reinman, 1984; Blair, 1994; Benjamin, 1995) and the peripheral toe distribution (Brodie, 1892; Kosinski, 1926) of the sural and superficial fibular nerves. Solomon et al. (2001) described five types additional to Kosinski's variants in their series of 68 feet. Adkinson et al. (1991) reported that 14% of 85 legs had the superficial fibular nerve located in the medial compartment, while in 12% this nerve divided deep to the deep fascia in the lateral compartment and then the medial dorsal cutaneous nerve of the foot passed into the anterior compartment (Adkinson, 1991).

Another variant of the superficial fibular nerve with more practical implications in the approach to the lateral malleolus was described by Blair and Botte (1994). These authors reported that in 16% of 25 cases the nerve branched deep, and the medial dorsal cutaneous nerve of the foot pierced the fascia anterior to the lateral malleolus, while the intermediate dorsal cutaneous nerve of the foot pierced the fascia posterior to the lateral malleolus and then crossed the bone to follow its course toward the dorsum of the foot.

The medial dorsal cutaneous nerve typically passes in front of the ankle joint and divides into two dorsal digital branches, one of which supplies the medial side of the hallux and the other supplies the adjacent side of the second and third toes. It communicates with the saphenous and deep fibular nerves. The intermediate branch traverses the dorsum of the foot laterally. It divides into dorsal digital branches that supply the contiguous sides of the third to fifth toes and the skin of the lateral aspect of the ankle, where it connects with the sural nerve. Some of the lateral branches of the superficial fibular nerve are frequently absent and are replaced by sural branches (Bergman, 1984, 1988; Williams, 2005; Mahadevan, 2008).

Accessory Fibular Nerves

An accessory superficial fibular nerve and an accessory deep fibular nerve have been described as variant branches of the superficial fibular nerve; both are probably the products of atypical branching of the main nerve deep to the crural fascia. The accessory deep fibular nerve was reported to be a common variant branch of the superficial fibular nerve. It participates in the innervation of the extensor digitorum brevis muscle, which can interfere with the differential diagnosis of fibular nerve lesions (Tzika, 2012). Rayegani et al. (2011) found the accessory deep fibular nerve to be present in 28 out of 230 patients (12%). In another study, Prakash et al. (2010) demonstrated the accessory deep fibular nerve as an additional branch of the superficial fibular nerve in 20 out of 60 specimens. The course of this nerve lay in the anterior compartment of the leg which then passed deep to the extensor retinaculum and supplied cutaneous innervation to the ankle and the dorsum of the foot. Paraskevas et al. (2013) also reported an accessory superficial fibular nerve, which arose from the superficial fibular nerve 0.89 cm proximal to its penetration of the crural fascia.

Tibial Nerve

The tibial nerve (medial popliteal nerve) (Fig. 11.2) is the larger component of the sciatic nerve. It is derived from the anterior divisions of the L4, L5, and S1-S3 ventral rami. From its origin at the apex of the popliteal fossa, it descends mid-line overlapped proximally by the hamstring muscles. It becomes more superficial in the popliteal fossa, where it is lateral to the popliteal vessels to the distal border of the popliteus. The nerve, artery, and vein are bound in a common neurovascular bundle. Proximally, the nerve is lateral to the popliteal artery, gradually moves superficial to it in the middle of the fossa, ending distally medial to the artery. The popliteal vein lies between the nerve and artery throughout the whole popliteal fossa. In the distal popliteal fossa, the junction of the two heads of the gastrocnemius overlaps it.

Within the popliteal fossa, it gives articular branches to the knee joint forming a plexus with a branch from the obturator nerve. The branches that innervate the gastrocnemius, plantaris, soleus, and popliteus arise proximally either independently or by a common trunk.

The nerve then passes anterior to the arch of the soleus and gastrocnemius, posterior to the tibialis posterior in a sheath with the posterior tibial vessels. It is solely contained within the posterior compartment of the leg. The tibial nerve descends until, in its distal third, it is posterior to the lower end of the tibia, covered only by skin and fasciae. Here, it is overlapped sometimes by the flexor hallucis longus. It extends under the flexor retinaculum and loops around the medial malleolus. It is first medial to, then posterior, ending lateral to the vessels at the ankle. In the leg, the tibial nerve gives off muscular branches to the tibialis posterior, the soleus, the flexor hallucis longus, and the flexor digitorum longus. In addition, it supplies the ankle joint with articular branches. Cutaneous innervation from the medial calcaneal branches supplies the medial aspect of the ankle and heel.

Apaydin et al. (2008b) examined the course and branching pattern of the tibial nerve in the deep posterior compartment of the leg and defined three particular types. Type I (55.6%): separate branches to each of the muscles in the deep posterior compartment of the leg. Type II (30.6%): two main branches of the tibial nerve that provide motor branches. Type III (13.8%): one main branch, giving rise to separate motor branches to each of the muscles. In 61.1% of their cases, the proximal and distal branches of the tibial nerve innervated the flexor hallucis longus. In 38.9%, this muscle was innervated only by one proximal branch. In all of their cases, the tibialis posterior was innervated by both the proximal and distal branches, and the flexor digitorum longus was innervated only distally (Apaydin, 2008b). The branch to the flexor hallucis longus accompanies the fibular vessels. It has an interosseous branch that descends near the fibula to reach the distal tibiofibular joint. It also gives off the medial calcaneal nerve, which perforates the flexor retinaculum to supply the skin of the heel and medial side of the sole. The medial calcaneal nerve can have two sets of branches, which reunite to form the rest of the nerve (Aasar, 1947).

The tibial nerve (Figs. 11.7 and 11.8) ends under the flexor retinaculum by dividing into the medial and lateral plantar nerves. Bareither et al. (1990) dissected 126 human cadaver lower extremities to determine

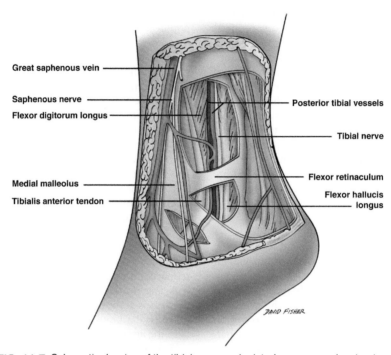

FIG. 11.7 Schematic drawing of the tibial nerve and related neuromuscular structures.

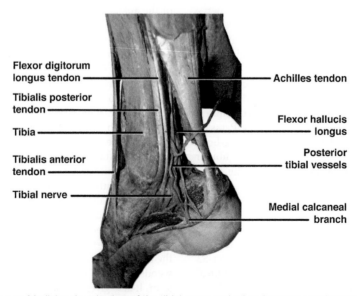

FIG. 11.8 Medial cadaveric view of the tibial nerve and related neuromuscular structures.

the level of division of the tibial nerve into medial and lateral plantar nerves (Figs. 11.9 and 11.10). They reported a considerable amount of variance in the level of division, documenting a higher incidence of division proximal to the usual description. This is deep to the flexor retinaculum between the calcaneus and medial malleolus.

The medial plantar nerve is the larger terminal division of the tibial nerve. The medial plantar artery accompanies it laterally. It originates under the flexor retinaculum and passes deep to the abductor hallucis. Between the abductor hallucis and flexor digitorum brevis it gives off a medial proper digital nerve to the hallux, and divides near the metatarsal bases into three common plantar digital nerves. Its cutaneous branches pierce the plantar aponeurosis between the abductor hallucis and flexor digitorum brevis to supply the skin of the sole of the foot.

Muscular branches supply the abductor hallucis, flexor digitorum brevis, flexor hallucis brevis, and the first lumbrical. The first two arise near the origin of the nerve and enter the deep surfaces of the muscles. The branch to the flexor hallucis brevis is from the

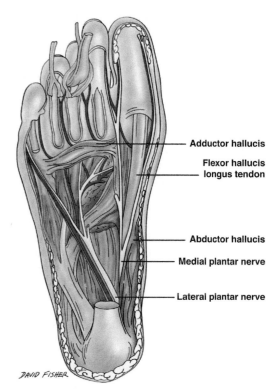

FIG. 11.10 Deeper anatomy of the medial and lateral plantar nerves.

medial digital nerve of the great toe, and that to the first lumbrical from the first common plantar digital nerve. Articular branches supply the joints of the tarsus and metatarsus. Three common plantar digital nerves pass between the slips of the plantar aponeurosis, each dividing into two proper digital branches. The first supplies adjacent sides of the hallux and second toe and the second supplies adjacent sides of the second and third toes; the third supplies adjacent sides of the third and fourth toes, and also connects with the lateral plantar nerve. The first gives a branch to the first lumbrical. Each proper digital nerve has cutaneous and articular branches: near the distal phalanges a dorsal branch supplies structures around the nail, and the termination of each nerve supplies the ball of the toe.

The lateral plantar nerve supplies the skin of the fifth toe, the lateral half of the fourth toe, and most of the deep muscles of the foot. It has superficial and deep branches. Before division, it supplies the flexor digitorum accessorius and abductor digiti minimi and gives rise to small branches that pierce the plantar fascia to supply the skin of the lateral part of the sole. The superficial branch splits into two common plantar digital nerves: the lateral

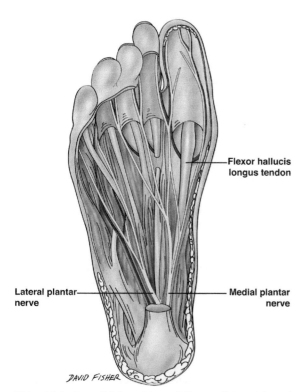

FIG. 11.9 Superficial anatomy of the medial and lateral plantar nerves.

supplies the lateral side of the fifth toe, the flexor digiti minimi brevis and the two interossei in the fourth intermetatarsal space; the medial connects with the third common plantar digital branch of the medial plantar nerve and divides into two to supply the adjoining sides of the fourth and fifth toes. The deep branch accompanies the lateral plantar artery deep to the flexor tendons and adductor hallucis and supplies the second to fourth lumbricals, adductor hallucis, and all the interossei (except those of the fourth intermetatarsal space). Branches to the second and third lumbricals pass distally deep to the transverse head of the adductor hallucis and curve round its distal border to reach them. The first and second lumbricals can receive branches from both the lateral and medial plantars. The branch of the lateral nerve to the second lumbrical courses forward, beneath the transversus (adductor hallucis), then turns backward over the transversus to reach the lumbrical muscle. Cruveilhier (1844) described a branch of the lateral plantar that pierced the transversus to reach the third lumbrical. The lateral nerve rarely provides a branch to the lateral head of the flexor hallucis brevis (Bergman, 1984, 1988).

Hallopeau's nerve is a branch of the lateral plantar nerve that supplies the flexor hallucis brevis muscle while also forming an anastomosis with the medial plantar nerve. In a study by Chou et al. (2008), this neural anastomosis was found in 4 out of 26 specimens.

Sural Nerve

The sural nerve (Fig. 11.5) is a cutaneous branch typically formed by the union of the lateral and medial sural communicating nerves, which originate from the common fibular and tibial nerves in the popliteal fossa 3–5 cm above the knee joint (Sunderland, 1978). After its formation, the sural nerve descends between the heads of the gastrocnemius, piercing the deep fascia proximally in the leg. It is not uncommon for the medial sural communicating branch to be joined at a variable level by the lateral sural communicating branch of the common fibular nerve after piercing the deep fascia. The sural nerve descends lateral to the calcaneal tendon, near the short saphenous vein, to the region between the lateral malleolus and the calcaneus and supplies the posterior and lateral skin of the distal third of the leg. It then passes distal to the lateral malleolus along the lateral side of the foot and little toe, supplying the overlying skin. It connects with the posterior femoral cutaneous nerve in the leg and with the superficial fibular nerve on the dorsum of the foot. The surface marking at the ankle is a line parallel to the calcaneal tendon halfway between the tendon and the lateral malleolus. However, its position is variable

(Webb et al., 2000; Apaydin, 2009). Apaydin et al. (2009) demonstrated that in 95.5% of their specimens the sural nerve was initially medial to the lateral border of the CT proximally and intersected with the lateral border of the CT at 55% of the mid-tendon line (Apaydin, 2009).

Several variations have been reported in the formation and distribution of branches of these nerves. The point of union of the two branches of the sural nerve is subject to wide variation. It can be high in the popliteal space or sometimes there is no union at all. The union can occur 3 cm below the origin of the fibular communicating nerve. The two branches of the sural nerve can arise 3 cm apart about 10 cm above the knee and pierce the medial head of the gastrocnemius muscle before joining the fibular communicating nerve. In some cases the two branches do not rejoin. The sural nerve sometimes supplies the dorsal cutaneous area of the lateral two-and-one-half toes. It can terminate at the lateral border of the foot without providing any digital branches. When the medial sural cutaneous nerve is joined by the fibular communicating nerve, the combined nerve is termed the sural nerve (Bergman, 1984, 1988).

Eid and Hegazi (2011) examined 24 specimens and noted a sural communicating nerve connected with the sural nerve in 87.5%. In 62%, the predominant site of union between these two nerves was in the lower one-third of the leg and ankle region. There were four types of pattern of innervation of the toes by the sural nerve. The predominant pattern was type I (45.8%), where the lateral side of the little toe was supplied by the sural nerve alone. The second most common pattern was type IV (29.2%), where the lateral 2 ½ toes were supplied by the sural nerve alone (Eid, 2011). Madhavi et al. (2005) determined the cutaneous pattern of distribution of the sural nerve on the dorsum of the foot in 260 Indian feet and demonstrated six patterns of innervation of the toes. The reported types did not differ from those reported by Kosinski in 1926. There was no association between the innervation pattern and side or sex. Two cases of anomalous innervation of the abductor digiti quinti muscle of the foot via the sural nerve have been described (Ragno, 1995). Amoiridis et al. (1997) reported motor fibers from the sural nerve innervating the abductor digiti minimi in 13 out of 207 individuals.

IMAGING

Sciatic nerve injuries are a common source of pain and reduced mobility in the lower extremities. Many forms of imaging allow for an increased accuracy of diagnosis.

Nerve Conduction Studies and Electromyography

Basic nerve conduction studies stimulate a specific nerve and record the ability of that nerve to translate an impulse to the muscle. These studies are used for localizing nerve lesions and determining pathological processes. They may be used to monitor both motor and sensory fibers of all major nerves and associated innervations in the lower extremity.

There are two methods for monitoring the sciatic nerve. (1) Yap and Hirota designed a method using two surface recording sites, the medial gastrocnemius and the laterally placed adductor digiti quinti muscles. These surface electrodes are placed 13–17 cm from the stimulating electrode at the apex of the popliteal fossa. A needle stimulating electrode is placed at the gluteal fold due to the depth of the sciatic nerve at that point.

2) Gassel and Trojaborg is essentially the same as Yap and Hirota except that the needle electrodes are the recording electrodes. The recording electrodes are placed in TA, gastrocnemius, soleus, extensor digitorum brevis, and abductor hallucis. The stimulating electrodes are placed (1) at the sciatic notch at the midpoint between the greater trochanter of the femur and the ischial tuberosity and (2) at the apex of the popliteal fossa.

Electromyography is similar to the nerve conduction study but measures the action potentials elicited by contraction of a specified muscle. These are usually performed in conjunction with one another.

Though these two methods allowed for a gross classification due to electrophysiology and distribution of nerve failure, they cannot give morphological details or changes within the nerve or its immediate surroundings. This is where imaging is indispensable.

Ultrasound

Ultrasound (US) is an imaging technique that uses sound waves to evaluate the structures beneath the skin surface in a "readily available, inexpensive high-resolution and dynamic technique" (Stoll, 2013). Waves are delivered by a transducer and are either absorbed, deflected, or reflected back to the transducer. Brightness of an image relates to the amount of sound waves reflected to the transducer; therefore, dark images absorb sound waves and are hypoechoic (e.g., fluid), whereas bright images reflect more waves and are hyperechoic (e.g., bone). The internal morphology of the sciatic nerve corresponds to the US image. The nerve is a tubular, hyperechoic structure, the epineurium, consisting of fascicles surrounded by a hypoechoic, connective tissue matrix. On US, this relates to two bright lines surrounding parallel hypoechoic lines (on long axis) or a honeycomb appearance on short-axis visualization. To visualize a superficial nerve, a higher frequency, linear probe, 7–18 MHz, may be used. This would include the sciatic nerve in the thigh or popliteal region. However, to image the sciatic nerve in the gluteal region, a curved probe, 2-5 or 4–7 MHz, must be used due to the increased depth of the nerve. The nerve may be distinguished from solid hyperechoic tendons and more hypoechoic muscles (Koenig, 2009). Currently, US is used for diagnosing nerve entrapments, trauma, and inflammation, as well as for guiding regional anesthesia and medications (Tsui, 2010; Tagliafico, 2010).

Magnetic Resonance Imaging

Magnetic resonance imaging of nerves, termed MR neurography, is used for depicting deep nervous tissue with excellent soft tissue differentiation. Evaluation of peripheral nerves is dependent on the morphological images of T1-weighted sequences and of signal changes of fluid-sensitive fat-suppressed heavily T2-weighted sequences. Damaged nerves and blood vessels appear as hyperintense on T2-weighted sequences (Stoll, 2013). Damaged nerves and blood vessels may further be discriminated by using gadolinium-DTPA contrast material (Stoll, 2013). MR neurography may aid in the identification of injured nerves, denervated muscles, disruptions in the blood-nerve barrier, nerve inflammation, nerve tumors, traumatic and compressive nerve lesions, entrapment neuropathies, inflammatory nerve disorders (Guillain-Barré syndrome, polyradiculoneuritis, and focal mononeuritis), and pure motor syndromes (Stoll, 2013).

PATHOLOGY/SURGICAL IMPLICATIONS
Intramuscular Injections

Intramuscular injections into the buttocks have been a common site of sciatic nerve injury since being documented in the 1920s (Mishra, 2010). These injuries may range from a transient sensory change to a permanent paralysis and paresthesia. A knowledge of the surface anatomy and underlying nerves enables the injection to be placed at a location that proves less morbid.

Sciatica

Sciatica is the common term for a number of back and leg symptoms associated with the sciatic nerve. The most common areas causing sciatica are due to disc rupture and osteoarthritic change at the L4/L5, L5/S1 and sometimes the L3/L4 levels. The prevalence of sciatica varies with the highest incidence of 40% most often in the 40s and 50s (Konstantinou, 2008).

Symptoms of sciatica include aching and sharp pain that begins in the buttocks and radiates down the distribution of nerve fibers. Traditionally unilateral due to the dorsolateral herniation of the nucleus pulposus compressing the spinal roots, the pain may be bilateral in lumbar stenosis and spondylolisthesis (Konstantinou, 2008). Common imaging studies, nerve conduction studies, and electromyography aid in the diagnosis. Surgical treatment includes decompression of the lumbar nerve root by unilateral hemilaminectomy. Other procedures include microdiscectomy and minimally invasive percutaneous techniques (Konstantinou, 2008).

Piriformis Syndrome

As the sciatic nerve exits the greater sciatic foramen in close proximity to the piriformis muscle, focal hyperirritability causing spasm, hypertrophy, or contracture of the muscle may cause entrapment. Symptoms mimic those of sciatica and are most often caused by trauma to the buttocks affecting the piriformis either directly or indirectly (Solheim, 1981). Diagnostic tests include Lasègue, Freiberg, and Pace signs. Lasègue's sign is localized pain with hip flexion and knee extension, applying pressure to the piriformis. Frieberg's includes passive internal rotation of the hip which elicits pain. Finally, Pace's sign reveals pain during hip flexion, adduction, and internal rotation. Treatment may include pharmacological therapy of NSAIDs, muscle relaxants, ice, rest, and muscle strength and stretching (Boyajian-O'Neill, 2008). In addition, acupuncture and trigger point injection of local anesthetic, steroids, or botulinum toxin type A may be used (Boyajian-O'Neill, 2008). Finally surgical decompression is the final option (Boyajian-O'Neill, 2008).

Other Injuries Involving the Sciatic Nerve and its Branches

Other injuries to the sciatic nerve and its branches include iatrogenic injuries (hip and knee arthroplasty), fractures (pelvic, femur, tibia, and fibula), compression of the nerves due to arterial aneurysm, and tarsal tunnel syndrome.

REFERENCES

Aasar, Y.H., 1947. Anatomical Anomalies. Fouad I University Press, Cairo, pp. 92–101.

Adkinson, D.P., Bosse, M.J., Gaccione, D.R., Gabriel, K.R., 1991. Anatomical variations in the course of the superficial peroneal nerve. J. Bone Jt. Surg. 73A, 112–114.

Amoiridis, G., Schols, L., Ameridis, N., Przuntek, H., 1997. Motor fibers in the sural nerve of humans. Neurology 49, 1725–1728.

Apaydin, N., Basarir, K., Loukas, M., Tubbs, R.S., Uz, A., Kinik, H., 2008a. Compartmental anatomy of the superficial fibular nerve with an emphasis on fascial release operations of the leg. Surg. Radiol. Anat. 30 (1), 47–52.

Apaydin, N., Loukas, M., Kendir, S., Tubbs, R.S., Jordan, R., Tekdemir, I., Elhan, A., 2008b. The precise localization of distal motor branches of the tibial nerve in the deep posterior compartment of the leg. Surg. Radiol. Anat. 30 (4), 291–295.

Apaydin, N., Bozkurt, M., Loukas, M., Vefali, H., Tubbs, R.S., Esmer, A.F., 2009. Relationships of the sural nerve with the calcaneal tendon: an anatomical study with surgical and clinical implications. Surg. Radiol. Anat. 1 (10), 775–780.

Arifoglu, Y., Sürücü, H.S., Sargon, M.F., Tanyeli, E., Yazar, F., 1997. Double superior gemellus together with double piriformis and high division of the sciatic nerve. Surg. Radiol. Anat. 19 (6), 407–408.

Babinski, M.A., Machado, F.A., Costa, W.S., 2003. A rare variation in the high division of the sciatic nerve surrounding the superior gemellus muscle. Eur. J. Morphol. 41 (1), 41–42.

Bareither, D.J., Genau, J.M., Massaro, J.C., 1990. Variation in the division of the tibial nerve: application to nerve blocks. J. Foot Surg. 29 (6), 581–583.

Beaton, L.E., Anson, B.J., 1938. The relation of the sciatic nerve and its subdivisions to the piriformis muscle. Anat. Rec. 70, 1–5.

Benjamin, A.C., TumaJr, P., Grillo, M.A., Ferreira, M.C., 1995. Revista do Hospital das Clinicas, vol. 50. Faculdade de Medicina de Sao Paulo, pp. 25–29.

Bergman, R.A., Thompson, S.A., Aww, A.K., Saddeh, F.A., 1988. Compendium of Human Anatomical Variations. Urban and Schwarzenburg, Baltimore, pp. 143–148.

Bergman, R.A., Thompson, S.A., Afifi, A.K., 1984. Catalogue of Human Variations. Urban & Schwarzenberg, Baltimore and Munich, pp. 158–161.

Blair, J.M., Botte, M.J., 1994. Surgical anatomy of the superficial peroneal nerve in the ankle and foot. Clin. Orthop. Relat. Res. 305, 229–238.

Boyajian-O'Neill, L., McClain, R., Coleman, M., Thomas, P., 2008. Diagnosis and management of piriformis syndrome: an osteopathic approach. J. Am. Osteopath. Assoc. 108, 657–664.

Brodie, G., Shaw, E.H., Macload, P., Harris, W.A., Fawcett, E., 1892. Collective investigation on the distribution of cutaneous nerve of the dorsum of the foot. J. Anat. Physiol. 26, 89–90.

Browne, J.A., Morris, M.J., 2007. Variant superficial fibular (peroneal) nerve anatomy in the middle third of the lateral leg. Clin. Anat. 20, 996–997.

Carare, R.O., Goodwin, M., 2008. A unique variation of the sciatic nerve. Clin. Anat. 21 (8), 800–801.

Chou, L.B., Choi, L.E., Ramachandra, T., Ma, G., 2008. Variation of nerve to flexor hallucis brevis. Foot Ankle Int. 29 (10), 1042–1044.

Cruveilhier, J., 1844. The Anatomy of the Human Body. Harper & Brothers, New York. Provided by Univ. of Mass Medical School, Lamar Soutter Library, archive.org.

Currin, S., Mirjalili, S., Meikle, G., Stringer, M., 2014. Revisiting the surface anatomy of the sciatic nerve in the gluteal region. Clin. Anat. 28, 144–149.

Dupont, G., Unno, F., Iwanaga, J., Oskouian, R.J., Tubbs, R.S., 2018. A variant of the sciatic nerve and its clinical implications. Cureus 10 (6), 6–8.

Eid, E.M., Hegazy, A.M., 2011. Anatomical variations of the human sural nerve and its role in clinical and surgical procedures. Clin. Anat. 24 (2), 237–245.

Franco, D., 2007. Manual of Regional Anesthesia, 83–84 and 92–100. www.Cook CountryRegional.com.

Gibbs, C.M., Ginsburg, A.D., Wilson, T.J., Lachman, N., Hevesi, M., Spinner, R.J., Krych, A.J., 2018. The anatomy of the perineal branch of the sciatic nerve. Clin. Anat. 31, 357–363.

Huban, T.R., Nayak, V.S., D'souza, A.S., 2012. A rare variation in the innervation of the gluteus maximus muscle. A case report. Glob. J. Adv. Res. 2, 1394–1396.

Huelke, D.F., 1958. Origin of the peroneal communicating nerve in adult man. Anat. Rec. 132, 81–92.

Kiros, M., Woldeyes, D., 2015. Anatomical variations in the level of bifurcation of the sciatic nerve in Ethiopia. J. Exp. Clin. Anat. 14, 1.

Koenig, R.W., Pedro, M.T., Heinen, C.P., Schmidt, T., Richter, H.P., Antoniadis, G., Kretschmer, T., 2009. High-resolution ultrasonography in evaluating peripheral nerve entrapment and trauma. Neurosurg. Focus 26, E13.

Konstantinou, K., Dunn, K.M., 2008. Sciatica: review of epidemiological studies and prevalence estimates. Spine 33, 2464–2472.

Kosinski, C., 1926. The course, mutual relations and distribution of the cutaneous nerves of the metazonal region of the leg and foot. J. Anat. Physiol. 60, 274–297.

Madhavi, C., Isaac, B., Antoniswamy, B., Holla, S.J., 2005. Anatomical variations of the cutaneous innervation patterns of the sural nerve on the dorsum of the foot. Clin. Anat. 18 (3), 206–209.

Mahadevan, V., 2008. Pelvic girdle and lower limb. In: Standring, S. (Ed.), Gray's Anatomy, fortyth ed. Elsevier, New York, pp. 1327–1429.

Mas, N., Ozeksi, P., Ozdemir, B., Kapakin, S., Sargon, M.F., Celik, H.H., Yener, N., 2003. A case of bilateral high division of the sciatic nerves, together with a unilateral unusual course of the tibial nerve. Neuroanatomy 2, 13–15.

Mirjalili, S., 2015. Nerves and Nerve Injuries, vol. 1. Elsevier, London.

Mishra, P., Stringer, M.D., 2010. Sciatic nerve injury from intramuscular injection: a persistent and global problem. Int. J. Clin. Pract. 64, 1573–1579.

Natsis, K., Totlis, T., Konstantinidis, G.A., Paraskevas, G., Piagkou, M., Koebke, J., 2014. Anatomical variations between the sciatic nerve and the piriformis muscle: a contribution to surgical anatomy in piriformis syndrome. Surg. Radiol. Anat. 36, 273–280.

Paraskevas, G.K., Natsis, K., Tzika, M., Ioannidis, O., 2013. Potential entrapment of an accessory superficial peroneal sensory nerve at the lateral malleolar area: a cadaveric case report and review of the literature. J. Foot Ankle Surg. 52, 92–95.

Patel, S., Shah, M., Vora, R., Zalawida, A., Rathod, S.P., 2011. A variation in the high division of the sciatic nevre and its relation with piriformis syndrome. Natl. J. Med. Res. 1 (2), 27–30.

Pokorny, D., Jahoda, D., Veigl, D., Pinskerova, V., Sonsa, A., 2006. Topographic variations of the relationship of the sciatic nerve and the piriformis muscle and its relevance to palsy after total hip arthroplasty. Surg. Radiol. Anat. 28, 88–91.

Prakash, Bhardwaj, A.K., Singh, D.K., Rajini, T., Jayanthi, V., Singh, G., 2010. Anatomic variations of superficial peroneal nerve: clinical implications of a cadaver study. Ital. J. Anat Embryol. 115 (3), 223–228.

Ragno, M., Santoro, L., 1995. Motor fibers in human sural nerve. Electromyogr. Clin. Neurophysiol. 35 (1), 61–63.

Raj, P.P., Parks, R.I., Watson, T.D., Jenkins, M.T., 1975. A new single-position supine approach to sciatic-femoral nerve block. Anesth. Analg. 54, 489–493.

Rayegani, S.M., Daneshtalab, E., Bahrami, M.H., Eliaspour, D., Raeissadat, S.A., Rezaei, S., Babaee, M., 2011. Prevalence of accessory deep peroneal nerve in referred patients to an electrodiagnostic medicine clinic. J. Brachial Plexus Peripher. Nerve Inj. 6 (1), 3.

Robards, C., Wang, R.D., Clendenen, S., Ladlie, B., Greengrass, R., 2009. Sciatic nerve catheter placement: success with using the Raj approach. Anesth. Analg. 109, 972–975.

Santanu, B., Pitbaran, C., Sudeshna, M., Hasi, D., 2013. Different neuromuscular variations in the gluteal region. IJAV 6, 136–139.

Sladjana, U.Z., Ivan, J.D., Bratislav, S.D., 2008. Microanatomical structure of the human sciatic nerve. Surg. Radiol. Anat. 30 (8), 619–626.

Small, S.P., 2004. Preventing sciatic nerve injury from intramuscular injections: literature review. J. Adv. Nurs. 47, 287–296.

Solheim, L.F., Siewers, P., Paus, B., 1981. The piriformis muscle syndrome. Sciatic nerve entrapment treated with section of the piriformis muscle. Acta Orthop. Scand. 52, 73–75.

Solomon, L.B., Ferris, L., Tedman, R., Henneberg, M., 2001. Surgical anatomy of the sural and superficial fibular nerves with an emphasis on the approach to the lateral malleolus. J. Anat. 199 (Pt 6), 717–723.

Stoll, G., Wilder-Smith, E., Bendszus, M., 2013. Imaging of the peripheral nervous system. Handb. Clin. Neurol. 115, 137–153.

Sunderland, S., 1978. Nerves and Nerve Injuries. Churchill Livingston, London.

Tagliafico, A., Bodner, G., Rosenberg, I., Palmieri, F., Garello, I., Altafini, L., Martinoli, C., 2010. Peripheral nerves: ultrasound-guided interventional procedures. Semin. Muscoskel. Radiol. 14, 559–566.

Tsui, B.C.H., Suresh, S., 2010. Ultrasound imaging for regional anesthesia in infants, children, and adolescents. Anesthesiology 112, 473–492.

Tubbs, R.S., Collin, P.G., D'Antoni, A.V., Loukas, M., Oskouian, R.J., Spinner, R.J., 2017. Sciatic nerve intercommunications: new finding. World Neurosurg. 98, 176–181.

Tzika, M., Paraskevas, G.K., Kitsoulis, P., 2012. The accessory deep peroneal nerve: a review of the literature. Foot 22 (3), 232–234.

Von Reinman, R., 1984. Uberzählige Nervi peronei beim Menschen. Accessory peroneal nerves in the human. Anat. Anzeiger 155, 257–267.

Watt, T., Hariharan, A.R., Brzezinski, D.W., Caird, M.S., Zeller, J.L., 2014. Branching patterns and localization of the common fibular (peroneal) nerve: an anatomical basis for planning safe surgical approaches. Surg. Radiol. Anat. 36, 821–828.

Webb, J., Moorjani, N., Radford, M., 2000. Anatomy of the sural nerve and its relation to the Achilles Tendon. Foot Ankle Int. 21, 475–477.

Williams, A., 2005. Pelvic girdle and lower limb. In: Standring, S. (Ed.), Gray's Anatomy, thirtninth ed. Elsevier, New York, pp. 1456–1499.

CHAPTER 12

Microanatomy of the Distal Sciatic Nerve in Six Mammalian Species

ANNA SERVER • MARIELLE ESTEVES COELHO • ANTONIA MATAMALA-ADROVER •
ANDRÉ P. BOEZAART • XAVIER SALA-BLANCH • MIGUEL A. REINA

INTRODUCTION

Translational research is relatively new in biomedical research. Its aim is to transfer or extrapolate knowledge from experimental animals to humans. Various experimental animal models have been used for studying peripheral nerve blocks—specifically, iatrogenic nerve injury during attempted nerve blocks. Because of its ease of access, the sciatic nerve, in particular, has traditionally been studied extensively in animal models. The aim of this chapter is to compare the microanatomic architectural features of the sciatic nerves of different mammalian species. Light microscopic images were analyzed in Wistar rats, New Zealand rabbits, hybrid pigs, Ripollesa sheep, beagles, and humans. The sciatic nerves were dissected from the posterior compartment of the leg at the division into its two terminal branches (the tibial and common peroneal nerves).

The resulting dissections are depicted in Figs. 12.1−12.4. Under microscopic examination, the number, shape, and size of fascicles differed widely from one species to another. There was a distinction between so-called oligofascicular species (rat, rabbit, and dog) and multifascicular species (pig, sheep, and human). Fascicle areas also varied widely, ranging from 0.043 mm^2 (pig) to 0.941 mm^2 (dog). There were also great differences between the circumferences and radii of the nerves and fascicles. All results are shown in Figs. 12.5−12.24. Successive cross-sections show the proximal to distal areas of the sciatic nerves of rats (Figs. 12.5−12.8), rabbits (Figs. 12.9−12.12), dogs (Figs. 12.13−12.16), pigs (Figs. 12.17−12.20), sheep (Figs. 12.21−12.23), and humans (Fig. 12.24).

The results indicated vast differences in nerve architectures in terms of the metrics studied, especially in the proportion of intrafascicular tissue versus interfascicular tissue ranges.

The similarities or dissimilarities between species may vary depending on the focus of a specific study. Also, it would be essential to consider the area, circumference, and radii of fascicles (Moayeri and Groen, 2009; Hagan et al., 2012; Asato et al., 2000; Rigaud et al., 2008; Ceballos et al., 1999) when studying the effects and toxicity of local anesthetic agents on peripheral nerves. The proportion of fascicular neural and nonneural tissues should also be taken into consideration when studying physical nerve lesions caused by direct nerve trauma.

The validity of the model should probably be based purely on the resemblance to the microanatomic characteristics of humans (Fig. 12.24).

CONCLUSION

Sciatic nerve architecture differs widely between species of experimental models, from the oligofascicular species (rat, rabbit, and dog) to the multifascicular species (sheep, pig, and human) (Server et al., 2018). The variances do not only refer to topograms but also to size—the smallest being the rat and the biggest being the sheep and human—size and number of fascicles, and neural-to-nonneural tissue ratios.

The nerves of the dog and rat, which are most often used to study toxicity and nerve injury, are the most unlike human nerves, while the nerves of the pig and sheep—arguably studied the least often—are the closest.

We have not had the opportunity to study nerves of nonhuman primates, but that should—in theory, at least—resemble the nerve architecture of humans closest. We believe it remains not only necessary but also essential and mandatory to choose the most suitable experimental model to conduct meaningful and relevant translational studies in the field of regional anesthesia.

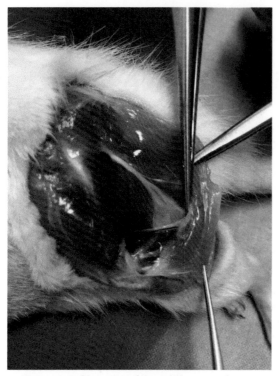

FIG. 12.1 Dissection of the sciatic nerve of a rat.

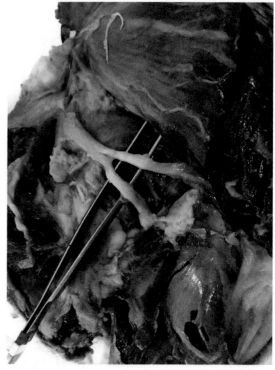

FIG. 12.3 Dissection of the sciatic nerve of a pig.

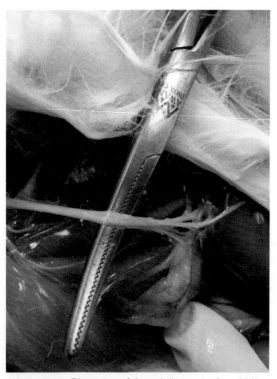

FIG. 12.2 Dissection of the sciatic nerve of a rabbit.

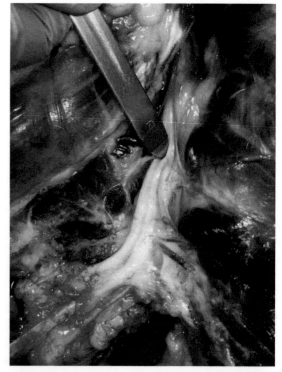

FIG. 12.4 Dissection of the sciatic nerve of a sheep.

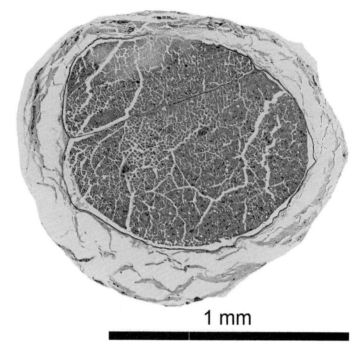

1 mm

FIG. 12.5 Cross-section of a sciatic nerve obtained from a rat. Stained with hematoxylin and eosin. Bar = 1 mm.

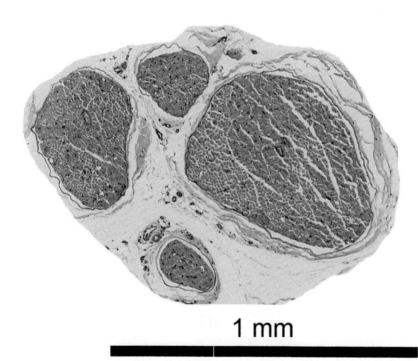

1 mm

FIG. 12.6 Cross-section of a sciatic nerve obtained from a rat. Stained with hematoxylin and eosin. Bar = 1 mm.

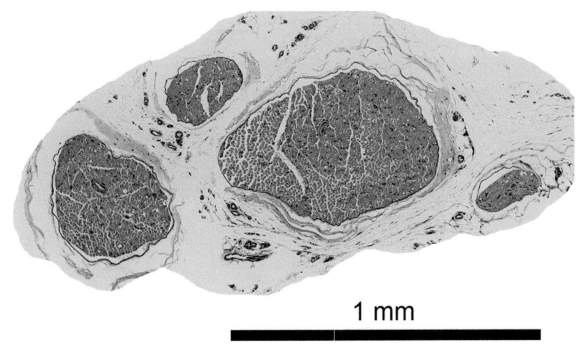

FIG. 12.7 Cross-section of a sciatic nerve obtained from a rat. Stained with hematoxylin and eosin. Bar = 1 mm.

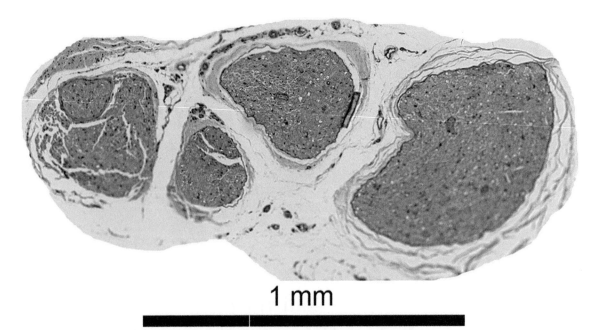

FIG. 12.8 Cross-section of a sciatic nerve obtained from a rat. Stained with hematoxylin and eosin. Bar = 1 mm.

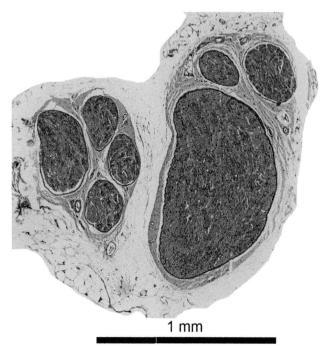

1 mm

FIG. 12.9 Cross-section of a sciatic nerve obtained from a rabbit. Stained with hematoxylin and eosin. Bar = 1 mm.

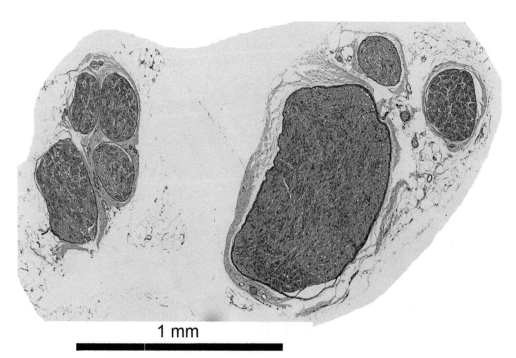

1 mm

FIG. 12.10 Cross-section of a sciatic nerve obtained from a rabbit. Stained with hematoxylin and eosin. Bar = 1 mm.

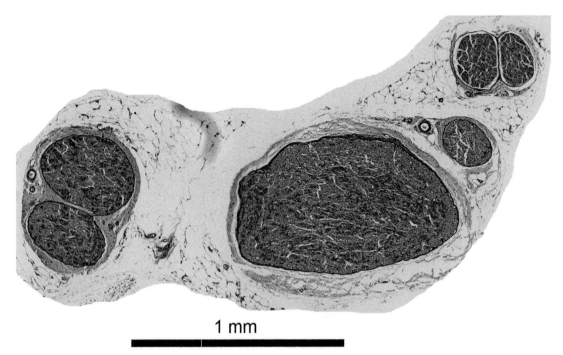

FIG. 12.11 Cross-section of a sciatic nerve obtained from a rabbit. Stained with hematoxylin and eosin. Bar = 1 mm.

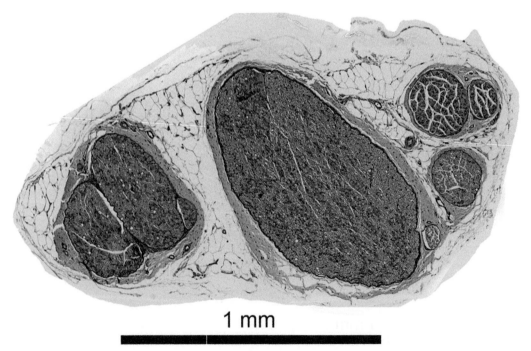

FIG. 12.12 Cross-section of a sciatic nerve obtained from a rabbit. Stained with hematoxylin and eosin. Bar = 1 mm.

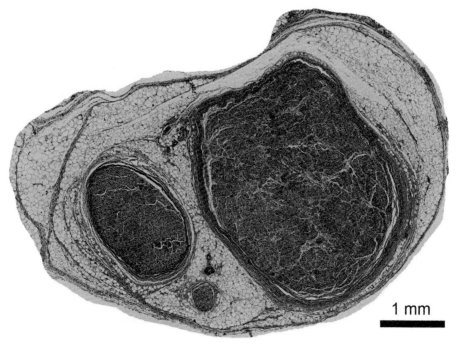

FIG. 12.13 Cross-section of a sciatic nerve obtained from a dog. Stained with hematoxylin and eosin. Bar = 1 mm.

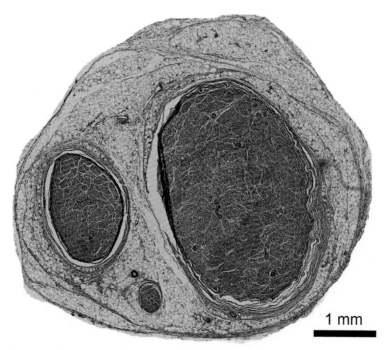

FIG. 12.14 Cross-section of a sciatic nerve obtained from a dog. Stained with hematoxylin and eosin. Bar = 1 mm.

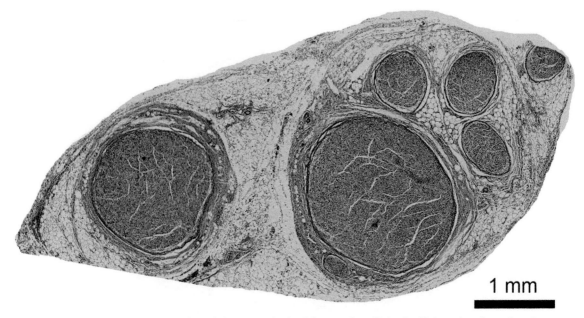

FIG. 12.15 Cross-section of a sciatic nerve obtained from a dog. Stained with hematoxylin and eosin. Bar = 1 mm.

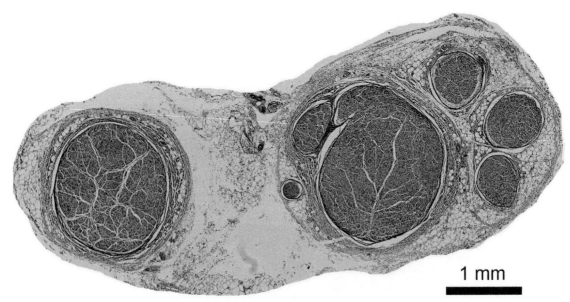

FIG. 12.16 Cross-section of a sciatic nerve obtained from a dog. Stained with hematoxylin and eosin. Bar = 1 mm.

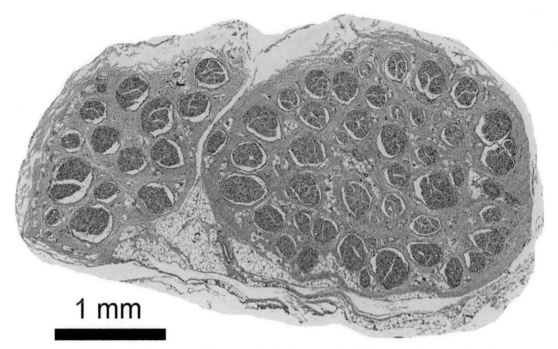

FIG. 12.17 Cross-section of a sciatic nerve obtained from a pig. Stained with hematoxylin and eosin. Bar = 1 mm.

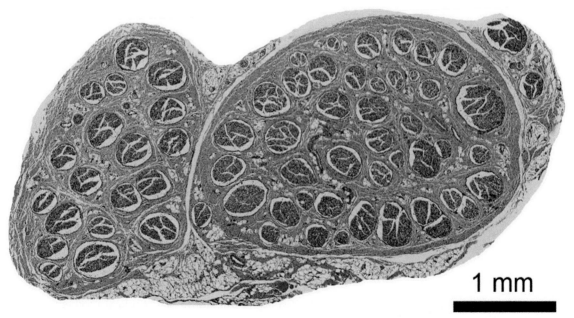

FIG. 12.18 Cross-section of a sciatic nerve obtained from a pig. Stained with hematoxylin and eosin. Bar = 1 mm.

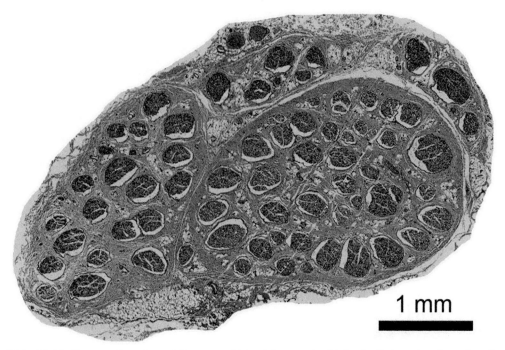

FIG. 12.19 Cross-section of a sciatic nerve obtained from a pig. Stained with hematoxylin and eosin. Bar = 1 mm.

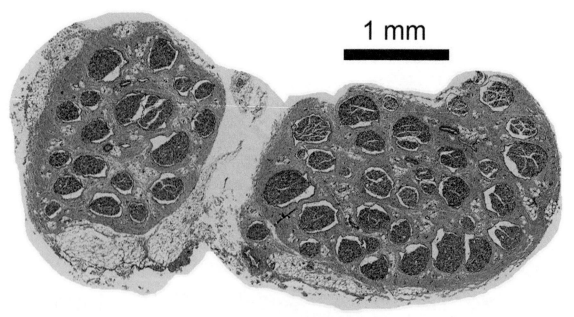

FIG. 12.20 Cross-section of a sciatic nerve obtained from a pig. Stained with hematoxylin and eosin. Bar = 1 mm.

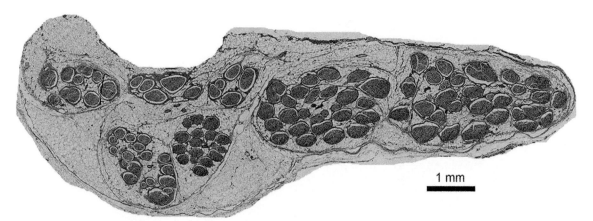

FIG. 12.21 Cross-section of a sciatic nerve obtained from a sheep. Stained with hematoxylin and eosin. Bar = 1 mm.

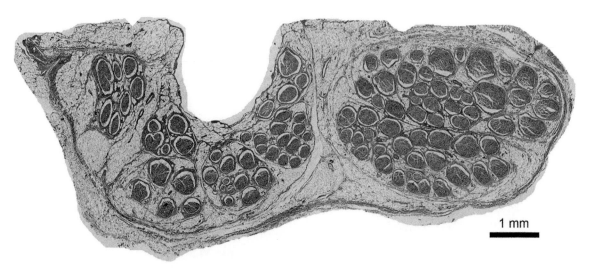

FIG. 12.22 Cross-section of a sciatic nerve obtained from a sheep. Stained with hematoxylin and eosin. Bar = 1 mm.

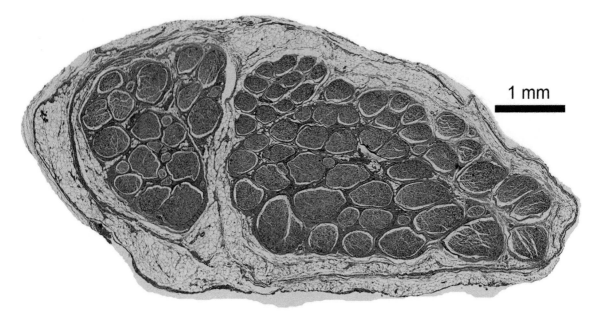

FIG. 12.23 Cross-section of a sciatic nerve obtained from a sheep. Stained with hematoxylin and eosin. Bar = 1 mm.

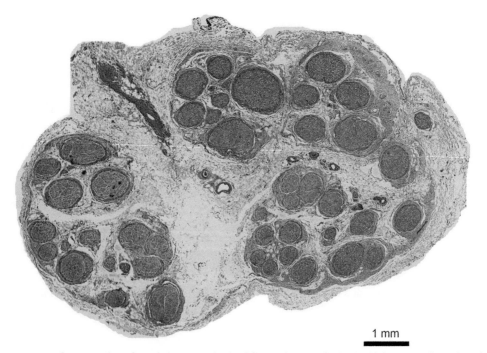

FIG. 12.24 Cross-section of a sciatic nerve obtained from a human. Stained with hematoxylin and eosin. Bar = 1 mm.

REFERENCES

Asato, F., Butler, M., Blomberg, H., Gordh, T., 2000. Variation in rat sciatic nerve anatomy: implications for a rat model of neuropathic pain. J. Peripher. Nerv. Syst. 5, 19–21.

Ceballos, D., Cuadras, J., Verdu, E., Navarro, X., 1999. Morphometric and ultrastructural changes with ageing in mouse peripheral nerve. J. Anat. 195, 563–576.

Hagan, C.E., Bolon, B., Keene, D., 2012. Nervous system. In: Treuting, P.M., Dintzis, S.M. (Eds.), Comparative Anatomy and Histology. A Mouse and Human Atlas. Elsevier, Amsterdam.

Moayeri, N., Groen, G.J., 2009. Differences in quantitative architecture of sciatic nerve may explain differences in potential vulnerability to nerve injury, onset time, and minimum effective anesthetic. Anesthesiology 111, 1128–1134.

Rigaud, M., Gemes, G., Barabas, M.E., et al., 2008. Species and strain differences in rodent sciatic nerve anatomy: implications for studies of neuropathic pain. Pain 136, 188–201.

Server, A., Reina, M.A., Boezaart, A.P., Prats-Galino, A., Esteves Coelho, M., Sala-Blanch, X., 2018. Microanatomical nerve architecture of six mammalian species: is trans-species translational anatomic extrapolation valid? Reg. Anesth. Pain Med. 43, 496–501.

CHAPTER 13

The Pelvic Splanchnic Nerves

SANTIAGO GUTIERREZ • R. SHANE TUBBS

INTRODUCTION

History and Introduction to the Surgical Relevance of the Pelvic Splanchnic Nerves

The pelvic splanchnic nerves (PSN) (Fig. 13.1) were first described by Eckhardt as "Nervi erigentes" in 1863, but such nerves had been mentioned earlier under other denominations: the "nerve for urinary bladder" by Galen c173, "middle hemorrhoidal nerves" by Meckel in 1817, "hypogastric branches of sacral nerves" by Cruveilhier in 1836, among others

(Swanson, 2015). They were described in macrodissected cadaveric human specimens as thin bundles arising from the second, third, and fourth ventral rami of the sacral nerves that carry sacral branches connecting to the pelvic or inferior hypogastric plexus (IHP) (Yamashita et al., 2017). However, the function and nature of those branches were unclear when they were described. Current opinion suggests that this network is responsible for both the autonomic parasympathetic and sympathetic innervation of the

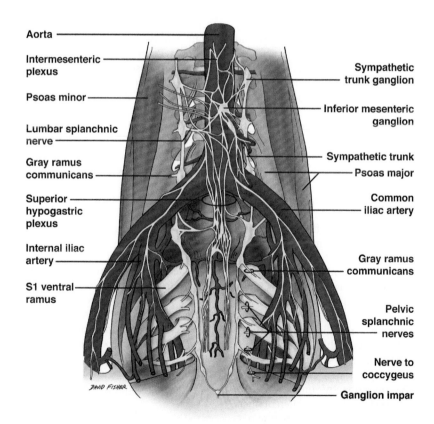

Aorta
Intermesenteric plexus
Psoas minor
Lumbar splanchnic nerve
Gray ramus communicans
Superior hypogastric plexus
Internal iliac artery
S1 ventral ramus

Sympathetic trunk ganglion
Inferior mesenteric ganglion
Sympathetic trunk
Psoas major
Common iliac artery
Gray ramus communicans
Pelvic splanchnic nerves
Nerve to coccygeus
Ganglion impar

DAVID FISHER

FIG. 13.1 Schematic drawing illustrating the pelvis splanchnic nerves and their neurovascular relationships.

Surgical Anatomy of the Sacral Plexus and Its Branches. https://doi.org/10.1016/B978-0-323-77602-8.00013-1

rectum, bladder, genitalia, prostate, and uterus (Ali et al., 2004; Jang et al., 2015). Thus, IHP and PSN functions are essential for the control of micturition, defecation, and sexual performance.

Since these functions have been recognized, complete understanding of the anatomical pathways remains a main focus for surgical scientific development. The preservation of these branches is vital for obtaining satisfactory functional outcomes in pelvic surgery, including in spine, urological, and gynecological procedures, while accomplishing the surgical objectives. This chapter will provide a comprehensive depiction of current knowledge regarding the nuclear origin and the anatomical structure of the PSN and their development, highlighting the essential functions regarding each body system related to it and their importance in clinical and surgical procedures.

A General Overview of the Autonomic Nervous System

The autonomic nervous system (ANS) is responsible for regulating the visceral functions of the body (Cramer and Darby, 2013). This set of automatic and partially voluntary features helps to sustain homeostasis and regulate variables such as blood pressure, digestive peristalsis, gastrointestinal secretions, bladder and rectal voiding, body temperature, and many other functions that are mostly under its full or partial domain (Hall and Guyton, 2011). The ANS is a complex neural and endocrine network comprising three components: the parasympathetic autonomic nervous system (PANS), sympathetic autonomic nervous system (SANS), and enteric nervous system (ENS). Earlier understanding and the literature about these systems described them as individually functioning compartments with distinct characteristics that were to an extent mutually antagonistic, as if they worked in an "on-off" fashion. They are now recognized as a set of complementary elements that sustain equilibrium among the body systems' vital functions by responding to each other. Thus, the ANS continually maintains homeostasis, balancing its forces through its structural components (Bankenahally and Krovvidi, 2016).

Every system of the body is supplied by elements of the ANS, which have been thoroughly described in the literature. Like any communication system, the ANS can be compared with a computer that combines input, central control, and output arms. Information derived from sensory visceral, special, and general afferent fibers constitutes the input arm of the system; the central nervous system (spinal nucleus, brainstem, and hypothalamus) represents the integratory center; and the output arm comprises a set of efferent nerves that stimulate glands, smooth muscle, and cardiac muscle through neurotransmitters and hormones (Catala and Kubis, 2013). These effectors trigger the cellular machinery to initiate the designated biological functions in the target tissues. All these mechanisms interact with each other through visceral reflexes that are, in the end, the "modus operandi" of the ANS. It now seems clear that the ANS relies not only on efferent motor nerve fibers to maintain homeostasis, but also on coordination with the endocrine and the immunological systems among many others. However, it is not the aim of the present chapter to describe those relationships.

As stated earlier, the efferent arm of the ANS is represented by the PANS and the SANS. The main central integratory centers for sympathetic information are located in the posterior hypothalamus. The SANS finds its peripheral origins in the lateral gray column of the thoracolumbar spinal cord, and the paravertebral ganglia chain. In contrast, the PANS follows a craniosacral distribution; the information related to this efferent arm is located within the anterior hypothalamus, the brainstem nuclei, and the sacral gray matter of the spinal cord. Recent studies have challenged the traditional autonomic distribution, as will be explained in the embryology section (Espinosa-Medina et al., 2016).

Structurally, the autonomic efferent arm consists of two neurons, the preganglionic and the postganglionic, the fibers of which reach the target organs through different pathways. The PSN, IHP, and HGN represent the efferent arms of the ANS within the pelvis. Detailed descriptions of the other components of the ANS that reside in the pelvis are beyond the scope of this chapter and will be undertaken elsewhere.

EMBRYOLOGY

The development of the spinal cord sacral segments, PSN, and pelvic plexus and the differentiation of the ANS into sympathetic and parasympathetic compartments, is intricate. Knowledge of it is necessary for understanding the functional relevance of the PSN. In this section, each aspect of it will be studied separately to reveal the complexity of the ANS within the abdominal and pelvic visceral structures, emphasizing the development of the sacral spinal segments, the ANS, and the PSN themselves.

Overview of Sacral Spinal Cord Development

The vertebrate spinal cord develops throughout a well-described series of embryological steps comprised under the label neurulation (Schoenwolf and Smith, 1990; Yang et al., 2003). After neural induction is complete, the primary neurulation process, which includes the closing of the neural groove, starts at the 10th Carnegie stage. The craniocervical portion closes and then passes through a ziplike "continuous closing model" both cranially to the rostral neuropore at stage 11 (24 days approximately) and caudally to the caudal neuropore. Established understanding of the closing of the neural groove has been challenged recently, and other models such as the "multisite closure model" have been proposed. Primary neurulation finishes at the level of the future somitic pair 31, which in turn corresponds to the future second sacral vertebra with its corresponding spinal cord segments (Donkelaar and Vilet, 2006).

A less well-understood process then begins. During secondary neurulation, the sacral and coccygeal segments are formed along with their ventral and dorsal roots (Shimokita and Takahashi, 2011; Lee et al., 2017). In human embryos, secondary neurulation begins at Carnegie stage 12 (around day 26) after closure of the caudal neuropore. It involves the differentiation of the caudal part of the neural tube from the caudal eminence without the intermediate phase of a neural plate (Donkelaar and Vilet, 2006). Derivatives from the caudal eminence include the coelom, alimentary canal, blood vessels, notochord, somites, and spinal cord. At this stage, the caudal eminence condenses into a densely populated structure called the neural cord. This later gives rise to neural structures in the caudal part of the body including somitic pairs 32 and below. Therefore, the secondary neurulation process drives the formation of the future third to fifth sacral vertebrae with their respective neural segments.

As previously indicated, the autonomic structures in the PANS such as the autonomic ganglia, plexuses, and their prolongations are derived from neural crest differentiation. Given the foregoing information, the sacral segments are formed during both primary and secondary neurulation. However, there is little consensus about the exact structural somitic limits that are formed during each of these two processes. For some authors such as Muller and O'Rahilly, secondary neurulation includes the formation of the whole lumbosacral region; for others such as Nievelstein, the process includes only the caudalmost part of the sacral segment and coccyx (Schoenwolf and Delongo, 1980; Nievelstein et al., 1993). The process is then complete when, around day 38 of embryonic life, the cell mass and central lumen of the caudal neural tube diminish as a result of apoptosis (retrogressive differentiation).

Development of the ANS for the Sacral Segments; Controversies

The ANS is then differentiated into specific cellular lineages within the spinal cord and neural crest via the action of specifically expressed transcription factors (Rohrer, 2011). BMP gene signaling stimulates the production of transcription factors Mash1 and the glial-derived neurotrophic factor GNDF along with its receptor subunits Phox2a and Phox2b, which are essential for the proper formation of all autonomic ganglia and neural crest derivatives (Pattyn et al., 1999). For example, Phox2b is needed for the expression of the GDNF-receptor subunit Ret and for maintaining Mash1 expression. Mutant expression of Phox2b also results in failure to express the genes encoding noradrenaline, dopamine-β-hydroxylase (DBH), and tyrosine hydroxylase (TH). Therefore, its homeodomain regulates the noradrenergic and sympathetic phenotype in vertebrates. Other transcription factors expressed almost exclusively by the sympathoadrenal lineage such as Islet1, Gata3, and Hand1 have been identified. The parasympathetic cells also express Phox2 factors but choline-acetyltransferase (ChAT) expression predominates over DBH and TH. However, as both sympathetic and parasympathetic systems have cholinergic and catecholaminergic transmission, the neurotransmitter phenotype does not help to distinguish between them. Parasympathetic fibers seem to be recognized by their lack of all the other mentioned transcription factors (Islet, Gata, and Hand) while they are positive for other paralogous homeobox genes such as Hmx2 and Hmx3 (Espinosa-Medina et al., 2016).

Espinosa-Medina et al. hypothesized that the cells within the thoracic and sacral autonomous nuclei, the PSN and the pelvic plexus expressed characteristics of sympathetic autonomic cells, so the sacral outflow was sympathetic (Espinosa-Medina et al., 2016, 2018). The debate arising from these findings has not been closed as several other authors such as Horn and Neuhuber have obtained conflicting results, suggesting that the phenotypes common to the sacral and thoracic segments are derived from an intrinsic spinal somitic identity rather than a sympathetic autonomic identity per se (Neuhuber et al., 2017; Horn, 2018).

Development of the Pelvic Splanchnic Nerves and Inferior Hypogastric Plexus

Development of the PSN is closely related to the development of the pelvic plexus or the IHP. Thus, both subjects should be studied together for proper understanding. In 1958, Kimmel and McCrea presented a detailed description of the development of the pelvic plexuses and their related nerves (Kimmel and McCrea, 1958). These authors showed that the IHP could be observed only from the 12-mm embryo stage, containing cells of neural origin and many primitive small cells, as the incipient PSN were found to contribute to IHP formation. Prolongations of the PSN arise from the proximal aspects of the anterior rami of the second, third, and fourth sacral nerves coursing medially along with the ventral aspects of the sacral vertebrae (Kimmel and McCrea, 1958). The distribution of their origins depends on the future targets of their functional output. For example, some prolongations of the third and fourth sacral rami are distributed directly toward the hindgut, whereas others from the second, third, and fourth sacral nerves extend ventrally within the pelvic mesenchyme. Within the latter, the relationship between the position of each prolongation and the anterior division of the hypogastric vein determines its endpoint. For instance, most prolongations lying medial to the vein enter the intermediate portion of the IHP, while a few join those that run laterally to the vein. These lateral projections approach the IHP through its anterior aspect surrounding the primordia of the urethra, the urinary trigone, and the caudal end of the ureter. Lastly, the ventral branches supply parasympathetic information to the urogenital organs (Kimmel and McCrea, 1958).

By the 23-mm stage, the IHP expands while the rostral and caudal prolongations penetrate the wall of the hindgut to initiate the formation of the submucosal and myenteric plexuses. Also, the extensions enter the rectum at the level of the ampulla and migrate caudally to penetrate the wall of the gut between the internal and external anal sphincters, coursing caudally to innervate mostly the autonomic element of the myenteric plexus.

In 2015, Jang et al. presented a study of the composition of the PSN and the hypogastric nerve (HGN) in elderly human cadaveric specimens. They investigated the autonomic phenotypes of the PSN using nitric oxide synthase (NOS), vasoactive intestinal peptide (VIP), and tyrosine hydroxylase (TH) labeling and found that the PSN had mixed fibers with the sympathetic phenotype (VIP+, NOS +, TH+) dominant in both the PSN and HGN. The PSN also had VIP+ cells, most probably related to Onuf's nucleus (ON). The authors hypothesized that the VIP+ cells could be postganglionic and could go upward or downward along the sacral sympathetic trunk and sacral plexus (Jang et al., 2015). This implies that the PSN could not only carry parasympathetic information, as traditionally believed, but also be the means of transport for mixed autonomic fibers with different origins within the spinal cord.

The neural pathways of the PSN include fibers that flow centrifugally from the spinal cord and others that ascend to the abdominal cavity to support the abdominal splanchnic nerves (see below for anatomical description). Hence, the rigidly segmented perspective on the nervous system as previously understood is becoming obsolete in the light of new advances in neuroscience (Jang et al., 2015; Espinosa-Medina et al., 2016; Horn, 2018).

ANATOMY AND RELATIONSHIPS
Nuclear Origin of the Pelvic Splanchnic Nerves

The pelvic parasympathetic pathways originate within the sacral parasympathetic nuclei. Those neural populations are located in the lateral and anterior horns of the second, third, and fourth sacral segments. Their location and nature have long been a source of debate, and it is clear, for instance, that there are four locations for the nuclear origin of the parasympathetic information of the sacral segments: the intermediolateral nucleus, the ventral nucleus (ON), the ventromedial nucleus, and the ventrolateral nucleus (Rexed, 1954; Schroder, 1981; Morita et al., 1984; Pullen et al., 1992). Retrograde tracing techniques using horseradish peroxidase (HRP) injected into specific pelvic structures to label neurons that are traced back into the spinal cord nuclei have provided ample information regarding the particular structures innervated by each cellular population, as explained in detail below.

Nucleus intermediolateralis sacralis

The intermediolateral column or nucleus intermediolateralis sacralis (NIL) has been described as a gray matter region forming a swelling on the lateral edge of the intermediate spinal zone throughout the thoracolumbar and sacral spinal cord. However, in the sacral segments, it appears cranially in S2 and ends caudally in S4. Although it was first mentioned in the literature in 1840 (Swanson, 2015), the cellular formation located medioventrally to the lateral motor group of the ventral horn was fully described and named NILs in Rexed's study of the cytoarchitectonic structure of cat spinal cords (Rexed, 1954). These cellular populations are very well differentiated from the anterior horn motor population because the cells are significantly smaller than those with a predominantly somatic function (Rexed, 1954). Yamamoto et al. (1978) and Morita et al. (1984) found that neurons were more strongly labeled with HRP in the ILNs at S2 after upper rectal injections, at S3 after injections in the apex or the corpus of the urinary bladder, and from S1 to S3 after injections into the urethral sphincter or the descending colon in cats (Yamamoto et al., 1978; Morita et al., 1984; Dorofeeva et al., 2009). Thus, the outflow innervation from the ILNs is predominantly directed to smooth muscle and is therefore autonomic.

The ventromedial nucleus

This cellular population is located in the anterior horn of the spinal anterior gray matter and Rexed's laminae VII and VIII (Rexed, 1954). It lies in the medial and ventral aspect of the anterior horn, sharing borders with the anterior funiculus (Pullen et al., 1992). Previous papers describing the sacral spinal innervations of the pelvic organs using HRP staining revealed that this nucleus innervates the rectum wall and the external anal sphincter predominantly on its S2 segment, the bladder on its S3 segment, and the urethral sphincter on its S1 to S3 segments. As will be discussed below, this cellular population innervates both striated and smooth muscles, a characteristic common to ON, which has a dual innervation character.

Onuf's nucleus

Bronislav Onufrowicz (Marcinowski, 2019) and the neurologist Joseph Collins studied the sacral autonomic structures within human spinal cords and described a neural nucleus that was predominantly located in lamina IX of S1-2 to S3-4 (Jang et al., 2015). They called this structure "nucleus X" and hypothesized that it was related to the activity of striated muscles associated with erection and ejaculation, and with the erector clitoridis and the bulbocavernosus or sphincter vaginae muscles. Their conjecture was largely accurate, but they affirmed its exclusively somatic nature and incorrectly ruled out its involvement with the urethral and anal sphincters. Moreover, Jacobsohn-Lask in 1931 assumed that the ON was intrinsically autonomic but stated, contradictorily, that it was related to the sympathetic nervous system.

The attribution of a somatic nature to the ON derived from retrograde tracing experiments on animals that revealed its relationship to the striated muscles of the pelvic sphincters. However, later observations led to two striking conclusions: (1) In patients with motor neuron diseases (MNDs), Werding-Hoffmans syndrome, Duchenne's muscular dystrophy, spinal muscular atrophy, and ALS, the ON was spared, whereas sacral motor neurons degenerated (Mannen et al., 1977); (2) In diseases such as Shy-Drager syndrome, Fabry's disease, and multiple system atrophy, both ON and the parasympathetic nucleus

degenerated, while other somatic nuclei were spared (Chalmers and Swash, 1987). This dissociation between MNDs (somatic) and other visceromotor neuronal malfunction diseases in respect of the sparing of the nucleus led to the conclusion that the ON and the ILNs were autonomic. Schroeder et al. presented a case series of human specimens studying ON specifically and found that it contained subpopulations of cells that were called the cranial group superiorly, the ventrolateral division, and the dorsomedial division. This finally supported the dual nature of the ON (Schroder, 1981).

Pullen et al. (1992) studied the ultrastructural architecture of the ON in human specimens and compared the cellular distributions within the anterior horn between a control group and an MND group (Pullen et al., 1992). Throughout their work, they found four significant cell populations in the ventral horn of the S2 segments: an intermediolateral nucleus (parasympathetic nucleus), a ventrolateral group, a ventromedial group, and a discrete ventral group. The ventral population was consistent with the ON previously described by Onufrowicz and was significantly better preserved in the MND patients while the other cell groups were diminished. These findings are consistent with the previous hypothesis that the nucleus is autonomic. Moreover, they showed that the ILNs have a different location from the ON, a conclusion that enriches the debate about previous claims that the ON is the cranial prolongation of the ILNs (Rexed, 1954). Therefore, the authors concluded that taking into account the location of the ON within the anterior horn (of S2 and S3), and its control of striated muscles of the external anal sphincter as well as the smooth muscles of bladder and rectum, its dual character can be affirmed, as previously indicated by Yamamoto and Schroder (Yamamoto et al., 1978; Schroder, 1981).

The Anatomical Situation of the PSN

The autonomic fibers of the lateral gray matter of the spinal cord join the sacral segments and their rami that exit the spinal cord through the conus medullaris and the structure named epiconus. Anatomically, the epiconus comprises the cord segments from L4 to S1, corresponding to the T12 and L1 vertebrae, while the conus medullaris includes the spinal segments between S2 and S5 together with the coccygeal segments. The anatomical delimitation of the epiconus, conus medullaris, and cauda equina is important because it correlates with clinical neurological syndromes that pertain to each structure. This will be discussed in the "clinical significance" section (Toribatake et al., 1997).

After leaving spinal segments S2 to S4, the bundles travel through the cauda equina embedded in the subarachnoid space. The subarachnoid course of the spinal nerves describes a vertical decline from their emergence in front of the L1-L2 vertebral segments until they pierce the dura at the height of their corresponding exit via the sacral foramina (Testut et al., 1977; Gray et al., 1995; Latarjet et al., 2004). The PSN detach from the spinal nerves as soon as they exit the sacral foramina and then enter the presacral tissue as a highly intertwined bundle of fibers. Possover et al. presented a detailed surgical description of the location of the PSN (Possover et al., 2007). They found that laparoscopic dissection of the pararectal space lateral to the sacral hypogastric fascia allows sacral nerve roots S1-S4 and the PSN nerve roots arising from S2 to S4 to be directly exposed.

The PSN then distribute in three main ways, as previously described by Kimmel et al. Most of the fibers run anterolaterally into the IHP to supply the pelvic viscera (Kimmel and McCrea, 1958). Others join the IHP directly to generate an ascendant pathway to the abdominal cavity, supplying the inferior mesenteric artery; and a minority of fibers lie superolaterally within the presacral tissue, over the pelvic brim anterior to the left iliac vessels, to enter the retroperitoneum and innervate the mesentery of the sigmoid and descending colon (Kimmel and McCrea, 1958; Gray et al., 1995; Cramer and Darby, 2013). The PSN, carrying the preganglionic parasympathetic fibers, join the sacral splanchnic nerves emerging from the sacral sympathetic trunks to join the IHP (Haroun, 2018).

Inferior Hypogastric Plexus

A detailed anatomical account of the IHP is mandatory for correct assessment of the PSN because it is in this critical structure that the sympathetic and the parasympathetic arms of the nervous system, carried by the PSN and the HGN, come together to provide the autonomic supply to the pelvic viscera. The IHP is a nervous laminar structure oriented anteroposteriorly; this lamina has a square appearance with irregular borders. It is found within a thin layer of extraperitoneal connective tissue applied to the pelvic side wall and anterolateral to the mesorectum (Gray et al., 1995). The anatomical position of the plexus differs between the sexes. In males, it is neighbored laterally by the internal iliac vessels, the middle rectal artery, the inferior bladder artery, and the attachments of the levator ani and the obturator internus muscles; medially, it lies against the rectum and prostate; superiorly, against the peritoneum of the rectovesical pouch, the umbilical artery, and the ureter; and anteriorly, it reaches the posterior aspect of the prostate. In females, the IHP is applied laterally to the uterine cervix, vaginal fornix, and the posterior aspect of the urinary bladder and its superior border is found where the uterine artery crosses the ureter at the base of the broad ligament (Gray et al., 1995). Ali et al. reported that the plexus is consistently found one-third of the way along and deep to a line drawn from the presumptive rectosigmoid junction at the level of the third sacral vertebra and the palpable posterior-superior surface of the pubic symphysis (Ali et al., 2004; Johnson, 2012).

As stated above, the plexus has a mixed fiber composition and derives from the pelvic splanchnic, sacral splanchnic, and lower lumbar ganglia (Kepper and Keast, 1995; Baader and Herrmann, 2003). The HGNs constitute a bridge between the superior and inferior hypogastric plexuses. Both descending pathways from the superior hypogastric plexus and ascending pathways from the PSN and IHP carry mixed autonomic information.

THE ROLE OF THE PSN IN SPECIFIC PELVIC ORGANS AND ITS PHYSIOLOGICAL IMPLICATIONS

The PSN supply a wide number of pelvic organs, and their relevance lies in the physiological functions that depend on them. Nerve-sparing techniques in surgery help to mitigate iatrogenic lesions of the pelvic nerves, avoiding a negative effect on patient functionality (Baader and Herrmann, 2003).

Rectum

The rectum receives double innervation: an autonomic innervation and a somatic sphincteric supply deriving from the spinal nerves. The PSN reach the organ through the mesorectum, covered by the parietal fascia; they pierce the endopelvic fascia, cross the retrorectal space, and form branches into the lateral ligaments of the rectum (Chew et al., 2016). The autonomic innervation derives from the IHP, the SHP, and directly from the PSN, predominantly from the S2 segment (Latarjet et al., 2004; Dorofeeva et al., 2009). The same distribution holds for the descending colon, though the representation of the PSN is stronger in the rectum (Dorofeeva et al., 2009). In nearly 50% of specimens, the rectum was innervated by the IHP (Baader and Herrmann, 2003). A somatotopic distribution within the IHP has been reported, showing that the posterior aspect of the IHP supplies the superior part of the rectum, whereas its anteroinferior part innervates the inferior aspect of the rectum. Furthermore, fibers from the perivascular plexus of the middle rectal artery penetrate the IHP and provide further innervation to the rectum. The fact that the rectum was always innervated on its lateral aspect but never on its posterior aspect is surgically important (Baader and Herrmann, 2003).

Rectal examination in vivo enables the 10−12 inferior centimeters of the rectum to be assessed. It is vital to evaluate sphincter contraction and the rectal wink to assess the integrity of its innervation. These clinical signs are important in the context of spinal trauma involving the spinal cord and Iatrogenic lesions.

Urinary System

Innervation of the urinary system is one of the most complex networks, comprising all cellular types. Uniquely, it functions as an afferent, peripheral control, central control, and efferent system that, like the fecal system, includes both central and peripheral neural arcs that translate into a complex coordinated blend of volitional and automatic control. The central sensorimotor pathways related to micturition and sphincter control comprise (1) the corticospinal pathways for the voluntary control of voiding; (2) the urethral reflex loop, from urethral afferents to pudendal motor neurons, which maintains the sphincter tone when the detrusor is inactive; (3) the detrusor reflex loop, from detrusor afferents to pudendal motor neurons, which causes sphincter relaxation when the detrusor is active; (4) the cord loop, from Barrington's nucleus located in the pontine tegmentum to the conus medullaris and the L-region of the brainstem, for coordinating the detrusor muscles and sphincter contraction and relaxation; and (5) the cerebral loop, including brainstem, cerebral cortex, and basal ganglia structures, which initiates and inhibits switching between the filling and voiding states (Brazis and Masdeu, 2011). The PSN are involved in both the afferent and efferent modalities of micturition, traveling through the IHP and then migrating into its anterior aspect called the vesical plexus (Sasaki, 2005; Cramer and Darby, 2013).

The peripheral nervous system reaches the bladder through its posterior and lateral aspects, leaving its anterior face free of innervating fibers (Baader and Herrmann, 2003). A case series published in 2003 demonstrated that the urinary bladder was innervated by the IHP in 79% of the hemipelves studied and the neural supply was lateral to the neck of the bladder and along the inferior vesical artery and ureter (Baader and Herrmann, 2003). There were no sex differences in these findings regarding the lower urinary tract. The parasympathetic component of the PSN is believed to be active during micturition, exciting the detrusor muscle (Cramer and Darby, 2013).

Sex-Specific Organs
Uterus

The uterus receives its autonomic innervation from the PSN and a portion of the IHP called the uterovaginal plexus (Rozycki and Wozniak, 1982). These fibers reach the organ from the rectouterine ligament and are situated in the parametrium and the cardinal ligament. There is a main group of lateral and posterior fibers and a more lateral and anterior secondary group. Some bundles reach the uterus following the mesosalpinx vessels and the ovarian ligament and terminate in the myometrium and endometrium (Latarjet et al., 2004). Baader found that innervation of the uterus derives directly from the IHP in 79% of cases and directly from the PSN in the rest. The authors also found that the uterosacral ligament, which is generally considered to contain only connective tissue, also contains nerve fibers that travel to the uterus. The parasympathetic information seems to be related to uterine inhibition and vasodilatation, but uterine behavior is mostly hormonally controlled (Baader and Herrmann, 2003; Standring, 2016).

Vagina

The innervation of the vagina is analogous to that of the penis; it is provided by the anterior portion of the IHP (a division called the vaginal plexus), the PSN, and the pudendal nerve. However, there is differential innervation of the upper third by the IHP and PSN, and the lower third is supplied by the pudendal nerve (Standring, 2016). Also, only 24% of specimens were reported to be innervated by the IHP, suggesting considerable variability in the autonomic innervation of the vagina (Baader and Herrmann, 2003). In addition, the PSN and its autonomous components innervate Skene's glands and the clitoris through the cavernous nerve of the clitoris to induce vasodilation and lubrication, analogous to stimulation of the penile glans and prostate (Santos and Taboga, 2006; Huynh et al., 2013). There is evidence that male ejaculation and female orgasm have similar mechanisms involving the IHP, which has mixed parasympathetic and sympathetic efferent arms.

Prostate and seminal vesicles

The prostatic plexus, an anterior division of the IHP, innervates the prostate. Both sympathetic and parasympathetic postganglionic fibers exit the prostatic plexus as the dorsolateral bundle, and the cavernous nerve innervates the erectile tissue of the penis and smooth muscle in the seminal vesicles, prostate, ductus deferens, and the nonstriated sphincter in the bladder (Cramer and Darby, 2013; Standring, 2016). However, parasympathetic innervation of the prostate is controversial (Rodrigues et al., 2002). After exiting the IHP, the prostatic nervous bundles reach the tips of seminal vesicles; they lie in the lateral endopelvic fascia close to Denonvillier's fascia, then they enter the periprostatic fibrous capsule to join the organ through its lateral sheets (Latarjet et al., 2004). Other fibers extend around the lateral prostatic surface to penetrate the surface of the bladder neck. Parasympathetic fibers activate secretomotor activity in the prostatic and seminal vesicles during the second phase (plateau) of sexual intercourse (Groat, 1980).

Penis

The penis receives sensory innervation from the genitofemoral and ilioinguinal nerves, branches from the lumbar plexus; the autonomic innervation derives from the IHP and the PSN. The latter is essential for eliciting erection, sending nerves through the bundles of Walsh including the cavernous nerves that run laterally outside Denonvillier's fascia (Chew et al., 2016). The PSN was named Eckhardt's nervi erigentes because of its involvement in erection (Swanson, 2015). Although erection depends mainly on parasympathetic stimuli, the sympathetic component (T12-L3) also makes a significant contribution. Erection depends mainly on two distinct central mechanisms, psychogenic and reflexogenic (Groat, 1980). The former is initiated by supraspinal centers in response to auditory, visual, olfactory, tactile, and imaginative stimuli, and its efferent (autonomic) limb can be either thoracolumbar or sacral. The latter is elicited exclusively by the parasympathetic pelvic nerves. This explains why psychogenic erections are abolished while reflexogenic erections persist in patients with spinal cord lesions above T12, while the opposite is observed in patients with lower motor neuron lesions that involve the sacral spinal cord, conserving the ability to elicit a psychogenic erection (Groat, 1980).

CLINICAL CONSIDERATIONS ABOUT THE PSN

Now that the historical, embryological, anatomical, and physiological aspects of the PSN and its related nervous structures have been described, the following sections of this chapter will present the noteworthy clinical aspects of the PSN. Clinical assessment and surgical

preservation of the autonomic nerves will be discussed in particular because they are crucial for obtaining optimal outcomes in several therapeutic modalities.

Several clinical and traumatic entities can affect the ANS. The main challenge for the clinician is to find evidence for the site of pathology, which can help to diagnose a peripheral or central disease or a systemic or local injury. For example, Guillain-Barre syndrome presents with autonomic dysfunctions including paralytic ileus and urinary retention owing to the involvement of the PSN. Sacral fractures and spinal cord injuries are examples of traumatic lesions to the PSN that cause cauda equina and conus medullaris syndromes. Other causes of autonomic neuropathy include amyloidosis, porphyria, diabetes mellitus, and Lambert Eaton myasthenic syndrome. Neoplastic lesions can involve the sacral autonomic innervation to the pelvic cavity through either local compression of the nerve fibers within the pelvic cavity or systemic paraneoplastic syndromes (Bankenahally and Krovvidi, 2016).

PELVIC SPLANCHNIC NERVES IN SURGERY

Although the PSN and IHP are clearly distinguished in the surgical field owing to their complex and fine structure and to the depth and narrowness of the pelvic cavity, sufficiently detailed knowledge of their topography can reduce the risk of iatrogenic lesions during surgery (Baader and Herrmann, 2003). Therapeutic interventions are increasingly being assessed by their effects on subsequent quality of life, so there should be a focus on establishing consistent surgical landmarks and nerve-preserving techniques (NPT) that could minimize postoperative morbidity (Maas et al., 1999; Shiozawa et al., 2010). However, the intrinsic variability of the pelvic nervous components makes this challenging to achieve.

The increasing interest in preserving the pelvic nerves during recent decades has led to several attempts to develop NPT in open, laparoscopic, and robotic surgery (Chew et al., 2016). General principles of preservation of the PSN are direct macroscopic visualization of the neural structures, the use of surgical anatomical landmarks, and neurostimulation when the nerves are dissected (Possover et al., 2007; Lemos et al., 2015). Two possible landmarks have been proposed for locating the IHP and the PSN (Ali et al., 2004). One is the "rectosigmoid junction," which has been described as overlying the third sacral vertebra and the posterior-superior aspect of the pubic symphysis. However, this is not an exact definition. The point where the mesenteric part of the large bowel becomes fixed and retroperitoneal is easily found at surgery, and this could serve as a surgical landmark for the third sacral vertebra (Ali et al., 2004). As the authors stated, the IHP is "consistently encountered one-third of the way along and deep to a line drawn from the presumptive rectosigmoid junction at the level of the third sacral vertebra and the palpable posterior superior surface of the pubic symphysis" (Ali et al., 2004).

Rectal Surgery

After radical rectal cancer surgery using total mesorectal excision (TME), the incidence of urinary dysfunction can be as high as 50% and sexual dysfunction can reach 85% (Chew et al., 2016; Wang et al., 2017). Low anterior resection syndrome (LARS), characterized by fecal incontinence, can be encountered in up to 70% with rectal cancers (Huang and Koh, 2019). The sympathetic nerves are easily injured when the mesorectum is dissected in the sacral and ventrolateral planes, while the parasympathetic nerves are often encountered during dissection of the lateral planes (Wang et al., 2017). With autonomic nerve preservation, the incidence of urinary dysfunction was between 2.1% and 24.4% and male sexual dysfunction ranged from 12% to 44.2% (Chew et al., 2016). Even though laparoscopic surgery allows loose clearance between the visceral and parietal fascia, the debate about laparoscopic versus open approaches in precluding urinary and sexual dysfunction has not been closed. Some reports claim that laparoscopic surgery is more likely than open approaches to cause urinary and sexual dysfunction, while others such as Liu's randomized trial have demonstrated a lower incidence of sexual dysfunction in laparoscopic TME with nerve preservation than in open procedures (11.6% vs. 16.9%) (Chew et al., 2016). The safety of robotic pelvic surgery with nerve-sparing TME has not been fully evaluated in respect of autonomic injuries, but the technique has shown promising preliminary results (Liang et al., 2007; Wang et al., 2017).

Gynecological Procedures

Radical surgery for endometriosis leads to urinary dysfunction in up to 17.5% of patients (Lemos et al., 2015), and in sacrocolpopexy there is an incidence of urinary incontinence in up to 44% and constipation in 26% due to injury to the PSN, HGN, and IHP (Shiozawa et al., 2010).

Radical hysterectomy is the classical surgical management for early-stage cervical carcinoma and has been used for more than a century. It involves resection of the uterus, cervix, and upper part of the vagina along with the parametrial tissues. The procedure has shown excellent outcomes in cancer treatment but has also led to high incidences of urinary, bowel, and sexual dysfunction. Bladder dysfunction occurs in 70%–80% of cases, bowel dysfunction in 43%, and sexual dysfunction due to the resection of the upper vagina. Different phases of the procedure can result in lesions to autonomic structures (Tseng et al., 2012). The PSN can be injured during the division of the deep uterine vein in the cardinal ligament, the HGNs during the resection of the uterosacral ligaments, the IHP during the division of the uterosacral and rectovaginal ligaments, and its bladder branch during resection of the vesicovaginal ligaments and paracolpium (Dursun et al., 2009; Kyo et al., 2016). Nerve-sparing procedures have decreased the risk of autonomic dysfunction, but there is no substantial support for evidence-based recommendations (Ito and Saito, 2004).

Urological Surgery

Radical prostatectomy (RP) is a very frequently used treatment for localized prostate cancer. It has increased the overall survival rate, but quality-of-life measures remain a critical concern for patients because of the high risk of post-prostatectomy urinary incontinence and sexual dysfunction (Bang and Almallah, 2016). Orgasmic pain or dysorgasmia has been reported in 14% of patients, climacturia in 21%–22% (Bang and Almallah, 2016), and only 40% recover erectile function. Moreover, long-term follow-ups have reported rates as high as 87% of erectile dysfunction (Faris et al., 2018). The advent of robotic approaches has improved postoperative sexual function, showing an odds ratio of 2.84 for potency at 1 year in comparison with open methods; however, there are no statistically significant differences from laparoscopic approaches (Faris et al., 2018). Techniques such as intrafascial nerve-sparing RP significantly increased the restoration of urinary continence in up to 92% of cases, and a pooled potency rate of 72% at 12 months follow-up. This technique is effective owing to the decreased traction or thermal injury and the preservation of the prostatic fascia and therefore of the neurovascular bundles.

Sacral Neuromodulation

During recent decades, sacral neuromodulation or sacral nerve stimulation (SNS) has emerged as an effective treatment for fecal incontinence, bladder dysfunction, and sexual dysfunction of various etiologies (Huang and Koh, 2019). It was described in 1995 by Matzel et al., and it has significantly reduced symptoms in patients. The technique consists of implanting a neurostimulator that provides impulses to the sacral nerves. The most common application is stimulation of the third sacral nerve, but others have been described. The aim is to stimulate the distal autonomic connections, including the PSN, to restore function. Etiologies for pelvic autonomic dysfunction that have been treated with SNS include obstetrical trauma, cauda equina syndrome, LARS, rectal resection, low anastomosis, and other pelvic surgeries. Recent reviews and meta-analyses have demonstrated a reduction from 9.5 to 3.1 fecal-incontinent episodes per week, and a reduction of up to 50% for overactive bladder (Hull, 2010).

CONCLUSION

The structural and molecular aspects of the PSN are complex and still under scientific investigation. Although knowledge of these critical structures has increased significantly, there is still much to research and learn about the composition, role, and nature of these nerves. PSN are involved in many physical functions that are directly related to the patient's quality of life. A broad understanding of the structural anatomical disposition of the nerves is paramount for obtaining surgical outcomes and developing nerve-preserving techniques that could help to minimize postoperative morbidities.

REFERENCES

Ali, M., Johnson, I.P., Hobson, J., Mohammadi, B., Khan, F., 2004. Anatomy of the pelvic plexus and innervation of the prostate gland. Clin. Anat. 17, 123–129.

Baader, B., Herrmann, M., 2003. Topography of the pelvic autonomic nervous system and its potential impact on surgical intervention in the pelvis. Clin. Anat. 16, 119–130.

Bang, S.L., Almallah, Y.Z., 2016. The impact of post-radical prostatectomy urinary incontinence on sexual and orgasmic well-being of patients. Urology 89, 1–5.

Bankenahally, R., Krovvidi, H., 2016. Autonomic nervous system: anatomy, physiology, and relevance in anaesthesia and critical care medicine. BJA. Educ. 16, 381–387.

Brazis, P.W., Masdeu, J.C., 2011. Localization in Clinical Neurology, sixth ed. Lippincott Williams & Wilkins, Philadelphia-PA, p. 663.

Catala, M., Kubis, N., 2013. Gross anatomy and development of the peripheral nervous system. In: Handbook of Clinical Neurology, first ed. Elsevier B.V., pp. 29–41

Chalmers, D., Swash, M., 1987. Selective vulnerability of urinary Onuf motoneurons in Shy-Drager syndrome. J. Neurol. 234, 259–260.

Chew, M., Yeh, Y., Lim, E., Seow-Choen, F., 2016. Pelvic autonomic nerve preservation in radical rectal cancer surgery: changes in the past 3 decades. Gastroenterol. Rep. 4, 173–185.

Cramer, G.D., Darby, S.A., 2013. Chapter 10: Neuroanatomy of the autonomic nervous system. In: Clinical Anatomy of the Spine, Spinal Cord, and ANS.

Donkelaar, H.J.T., Vilet, T van der, 2006. Overview of the development of the human brain and spinal cord. In: Clinical Neuroembriology: Development and Developmental Disorders of the Human Central Nervous System. Springer-Verlag Berlin Heidelberg, Berlin, pp. 1–40.

Dorofeeva, A.A., Panteleev, S.S., Makarov, F.N., 2009. Involvement of the sacral parasympathetic nucleus in the innervation of the descending colon and rectum in cats. Neurosci. Behav. Physiol. 39, 207–210.

Dursun, P., Ayhan, A., Kuscu, E., 2009. Nerve-sparing radical hysterectomy for cervical carcinoma. Crit. Rev. Oncol. Hematol. 70, 195–205.

Espinosa-Medina, I., Saha, O., Boismoreau, F., Brunet, J.F., 2018. The "sacral parasympathetic": ontogeny and anatomy of a myth. Clin. Auton. Res. 28, 13–21.

Espinosa-Medina, I., Saha, O., Boismoreau, F., Chettouh, Z., Rossi, F., Richardson, W.D., Brunet, J.-F., 2016. The sacral autonomic outflow is sympathetic. Science 354, 893–897.

Faris, A.E.R., Montague, D.K., Gill, B.C., 2018. Perioperative educational interventions and contemporary sexual function outcomes of radical prostatectomy challenges to quantifying sexual function. Sex. Med. Rev 7, 293–305.

Gray, H., Williams, P.L., Bannister, L.H., 1995. Gray's Anatomy. The Anatomic Basis of Medicine and Surgery, thirty eighth ed. Curchill Livingstone, New York, pp. 1256–1259.

Groat, W.C., 1980. Physiology of male sexual function. Ann. Intern. Med. 92, 329.

Hall, J.E., Guyton, A.C., 2011. Guyton and Hall Textbook of Medical Physiology.

Haroun, H.S., 2018. Clinical anatomy of the splanchnic nerves. MOJ. Anat. Physiol. 5, 87–90.

Horn, J.P., 2018. The sacral autonomic outflow is parasympathetic: langley got it right. Clin. Auton. Res. 28, 181–185.

Huang, Y., Koh, C.E., 2019. Sacral nerve stimulation for bowel dysfunction following low anterior resection: a systematic review and meta-analysis. Color. Dis. 21 (11), 1240–1248.

Hull, T.L., 2010. Sacral neuromodulation stimulation in fecal incontinence. Int. Urogynecol. J. 21, 1565–1568.

Huynh, H.K., Willemsen, A.T.M., Lovick, T.A., Holstege, G., 2013. Pontine control of ejaculation and female orgasm. J. Sex. Med. 10, 3038–3048.

Ito, E., Saito, T., 2004. Nerve-preserving techniques for radical hysterectomy. Eur. J. Surg. Oncol. 30, 1137–1140.

Jang, H.S., Cho, K.H., Hieda, K., Kim, J.H., Murakami, G., Abe, S., Matsubara, A., 2015. Composite nerve fibers in the hypogastric and pelvic splanchnic nerves: an immunohistochemical study using elderly cadavers. Anat. Cell. Biol. 48, 114.

Johnson, I.P., 2012. Colorectal and uterine movement and tension of the inferior hypogastric plexus in cadavers. Chiropr. Man. Ther. 20, 13.

Kepper, M., Keast, J., 1995. Immunohistochemical properties and spinal connections of pelvic autonomic neurons that innervate the rat prostate gland. Cell. Tissue. Res. 281, 533–542.

Kimmel, D.L., McCrea, L.E., 1958. The development of the pelvic plexuses and the distribution of the pelvic splanchnic nerves in the human embryo and fetus. J. Comp. Neurol. 110, 271–297.

Kyo, S., Kato, T., Nakayama, K., 2016. Current concepts and practical techniques of nerve-sparing laparoscopic radical hysterectomy. Eur. J. Obstet. Gynecol. Reprod. Biol. 207, 80–88.

Latarjet, M., Ruiz Liard, A., Pró, E., 2004. Anatomía Humana, fourth ed. Editorial Panamericana, Bogota Dc.

Lee, J.Y., Lee, E.S., Kim, S.P., Lee, M.S., Phi, J.H., Kim, S.K., Hwang, Y.I., Wang, K.C., 2017. Neurosphere formation potential resides not in the caudal cell mass, but in the secondary neural tube. Int. J. Dev. Biol. 61, 545–550.

Lemos, N., Souza, C., Marques, R.M., Kamergorodsky, G., Schor, E., Girão, M.J.B.C., 2015. Laparoscopic anatomy of the autonomic nerves of the pelvis and the concept of nerve-sparing surgery by direct visualization of autonomic nerve bundles. Fertil. Steril. 104, e11–e12.

Liang, J., Lai, H., Lee, P., 2007. Laparoscopic pelvic autonomic nerve-preserving surgery for patients with lower rectal cancer after chemoradiation therapy. Ann. Surg Oncol. 14, 1285–1287.

Maas, K., Moriya, Y., Kenter, G., Trimbos, B., van de Velde, C., 1999. A plea for preservation of the pelvic autonomic nerves. Lancet 354, 772–773.

Mannen, T., Iwata, M., Toyokura, Y., Nagashima, K., 1977. Preservation of a certain motoneurone group of the sacral cord in amyotrophic lateral sclerosis: its clinical significance. J. Neurol. Neurosurg. Psychiatry 40, 464–469.

Marcinowski, F., 2019. Bronislaw onuf-onufrowicz (1863–1928). J. Neurol. 266, 281–282.

Morita, T., Nishizawa, O., Noto, H., Tsuchida, S., 1984. Pelvic nerve innervation of the external sphincter of urethra as suggested by urodynamic and horse-radish peroxidase studies. J. Urol. 131, 591–595.

Neuhuber, W., Mclachlan, E., Jänig, W., 2017. The sacral autonomic outflow is spinal, but not "sympathetic". Anat. Rec. 300, 1369–1370.

Nievelstein, R.A.J., Hartwig, N.G., Vermeij-Keers, C., Valk, J., 1993. Embryonic development of the mammalian caudal neural tube. Teratology 48, 21–31.

Pattyn, A., Morin, X., Cremer, H., Goridis, C., Brunet, J.-F., 1999. The homeobox gene Phox2b is essential for the development of autonomic neural crest derivatives. Nature 399, 366–370.

Possover, M., Chiantera, V., Baekelandt, J., 2007. Anatomy of the sacral roots and the pelvic splanchnic nerves in women using the LANN technique. Surg. Laparosc. Endosc. Percutaneous Tech. 17, 508–510.

Pullen, A.H., Martin, J.E., Swash, M., 1992. Ultra structure of pre-synaptic input to motor neurons in Onuf's nucleus: controls and motor neuron disease. Neuropathol. Appl. Neurobiol. 18, 213–231.

Rexed, B., 1954. A cytoarchitectonic atlas of the spinal cord in the cat. J. Comp. Neurol. 100, 297–379.

Rodrigues, A.O., Machado, M.T., Wroclawski, E.R., 2002. Prostate innervation and local anesthesia in prostate procedures. Rev. Hosp. Clin. 57, 287–292.

Rohrer, H., 2011. Transcriptional control of differentiation and neurogenesis in autonomic ganglia. Eur. J. Neurosci. 34, 1563–1573.

Rozycki, Z., Wozniak, W., 1982. Topography and structure of the utero-vaginal plexus in human fetuses. Ginekol. Pol. 53, 837–844.

Santos, F.C.A., Taboga, S.R., 2006. Female prostate : a review about the biological repercussions of this gland in humans and rodents. Anim. Reprod. 3, 3–18.

Sasaki, M., 2005. Role of Barrington's nucleus in micturition. J. Comp. Neurol. 493, 21–26.

Schoenwolf, G.C., Delongo, J., 1980. Ultrastructure of secondary neurulation in the chick embryo. Am. J. Anat. 158, 43–63.

Schoenwolf, G.C., Smith, J.L., 1990. Mechanisms of neurulation: traditional viewpoint and recent advances. Development 109, 243–270.

Schroder, H.D., 1981. Onuf's nucleus X: a morphological study of a human spinal nucleus. Anat. Embryol. 162, 443–453.

Shimokita, E., Takahashi, Y., 2011. Secondary neurulation: fate-mapping and gene manipulation of the neural tube in tail bud. Dev. Growth. Differ. 53, 401–410.

Shiozawa, T., Huebner, M., Hirt, B., Wallwiener, D., Reisenauer, C., 2010. Nerve-preserving sacrocolpopexy: anatomical study and surgical approach. Eur. J. Obstet. Gynecol. Reprod. Biol. 152, 103–107.

Standring, S., 2016. Gray's Anatomy, fortyfirst edition. Elsevier.

Swanson, L., 2015. Neuroanatomical Terminology: A Lexicon of Classical Origins and Historical Foundations. Oxford University Press.

Testut, L., Latarjet, A., Devy, G., Dupret, S., 1977. Tratado de Anatomía Humana. Tomo 3. Meninges, Sistema Nervioso Periférico, Órganos de Los Sentidos, Aparato de La Respiracion y de La Fonacion, Glandulas de Secresion Interna, ninth ed. Salvat Editores, Barcelona.

Toribatake, Y., Baba, H., Kawahara, N., Mizuno, K., Tomita, K., 1997. The epiconus syndrome presenting with radicular-type neurological features. Spinal Cord 35, 163–170.

Tseng, C., Shen, H., Lin, Y., Lee, C., Wei-Cheng Chiu, W., 2012. A prospective study of nerve-sparing radical hysterectomy for uterine cervical carcinoma in Taiwan. Taiwan. J. Obstet. Gynecol. 51, 55–59.

Wang, G., Wang, Z., Jiang, Z., Liu, J., Zhao, J., Li, J., 2017. Male urinary and sexual function after robotic pelvic autonomic nerve-preserving surgery for rectal cancer. Int. J. Med. Robot. Comput. Assist. Surg. 13, e1725.

Yamamoto, T., Satomi, H., Ise, H., Takatama, H., Takahashi, K., 1978. Sacral spinal innervations of the rectal and vesical smooth muscles and the sphincteric striated muscles as demonstrated by the horseradish peroxidase method. Neurosci. Lett. 7, 41–47.

Yamashita, R., Isoda, H., Arizono, S., Furuta, A., Ohno, T., Ono, A., Murata, K., Togashi, K., 2017. Selective visualization of pelvic splanchnic nerve and pelvic plexus using readout-segmented echo-planar diffusion-weighted magnetic resonance neurography: a preliminary study in healthy male volunteers. Eur. J. Radiol. 86, 52–57.

Yang, H.J., Wang, K.C., Chi, J.G., Lee, M.S., Lee, Y.J., Kim, S.K., Cho, B.K., 2003. Neural differentiation of caudal cell mass (secondary neurulation) in chick embryos: hamburger and Hamilton stages 16–45. Dev. Brain Res. 142, 31–36.

CHAPTER 14

The Superior Hypogastric Plexus

GRAHAM C. DUPONT • R. SHANE TUBBS

INTRODUCTION

The pelvic autonomic plexuses are mazelike and invariably end up fusing or are closely interrelated. One of the main constituents of the pelvic plexuses is the hypogastric plexus, originally observed by Latarjet and Rochet (1926). It was thought of as a singular entity formed by anastomosing strands from the abdominal aorta plexus at the level of the aortic bifurcation. Ranson (1947) described sympathetic fibers from the plexus that split into two parts lying on either side of the rectum, yet in his work these fibers are referred to simply as the pelvic plexuses. As with many peripheral neurological structures, the superior hypogastric plexus (Figs. 14.1 and 14.2) is subject to variation in its course and morphological arrangement, with the most relevant study on its variations completed by Paraskevas et al. (2008). Preservation of the pelvic plexuses is also crucial in surgical approaches to the abdominopelvic region. The management of pelvic pain from pathologies such as prostate or ovarian cancer, trauma, endometriosis or severe dysmenorrhea, ectopic pregnancy (and other pregnancy-related pathologies) will also be examined in detail.

GENERAL ANATOMY AND VARIATIONS

The superior hypogastric plexus is a retroperitoneal structure, fixated anterior to the aortic bifurcation, bounded by left common iliac vein, median sacral vessels, fifth lumbar vertebrae, sacral promontory, and common iliac arteries. Authors and texts have referred to this plexus as the presacral *nerve*, however this is a network of nerves, and is also located prelumbar. The superior hypogastric plexus is found within the extraperitoneal connective tissue along the midline, and slightly leftward. It is formed from branches of the aortic plexus (sympathetic and parasympathetic), and lumbar splanchnic (sympathetic) nerves, and pelvic splanchnic (parasympathetic) nerves that project upward from the inferior hypogastric plexus via the hypogastric nerves. Visceral afferent nerves also traverse the superior hypogastric plexus. The intermediate portion of the ureteric plexus is formed from contributions of the superior hypogastric plexus and hypogastric nerve,

usually penetrating the muscular coat of the uterus or accompanying blood vessels to the adventitia (Standring, 2016). The superior hypogastric plexus supplies innervation to the pelvic wall of the rectum and internal anal sphincter, by way of following the inferior mesenteric and superior rectal arteries. The plexus also supplies parts of the perineum. This parasympathetic supply inhibits the rectal muscles and faciliatory to internal anal sphincter tone, thus providing resistance to defecation (Godlewski and Prudhomme, 2000).

The superior hypogastric plexus is most often plexiform in appearance, though there are deviations from plexiform appearance. The plexus may be formed from a singly thin, rounded nerve; a wide plexiform morphology; a broad, bandlike trunk with scattered nerve bundles; and two distinct nerves in close proximity to one another (Paraskevas et al., 2008).

Type I

This variation (17.14%) appears as a single thin rounded, nerve. Paraskevas et al. (2008) refer to this nerve in their study as the presacral nerve; however, in the current text, its contemporary denomination, the prelumbar nerve, will be used. The prelumbar nerve forms below the abdominal aortic bifurcation, traverses the left side of the body, anterior to left common iliac vein, and subsequently bifurcates into respective two hypogastric nerves. This nerve maintains close proximity to the superior rectal artery and peritoneum along its course.

Type II

This variation (28.57%) appears in the classical plexiform arrangement covering the area between the common iliac arteries.

Type III

This variation (22.85%) is a broader, quadrated, thicker trunk with nerve bundles intermingled with connective tissue. This trunk usually extends from the abdominal aorta bifurcation to the sacral promontory.

Surgical Anatomy of the Sacral Plexus and Its Branches. https://doi.org/10.1016/B978-0-323-77602-8.00014-3

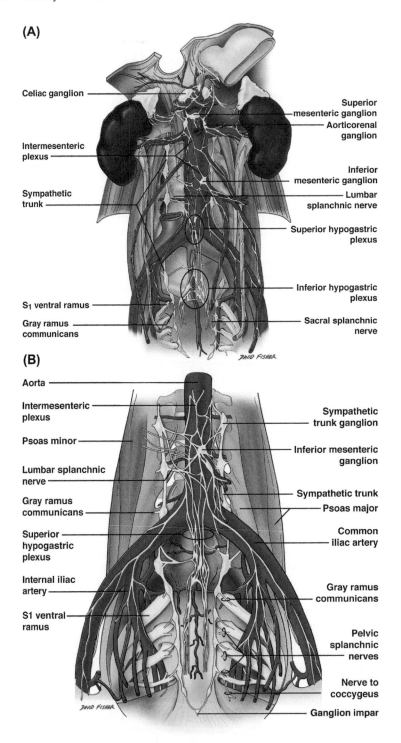

(A)

Celiac ganglion

Superior mesenteric ganglion

Aorticorenal ganglion

Intermesenteric plexus

Inferior mesenteric ganglion

Sympathetic trunk

Lumbar splanchnic nerve

Superior hypogastric plexus

Inferior hypogastric plexus

S₁ ventral ramus

Gray ramus communicans

Sacral splanchnic nerve

DAVID FISHER

(B)

Aorta

Intermesenteric plexus

Sympathetic trunk ganglion

Psoas minor

Inferior mesenteric ganglion

Lumbar splanchnic nerve

Gray ramus communicans

Sympathetic trunk

Psoas major

Superior hypogastric plexus

Common iliac artery

Internal iliac artery

Gray ramus communicans

S1 ventral ramus

Pelvic splanchnic nerves

Nerve to coccygeus

DAVID FISHER

Ganglion impar

FIG. 14.1 Schematic drawing of the autonomic nerves of the (A) abdomen and (B) pelvis noting the superior hypogastric plexus.

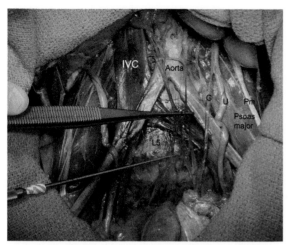

FIG. 14.2 Cadaveric view of the superior hypogastric plexus held up with forceps and traveling over the dissector probe. For reference, note the inferior vena cava (IVC), body of the L5 vertebra, gonadal vessel (G), ureter (U), and psoas minor tendon (Pm).

Type IV

This variation (31.44%) appears as two nerves that run alongside one another before separating. These two nerves run medially at the level of the fifth lumbar vertebrae and separate laterally at the first sacral vertebrae and then separate.

Though the superior hypogastric plexus is said to be bounded by the sacral promontory, a significant number of specimen (37.14%; $n = 35$) had the plexus extend up to 12.3 mm beyond the sacral promontory. The plexus may be situated as close as 6.1 mm to the right of the midline, be as wide as 41.2 mm, and as long as 98 mm (Paraskevas et al., 2008). Delmas and Laux, (1928) examined the configuration of the superior hypogastric plexus and found that the superior hypogastric plexus consistently received branches from the third and fourth sympathetic ganglion. The plexus is derived from three roots, two lateral and one intermediate, the former being from the pelvic visceral nerves, the latter being a continuation of the abdominal aorta plexus. Argentino (1934) describes one type of superior hypogastric plexus in which there were three distinct roots covered by a fibrous connective sheath. Savas (1958) dissected 126 cadavers, male and female, and found a common nerve trunk in 63.5% of specimen; thin striplike trunk in 23.8%; and a wide plexiform configuration in 12.7%. Furthermore, Savas (1958) was one of the first to assert that firstly, the presacral nerve was prelumbar, and that is does not in fact exist and is simply a part of the superior hypogastric plexus.

Paraskevas et al. (2008) also located sympathetic fibers stemming not only from the lumbar region, but also from thoracic sympathetics through the celiac plexus; major and minor splanchnics are also seen terminating at the superior hypogastric plexus.

EJACULATORY DISORDERS FROM LUMBAR INTERBODY FUSIONS

Male sexual function is governed by the superior hypogastric plexus, allowing for normal sperm transit through innervation of the smooth muscle of the vas deferens and seminal vesicle. Sympathetic innervation of the male structures from the plexus allow for contraction of the smooth muscle of the genital tract resulting in the emission of semen. Reflux of semen into the bladder is prevented by simultaneous sympathetic stimulation of urethral proximal muscles and sphincteric closure of the neck of the bladder (Paraskevas et al., 2008). Approaches to the spine for lumbar interbody fusion surgery result in noticeable incidence of retrograde ejaculation. Lindley et al. (2012) notes that while anterior lumbar interbody fusion (ALIF) has gained popularity, retrograde ejaculation occurred in 7.4% of patients undergoing ALIF, and 9.8% undergoing artificial disc replacement. Sasso et al. (2003) reported an incidence of retrograde ejaculation following ALIF ranging between 0.42% and 5.9%. The incidence of retrograde ejaculation may be lowered by using retroperitoneal exposure of the L4-L5 and L5-S1 disc spaces, as opposed to the transperitoneal approach which was reported to result in a 10 times higher incidence of retrograde ejaculation (Sasso et al., 2003). Accessing the disc space and vertebral bodies through the retroperitoneal tissue requires avoidance of the great vessels, lumbosacral plexus, while also paying close attention to avoiding the superior hypogastric plexus. Cutting through tissue without careful blunt dissection may sever the connections between the superior hypogastric plexus and the seminal vesicles, vas deferens, and other pelvic ejaculatory structures, and subsequently result in ejaculatory disorders.

SYMPATHETIC BLOCKADE AND NEUROLYSIS

The superior hypogastric plexus block is often used for nonmalignant as well as neoplastic pain originating from the pelvis. Examples of such nonmalignant indications are, but are not limited to: endometriosis, severe dysmenorrhea, pelvic inflammatory disease, proctalgia, testicular pain, and ilioinguinal neuralgia. The patient is positioned similar to a lumbar sympathetic plexus block, and a 22-gauge, 5-inch spinal needle is walked lateral to the anterior one-fifth of the vertebral body and advanced through the psoas fascia and into the retroperitoneal space. Anesthetic is then injected into the area of the plexus. Transdiscal, transvaginal, and transarterial techniques may also be used. There are severe complications with these procedures such as backache; retroperitoneal hematoma; epidural, subdural, or subarachnoid injection; bladder or ureteral injury; iatrogenic nerve damage; rectal perforation; discitis; and infection, thus knowledge of the relevant anatomy is vital (Rastogi et al., 2009). For patients with >50% pain relief from diagnostic blocks, therapeutic neurolytic blocks typically consisting of 10% phenol solution or absolute alcohol are indicated (Tharian et al., 2019).

REFERENCES

Argentino, A., 1934. Riceche morfologiche sul cosideto "nervo presacrale". Anat. Bericht 28, 7.

Delmas, J., Laux, G., 1928. Constitution, forme et rapports du nerf présacré. Anat. Bericht 12, 420.

Godlewski, G., Prudhomme, M., 2000. Embryology and anatomy of the anorectum. Surg. Clin. 80, 319–343.

Latarjet, A., Rochet, P.H., 1926. Le plexus hypogastrique chez la femme. Anat. Bericht 5, 427.

Lindley, E.M., McBeth, Z.L., Henry, S.E., Cooley, R., Burger, E.L., Cain, C.M., Patel, V.V., 2012. Retrograde ejaculation after anterior lumbar spine surgery. Spine 37, 1785–1789.

Paraskevas, G., Tsitsopoulos, P., Papaziogas, B., Natsis, K., Martoglou, S., Stoltidou, A., Kitsoulis, P., 2008. Variability in superior hypogastric plexus morphology and its clinical applications:a cadaveric study. Surg. Radiol. Anat. 30, 481–488.

Ranson, S.W., 1947. The Anatomy of the Nervous System: Its Development and Function. WB & Saunders Co., Philadelphia, p. 135.

Rastogi, R., Agarwal, S., Enany, N., Munir, M.A., 2009. Sympathetic blockade. In: Current Therapy in Pain, pp. 612–620.

Sasso, R.C., Kenneth, B.J., LeHuec, J.C., 2003. Retrograde ejaculation after anterior lumbar interbody fusion: transperitoneal versus retroperitoneal exposure. Spine 28 (10), 1023–1026.

Savas, A., 1958. Contribution in presacral nerve study. In: Proceedings of the Aristotle University of Thessaloniki, Greece, vol. 2, pp. 283–297.

Standring, S., 2016. Gray's Anatomy: The Anatomical Basis of Clinical Practice, fortyfirst ed. Elsevier Limited, Philadelphia.

Tharian, A.R., Kusper, T.M., Knezevic, N.N., 2019. Superior hypogastric plexus. Pain 851–854.

The Inferior Hypogastric Plexus

STEPHEN J. BORDES, JR. • R. SHANE TUBBS

ANATOMY

The inferior hypogastric, or pelvic, plexus is a meshwork of nerve branches consisting of pelvic splanchnic fibers and superior hypogastric plexus fibers (Figs. 15.1 and 15.2) (Hounnou et al., 2003). Although not part of the sacral plexus, the juxtaposition to the inferior hypogastric plexus makes knowledge of its anatomy important with any discussion on the sacral plexus. The superior hypogastric plexus consists of sympathetic fibers from the lumbar and thoracic regions (Röthlisberger et al., 2018). The preaortic part of the superior hypogastric plexus gives rise to the hypogastric nerves which course from its inferior portion in parallel to the internal iliac vessels along the posterolateral pelvic border and join a network of parasympathetic fibers coming from the sacral plexus (Röthlisberger et al., 2018; Sienkiewicz-Zawilinska et al., 2018). The inferior hypogastric plexus' superior border follows the posterior aspect of the internal iliac artery (Sienkiewicz-Zawilinska et al., 2018). The posterior, or dorsal, border lies next to the sacrum and receives sacral rami (Sienkiewicz-Zawilinska et al., 2018). The inferior, or caudal, border is formed by a line between the ureter's point of entry into the broad ligament and the S4 rami (Sienkiewicz-Zawilinska et al., 2018). The inferior hypogastric plexus controls micturition and erectile function (Röthlisberger et al., 2018). Its fibers innervate pelvic and sacral viscera via the uterovaginal, vesicoureteral, middle rectal, and cavernous plexi (Shoja et al., 2013; Spackman et al., 2007). Traditionally, the inferior hypogastric plexus is said to consist of S1-S5 ventral rami; however, studies show that S3 and S4 rami may contribute more heavily than the rest (Shoja et al., 2013). Disruption of the fibers at the level of the inferior vesicle vasculature or to the uterosacral ligament may result in significant loss of function of sacral and pelvic viscera (Shoja et al., 2013). Sympathetic fibers traveling through this plexus maintain sphincter continence and attenuate peristalsis by way of vasomotor innervation of smooth muscle (Shoja et al., 2013). These fibers also carry afferent nociceptive fibers

from sacral and pelvic organs with the vagina, cervix, bladder, and rectum serving as exceptions as they travel with parasympathetic fibers (S2-S4) (Shoja et al., 2013; Mitchell, 1953). Pelvic parasympathetic innervation of the genitourinary and distal digestive systems provides visceromotor, secretomotor, and vasodilator effects (Mitchell, 1953). The distal colon, rectum, bladder, prostate, urethra, seminal vesicles, vas deferens, epididymis, fallopian tubes, uterus, vagina, erectile tissue, bulbourethral glands, vestibular glands, renal pelvis, and ureter exhibit such parasympathetic effects (Mitchell, 1953). Autonomic fibers from the inferior hypogastric plexus traveling around the bladder and seminal vesicles exhibit sympathetic dominance, whereas autonomic fibers traveling inferolaterally near the rectum and prostate exhibit parasympathetic dominance (Muraoka et al., 2018). Such a finding can be demonstrated by immunohistochemical staining of nerve fibers for vasoactive intestinal peptide (VIP), tyrosine hydroxylase (TH), and nitric oxide synthase (nNOS) (Muraoka et al., 2018). VIP and nNOS are markers of parasympathetic nerves and acetylcholine release, while TH is a marker for sympathetic nerves as norepinephrine is a major neurotransmitter and metabolite of phenylalanine (or tyrosine) in this pathway (Muraoka et al., 2018). As a result, it can be seen that the inferior hypogastric plexus is a complex system comprising both cholinergic and adrenergic fibers (Alsaid et al., 2009).

In females, the uterovaginal plexus is an analog of the deferential and prostatic plexus in males (Sienkiewicz-Zawilinska et al., 2018). It extends from inferior hypogastric nerves supravaginally and on either side of the uterus (Shoja et al., 2013). This subdivision contains the lateral vasomotor nerves of Laterjet and Rochet and communicates with the ovarian and ureteric plexi (Shoja et al., 2013). This plexus is located laterally to the uterosacral ligament on either side (Shoja et al., 2013). Nerve fibers in this plexus run with uterosacral and cardinal ligaments as well as uterine arteries. The uterosacral plexus innervates the uterus, vaginal wall,

Surgical Anatomy of the Sacral Plexus and Its Branches. https://doi.org/10.1016/B978-0-323-77602-8.00015-5

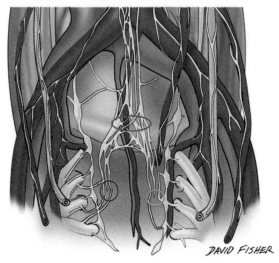

DAVID FISHER

FIG. 15.1 Schematic drawing of the formation of the inferior hypogastric plexus from the superior hypogastric plexus above (*blue oval*), the pelvic splanchnic nerves (*red circle*), and sacral splanchnics (*green circle*).

vestibular bulbs, greater vestibular glands, and clitoris (Shoja et al., 2013; Spackman et al., 2007; Mitchell, 1953). Anterior extensions of vaginal nerves are also known as cavernous nerves (Sienkiewicz-Zawilinska et al., 2018). As such, these nerves heavily contribute to female sexual function. Sympathetic fibers originating from T10-L2 innervate the constituents of this plexus (Shoja et al., 2013). Pain returns to central structures via parasympathetic fibers (Mitchell, 1953).

The vesicoureteral plexus gives off superior and inferior vesicle nerves which primarily innervate the bladder, internal urethral sphincter, distal ureters, seminal vesicles, and urethra (in men) and joins the uterovaginal plexus (in women) (Sienkiewicz-Zawilinska et al., 2018). Parasympathetic fibers result in contraction of the detrusor muscle while sympathetic fibers, primarily innervating the trigone, inhibit the micturition reflex and function to maintain continence (Shoja et al., 2013; Mitchell, 1953). The somatic system also contributes to the micturition reflex via the pudendal nerve which enables the pelvic diaphragm and external urethral sphincter to relax (Shoja et al., 2013). Sympathetic and parasympathetic fibers carry sensory afferents; however, pain is relayed through the sympathetic system (Shoja et al., 2013; Mitchell, 1953).

The middle and inferior rectal plexuses, a collection of six to eight nerve branches from the posterior inferior hypogastric plexus, travel primarily with the middle and inferior rectal arteries and provide autonomic innervation to the middle and inferior rectum

(Sienkiewicz-Zawilinska et al., 2018; Shoja et al., 2013). Parasympathetic nerves carry afferent pain signals from this organ (Shoja et al., 2013). This plexus also receives input from the pudendal nerve (Sienkiewicz-Zawilinska et al., 2018).

The prostatic plexus is a branch of the inferior hypogastric plexus that courses around the prostate inferolaterally (Sienkiewicz-Zawilinska et al., 2018). The deferential plexus is a small amalgamation of nerves from the prostatic, inferior hypogastric, and vesicoureteral plexuses. It innervates the vas deferens and seminal vesicles (Sienkiewicz-Zawilinska et al., 2018).

The cavernous plexus, in males, is an anterior extension of the prostatic plexus and innervates erectile tissues of the penis after forming anastomoses with the dorsal nerve of the penis (Sienkiewicz-Zawilinska et al., 2018). Stimulation of these nerves results in glans engorgement, penile lengthening, and increased blood flow to these organs (Shoja et al., 2013).

HISTOLOGY

The inferior hypogastric plexus can be stained and visualized using microscopy or 3D reconstruction. Sections of the nerve plexus can first be stained with hematoxylin and eosin (HE) or hematin-eosin-safran (HES) (Alsaid et al., 2009). S100 protein immune labeling is used as a nuclear marker for Schwann cells, and Luxol fast blue dye is used to stain myelin (Alsaid et al., 2009). A combination of different markers can be used to identify cholinergic and adrenergic fibers. Adrenergic fibers rely heavily on the neurotransmitter norepinephrine, a metabolite of phenylalanine, tyrosine, and dopamine. As a result, TH marker can identify this enzymatic and metabolic pathway in sympathetic fibers (Alsaid et al., 2009). Cholinergic fibers use acetylcholine as their major neurotransmitter. Vesicular acetylcholine transporter (VAChT) can be labeled as a result (Alsaid et al., 2009). Other studies have had success labeling cholinergic fibers with nNOS and VIP which are products secreted following acetylcholine release (Sienkiewicz-Zawilinska et al., 2018; Muraoka et al., 2018).

TOPOGRAPHY

The inferior hypogastric plexus is located at the level of the posterior pelvic floor and forms a triangular structure extending from a broad, posterior base to an anterior inferior point opposite the sacral concavity (Sienkiewicz-Zawilinska et al., 2018; Mauroy et al., 2003, 2007a, 2007b). The plexus has three edges: a posterior superior or dorsal cranial edge parallel to

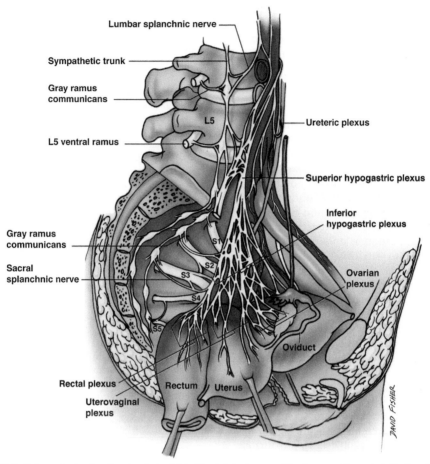

FIG. 15.2 Schematic drawing (hemisected pelvis) of the inferior hypogastric plexus and its parts in the female pelvis.

the internal iliac artery, a posterior inferior edge in contact with sacral roots, and a caudal edge extending from the fourth sacral ventral rami to the ureter at its point of entry into the broad ligament (Sienkiewicz-Zawilinska et al., 2018; Mauroy et al., 2007a). The plexus also contains three angles: a superior angle following the hypogastric nerve from the superior hypogastric plexus, a posterior angle in contact with the fourth sacral rami, and an anterior inferior angle in contact with the ureter and broad ligament (Sienkiewicz-Zawilinska et al., 2018; Mauroy et al., 2007a, 2007b). Blood vessels and viscera serve as landmarks for the inferior hypogastric plexus. The posterior margin of the internal iliac artery and inferior hypogastric artery serve as the superior border of the plexus, which lies approximately 10 mm inferior to it and covers the anterior sacrum (Sienkiewicz-Zawilinska et al., 2018; Mauroy et al., 2007a). The apex of the inferior hypogastric plexus lies adjacent to the point at which the ureter pierces the broad ligament; as a result, the ureter is an important visceral structure when determining location (Hounnou et al., 2003; Sienkiewicz-Zawilinska et al., 2018).

VARIATIONS

An irregular communicating branch may be found in some individuals. This branch connects the inferior hypogastric plexus with the pudendal nerve (Mauroy et al., 2003). In males, this branch can typically be found in the sacral concavity behind the vas deferens and ureter (Mauroy et al., 2003).

PATHOLOGY

Most pathologies involving the inferior hypogastric plexus and its efferent branches involve transection, compression, stretching, or coagulation of nerves due to surgical interventions such as prostatectomy, hysterectomy, orthopedic procedures involving the anterior lumbosacral approach, and childbirth (Sienkiewicz-Zawilinska et al., 2018; Spackman et al., 2007).

SURGICAL APPROACH

The inferior hypogastric plexus is often injured during radical surgical procedures to the prostate, uterus, and rectum (Hounnou et al., 2003). Lesions to this plexus can result in bladder incontinence and sexual dysfunction. Complications include erectile dysfunction, inability to ejaculate, loss of vaginal lubrication, and loss of the micturition reflex (Hounnou et al., 2003). Anterior approaches to the lumbosacral region increase risks of complication as does manipulation of pelvic organs due to stretching and coagulation (Hounnou et al., 2003; Alsaid et al., 2009). Some studies have shown favorable outcomes using a suprapubic approach for prostatectomy (Mauroy et al., 2003, 2007b). Nerve concentrations on the anterior prostate are typically low; as a result, lateral dissections tend to spare the nerves in this region (Huri et al., 2017). Others have shown that unilateral ligation of inferior hypogastric plexus afferent branches preserves sexual function and continence in the event nerves cannot be spared bilaterally (Mauroy et al., 2003). In the case of hysterectomy, laparotomy increases risks of urinary complications compared with vaginal hysterectomy (Mauroy et al., 2007b). Approximately, one-half of women with incontinent urinary sphincters have undergone anterior hysterectomy (Mauroy et al., 2007b). It is important to note that surgical dissection beneath the ureter and uterine artery risks transection of the vaginal nerve and its branches. Dissection and coagulation near the uterovesical junction risks insult to the vesical nerve which may denervate the anterior pelvic floor (Mauroy et al., 2007b). Immunohistochemical staining and microscopic visualization studies have decreased the incidence of iatrogenic injury during radical surgical procedures (Huri et al., 2017).

A transsacral approach may be used to anesthetize the inferior hypogastric plexus for the treatment, localization, or diagnosis of chronic pain involving the penis, vagina, bladder, rectum, anus, perineum, and lower pelvis (Schultz, 2007). Conditions involving these organs include endometriosis, malignancy, vulvodynia, tenesmus, enteritis, acute herpes zoster, and postherpetic neuralgia involving the sacral dermatomes (Mitchell, 1953; Schultz, 2007).

REFERENCES

Alsaid, B., Bessede, T., Karam, I., et al., 2009. Coexistence of adrenergic and cholinergic nerves in the inferior hypogastric plexus: anatomical and immunohistochemical study with 3D reconstruction in human male fetus. J. Anat. 214 (5), 645−654. https://doi.org/10.1111/j.1469-7580.2009.01071.x.

Hounnou, G.M., Uhl, J.F., Plaisant, O., Delmas, V., 2003. Morphometry by computerized three-dimensional reconstruction of the hypogastric plexus of a human fetus. Surg. Radiol. Anat. 25 (1), 21−31. https://doi.org/10.1007/s00276-002-0091-9.

Huri, E., Sargon, M., Tatar, I., Aydin, M., Ezer, M., Soylemezoglu, F., 2017. Novel anatomic mapping of pelvic plexus at prostatic and periprostatic region on fresh frozen cadaveric setting. Urol. J. 14 (6), 5064−5067.

Mauroy, B., Demondion, X., Drizenko, A., et al., 2003. The inferior hypogastric plexus (pelvic plexus): its importance in neural preservation techniques. Surg. Radiol. Anat. 25 (1), 6−15. https://doi.org/10.1007/s00276-002-0083-9.

Mauroy, B., Demondion, X., Bizet, B., Claret, A., Mestdagh, P., Hurt, C., 2007. The female inferior hypogastric (= pelvic) plexus: anatomical and radiological description of the plexus and its afferences − applications to pelvic surgery. Surg. Radiol. Anat. 29 (1), 55−66. https://doi.org/10.1007/s00276-006-0171-3.

Mauroy, B., Bizet, B., Bonnal, J.L., Crombet, T., Duburcq, T., Hurt, C., 2007. Systematization of the vesical and uterovaginal efferences of the female inferior hypogastric plexus (pelvic): applications to pelvic surgery on women patients. Surg. Radiol. Anat. 29 (3), 209−217. https://doi.org/10.1007/s00276-007-0195-3.

Mitchell, G., 1953. Anatomy of the Autonomic Nervous System. E&S Livingstone Ltd., London.

Muraoka, K., Morizane, S., Hieda, K., et al., 2018. Site-dependent differences in the composite fibers of male pelvic plexus branches: an immunohistochemical analysis of donated elderly cadavers. BMC Urol. 18 (1), 1−11. https://doi.org/10.1186/s12894-018-0369-9.

Röthlisberger, R., Aurore, V., Boemke, S., et al., 2018. The anatomy of the male inferior hypogastric plexus: what should we know for nerve sparing surgery. Clin. Anat. 31 (6), 788−796. https://doi.org/10.1002/ca.23079.

Schultz, D.M., 2007. Inferior hypogastric plexus blockade: a transsacral approach. Pain Physician 10 (6), 757−763.

Shoja, M.M., Sharma, A., Mirzayan, N., et al., 2013. Neuroanatomy of the female abdominopelvic region: a review with application to pelvic pain syndromes. Clin. Anat. 26 (1), 66−76. https://doi.org/10.1002/ca.22200.

Sienkiewicz-Zawilinska, J., Zawilinski, J., Kaythampillai, L., et al., 2018. Autonomic nervous system of the pelvis - general overview. Folia. Med. Cracov. 21−44. https://doi.org/10.24425/fmc.2018.124656.

Spackman, R., Wrigley, B., Roberts, A., Quinn, M., 2007. The inferior hypogastric plexus: a different view. J. Obstet. Gynaecol. 27 (2), 130−133. https://doi.org/10.1080/01443610601113839.

CHAPTER 16

Variations of the Sacral Plexus

NIHAL APAYDIN • R. SHANE TUBBS

The sacral plexus lies against the posterior pelvic wall anterior to the piriformis, posterior to the internal iliac vessels and ureter, and behind the sigmoid colon on the left. The sacral plexus is formed by the lumbosacral trunk, the first to third sacral ventral rami, and part of the fourth sacral ventral ramus (the remainder of which joins the coccygeal plexus). The upper four sacral ventral rami enter the pelvis by the anterior sacral foramina, the fifth between the sacrum and coccyx. The first and second sacral ventral rami are large, the third to fifth diminish progressively. Each receives a gray ramus communicans from a corresponding sympathetic ganglion. Visceral efferent rami leave the second to fourth sacral rami as the pelvic splanchnic nerves, containing parasympathetic fibers to minute ganglia in the walls of the pelvic viscera. The origins of the nerves forming the sacral plexus are highly variable depending on whether the plexus is prefixed, postfixed, or has the usual pattern (Fig. 16.1). The range of these variations was extensively defined by Eisler (1892), providing the basis for different classification systems that are still used today (Table 16.1).

NERVE TO PIRIFORMIS

The nerve to the piriformis usually arises from the dorsal branches of the S1-S2 ventral rami and enters the anterior surface of the piriformis. It sometimes arises from only the S2 ventral ramus (Bergman et al., 1984, 1988; Williams, 2005; Mahadevan, 2008). It can be a single or doubled nerve. An additional branch can arise from the superior gluteal nerve (SGN).

NERVE TO OBTURATOR INTERNUS

The nerve to the obturator internus and gemellus superior arises from the L5-S1 and S2 ventral rami. It leaves the pelvis via the greater sciatic foramen below the piriformis. It gives a branch to the upper posterior surface of the gemellus superior, crosses the ischial spine, and then reenters the pelvis via the lesser sciatic foramen running on the pelvic surface of the obturator internus. Aung et al. (2001) examined the innervation patterns of the obturator internus, superior and inferior gemelli, and quadratus femoris muscles in 101 pelvic halves of 60 human cadavers and found that the quadratus

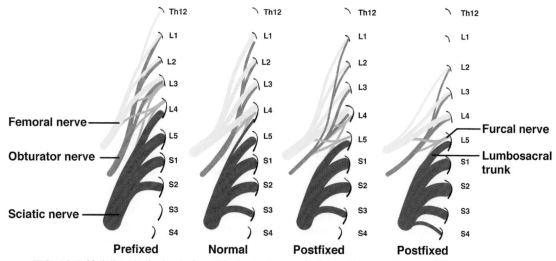

FIG. 16.1 Variations in the level of contribution to the sacral plexus. (After von Lanz and Wachsmuth (1972).)

Surgical Anatomy of the Sacral Plexus and Its Branches. https://doi.org/10.1016/B978-0-323-77602-8.00016-7

TABLE 16.1
Range of Variation of Sacral Plexus.

Nerve	Prefixed Plexus (High Form)	Usual Pattern	Postfixed Plexus (Low form)
Lumbosacral trunk	L4	L4	L4
Nerve to quadratus femoris	L4, L5	L4, L5, S1	L5, S1
Nerve to obturator internus	L4, L5, S1, S2	L5, S1, S2	S1, S2, S3
Tibial	L3, L4, L5, S1, S2	L4, L5, S1, S2, S3	L5, S1, S2, S3, S4
Superior gluteal	L4, L5, S1	L4, L5, S1, S2	L5, S1, S2
Inferior gluteal	L4, L5, S1	L5, S1, S2	(L5), S1, S2
Nerve to piriformis	L5, S1, S2	S1, S2	S1, S2, S3
Common fibular	L3, L4, L5, S1	L4, L5, S1, S2	L5, S1, S2, S3
Posterior femoral cutaneous	L5, S1, S2	S1, S2, S3	S2, S3, S4
Pudendal	L5, S1, S2, S3	S1, S2, S3, S4	S1, S2, S3, S4
EXTREME RANGE OF VARIATIONS			
Lumbosacral trunk	L3 or L3, L4	L4	L4, L5 or L5
Common fibular	L3, L4, L5, S1, S2	L4, L5, S1, S2	L4, L5, S1, S2, S3, S4
Tibial	L3, L4, L5, S1, S2	L4, L5, S1, S2, S3	L4, L5, S1, S2, S3, S4
Posterior femoral cutaneous	L5, S1, S2, S3	L5, S1, S2, S3, S4	L5, S1, S2, S3, S4

Source: Eisler, P., 1892. Der Plexus lumbosacralis des Menschen. Halle.

femoris and obturator internus nerves formed a common trunk in 84.6%. There was also frequently communication between the obturator internus and quadratus femoris nerves. The obturator internus nerve arose from the ventral surface of L5, S1, S2, and S3 in 84.6% (Aung et al., 2001).

SUPERIOR GLUTEAL NERVE

The SGN arises from the dorsal branches of the L4-L5 and S1-S2 ventral rami. It is accompanied by the superior gluteal vessels and leaves the pelvis via the greater sciatic foramen above the piriformis. It then divides into superior and inferior branches. The superior branch accompanies the upper branch of the deep division of the superior gluteal artery and innervates the gluteus medius and occasionally the gluteus minimus. The inferior branch runs with the lower ramus of the deep division of the superior gluteal artery across the gluteus minimus and innervates the gluteus medius and minimus. It then ends in the tensor fasciae latae (Williams, 2005; Mahadevan, 2008). This nerve can receive fibers from the S2 spinal nerve. A branch to the piriformis can arise from the lowest root of this nerve (Bergman et al., 1984, 1988).

The branching pattern and the course of the SGN was classified into two types by Jacobs and Buxton (1989): (1) transverse neural trunk pattern, in which the branches arose separately in parallel to each other and (2) spray pattern, in which the SGN had branches that fanned out along the intermuscular plane between the gluteus medius and minimus. In most of their cases (80%), they observed the spray pattern. However, a more recent study by Apaydin et al. (2013) revealed the "transverse neural trunk pattern" in 85.7% of the specimens and the "spray pattern" in 14.3%.

INFERIOR GLUTEAL NERVE

The inferior gluteal nerve arises from the dorsal branches of the L5, S1, and S2 ventral rami. It leaves the pelvis via the greater sciatic foramen below the piriformis and divides into branches that enter the deep surface of the gluteus maximus (Williams, 2005; Mahadevan, 2008). It can also be joined with the nerve to the short head of the biceps femoris. The inferior gluteal nerve frequently provides a communicating branch that joins the posterior femoral cutaneous nerve (Bergman et al., 1984, 1988). The motor branches of the inferior gluteal nerve, after branching from the main trunk, spread in a large area curving medially and dorsally and entering the deep surface of the gluteus maximus (Apaydin et al., 2009a).

NERVE TO QUADRATUS FEMORIS

This arises from the ventral branches of the L4-S1 ventral rami. It leaves the pelvis via the greater sciatic foramen below the piriformis; descends on the ischium deep to the sciatic nerve, the gemelli, and the tendon of the obturator internus; and innervates the gemellus inferior, quadratus femoris, and the hip joint (Williams, 2005; Mahadevan, 2008). Wilson (1889) was probably the first to report an abnormal distribution of the nerve to the quadratus femoris, in which the nerve was longer than usual and entered the anterior aspect of the adductor magnus supplying it. Bergman also noted this nerve to give branches to the upper part of the adductor magnus and superior gemellus. Bardeen and Elting (1901) suggested there could be numerous communicating branches between the nerve and the quadratus femoris, obturator internus, and piriformis because of their close positional relationship. The branch to the superior gemellus is sometimes this muscle's only nerve supply (Aasar, 1947; Bergman et al., 1984, 1988). Kikuchi (1987) described the superior gemellus as supplied not only by the nerve to the obturator internus (obturator internus nerve) but also by that to the quadratus femoris (quadratus femoris nerve). He inferred that the superior gemellus has two different embryological origins. Honma et al. (1998) reported a communication between a branch to the inferior gemellus from the quadratus femoris nerve and a branch of the obturator internus nerve within the obturator internus muscle and recognized these muscles as part of the same muscle mass. Aung et al. (2001) reported in their series of 101 specimens that the quadratus femoris nerve arose from the ventral surface of L4, L5, and S1 in 79.4%. This nerve and the nerve to the obturator internus can be united in their early course (Piersol 1918).

POSTERIOR FEMORAL CUTANEOUS NERVE

This is also known as the posterior cutaneous nerve of the thigh. It is not a branch of the sciatic nerve. Its branches are all cutaneous and are distributed to the gluteal region, perineum, and the flexor aspect of the thigh and leg. It arises from the dorsal branches of S1, S2, and the ventral branches of S2, S3. It typically leaves the pelvis via the greater sciatic foramen below the piriformis, first medial and then superficial to the sciatic nerve. It descends under the gluteus maximus with the inferior gluteal vessels, lying posterior or medial to the sciatic nerve. It runs down superficial to the long head of the biceps femoris, deep to the fascia lata. It pierces the deep fascia behind the knee and becomes superficial, accompanying the short saphenous vein. Its terminal twigs connect with the sural nerve. Three or four gluteal branches curl around the lower border of the gluteus maximus to supply the skin over the inferolateral portion of the muscle. The perineal branch supplies the superomedial skin in the thigh. It communicates with the inferior rectal and posterior scrotal or labial branches of the perineal nerve and gives numerous branches to the skin of the back and medial sides of the thigh, the popliteal fossa, and the proximal part of the back of the leg (Williams, 2005; Mahadevan, 2008).

A number of variations in the course and distribution of this nerve have been reported. It can originate as two trunks from the common fibular and tibial nerves after they separate from the sciatic nerve. In such cases, the ventral trunk accompanies the tibial nerve below the piriformis and provides the perineal and medial femoral branches of the posterior femoral cutaneous nerve. The dorsal trunk accompanies the common peroneal nerve beneath the piriformis and provides the gluteal and femoral branches of the posterior femoral cutaneous nerve. The posterior femoral cutaneous nerve can be joined with a branch from the sciatic nerve. A perineal branch sometimes pierces the sacroiliac ligament. In some cases, the posterior femoral cutaneous ends behind the knee and can be replaced in the leg by a branch from the sural nerve (Bergman et al., 1984, 1988). The communicating branches from the sciatic nerve to the posterior femoral cutaneous nerve can innervate the long head of the biceps femoris (Aasar, 1947). Two posterior femoral cutaneous nerves may be present (Huban et al., 2012).

Tubbs et al. (2009) reported the perineal branch of the posterior femoral cutaneous nerve to arise directly from the posterior femoral cutaneous nerve in 55% of sides and from the inferior cluneal nerve in 30%. It was absent in 15%. It was found to pierce the sacrotuberous ligament and give two to three branches to the medial thigh that continued on to the scrotum or labia major. Communications between this branch and the perineal branch of the pudendal nerve were common. Tunali et al. (2011) reported a communicating branch between the posterior femoral cutaneous nerve and the sciatic nerve, 11 cm below the infrapiriform foramen.

PERFORATING CUTANEOUS NERVE

When present, the perforating cutaneous nerve usually arises from the posterior aspects of the S2 and S3 ventral rami. It pierces the sacrotuberous ligament, curves round the inferior border of the gluteus maximus, and supplies the skin over the inferomedial aspect of this muscle. Instead of piercing the sacrotuberous ligament, it sometimes accompanies the pudendal nerve or passes between the ligament and the gluteus maximus. It can arise from the pudendal nerve or be absent, in which case it can be replaced by a branch from either the posterior femoral cutaneous nerve or the third and fourth, or fourth and fifth, sacral ventral rami. It is sometimes joined with the pudendal nerve at its origin. Its prevalence has been reported as 64% (Aasar, 1947; Bergman et al., 1984, 1988).

SCIATIC NERVE

This is the largest nerve in the body. It is almost 2 cm wide at its origin near the sacral plexus. It originates from the ventral rami of spinal nerves L4-L5, S1-S3. The greater part of S2 and S3 converge on the inferomedial aspect of the lumbosacral trunk in the greater sciatic foramen to form the sciatic nerve. The ventral and dorsal divisions of the nerve do not separate physically from each other, but their fibers remain separate within the rami. The ventral and dorsal divisions of each contributing root join within the sciatic nerve. The fibers of the dorsal divisions go on to form the common fibular nerve and those of the ventral division form the tibial nerve. The sciatic nerve occasionally divides into common fibular and tibial nerves inside the pelvis. In these cases the common fibular nerve usually runs through the piriformis. The sciatic nerve typically comes out of the pelvis through the greater sciatic foramen, entering the gluteal region anterior to the piriformis muscle. After reaching the lateral aspect of the ischial tuberosity, it turns vertically downward to run between the ischium medially and the greater trochanter laterally. For most of its trajectory in the gluteal region it runs parallel to the midline. Superiorly it lies deep to gluteus maximus, resting first on the posterior ischial surface with the nerve to the quadratus femoris between them. It then crosses posterior to the obturator internus, gemelli, and quadratus femoris, separated by the latter from the obturator externus and the hip joint. The posterior femoral cutaneous nerve and the inferior gluteal artery usually accompany it medially. The nerve then enters the thigh behind the adductor magnus and is crossed posteriorly by the long head of the biceps femoris. It corresponds to a line drawn from just medial to the midpoint between the ischial tuberosity and greater trochanter to the apex of the popliteal fossa. It gives articular branches to the posterior aspect of the hip joint. These branches are sometimes derived directly from the sacral plexus. Muscular branches are distributed to the biceps femoris, semitendinosus, semimembranosus, and the ischial part of the adductor magnus.

The sciatic nerve has two main terminal branches: the tibial nerve and the common fibular nerve. The tibial nerve arises from its medial side, being derived from the anterior divisions of the ventral rami of L4-L5, S1-S3, and the common peroneal nerve arises from its lateral side, being derived from the posterior divisions of the ventral rami of L4-L5, S1-S2. However, the point of division of the sciatic nerve into its major components (tibial and common fibular) is very variable. The most common site is at the junction of the middle and lower thirds of the thigh, near the apex of the popliteal fossa, but the division can occur at any level above this point, or, more rarely, below it. It is also possible for these components to leave the sacral plexus separately, in which case the common fibular component usually passes through the piriformis at the greater sciatic notch while the tibial passes below the muscle (Bergman et al., 1984, 1988; Williams, 2005; Mahadevan, 2008).

The tibial and common peroneal components can easily be identified as two separate nerves throughout their trajectory in about 11% of cases. However, even in those cases a common sheath of connective tissue surrounds the two components. The sciatic nerve can be readily divided artificially back to the spinal nerves. It is therefore important not to confuse this with a true separation of the components, which generally takes place in the popliteal fossa. Upon entering the popliteal fossa, the two nerve components (peroneal and tibial) finally diverge from each other, having never mixed their fibers. The tibial nerve continues to run posteriorly in the direction of the main trunk, at the center of the popliteal fossa. The common peroneal component turns laterally to run just medial to the biceps tendon.

A number of variations in the course and distribution of the sciatic nerve have been reported. The main variations concern the relationship of the nerve to the piriformis. Beaton and Anson classified variations in the relationship of the sciatic nerve and its subdivisions to the piriformis muscle in 120 specimens in 1937, and in 240 specimens in 1938. Their classification, known as the Beaton and Anson classification, is as follows:
- Type 1: undivided nerve below undivided muscle;
- Type 2: divisions of nerve between and below undivided muscle;
- Type 3: divisions above and below undivided muscle;
- Type 4: undivided nerve between heads;
- Type 5: divisions between and above heads; and
- Type 6: undivided nerve above undivided muscle.

Patel et al. (2011) reported two other types, which were not previously defined by Beaton and Anson. These were a sciatic nerve (1) already divided in the pelvis, its two divisions traveling out below the piriformis; and (2) already divided in the pelvis, its two divisions leaving the pelvis differently (the common fibular nerve coming out after piercing the piriformis and the tibial nerve coming out below the piriformis). Additionally, Arifoglu et al. (1997) reported a case with a double superior gemellus and double piriformis associated with a high-dividing sciatic nerve, which passed between the two piriformis muscles in the same lower extremity. Carare and Goodwin (2008) observed the common peroneal nerve and the tibial nerve to originate independently from the lumbosacral plexus in one case. Furthermore, in their case, the two roots of the common peroneal nerve joined only at the inferior end of the piriformis muscle, after one of the roots pierced the muscle.

The sacral nerve can bifurcate into its two major divisions (common peroneal and tibial) anywhere between the sacral plexus and the lower part of the thigh. The two terminal branches can arise directly from the sacral plexus (Santanu et al., 2013). The division into terminal branches has been reported to occur below the popliteal space. The nerve to the short head of the biceps femoris sometimes arises directly from the sacral plexus. In one study of 420 limbs, the sciatic nerve passed beneath the piriformis in 87.5%, through it in 12% (peroneal division), and above it in 0.5%. In another study of 138 subjects, the sciatic passed beneath the piriformis in 118 cases (85.5%), the peroneal division passed through it in 17 (12.3%), and the entire sciatic passed through it in 3 (2.2%) (Bergman et al., 1984, 1988). Babinski et al. (2003) described another anatomical variation in which the common fibular nerve passed superior, and the tibial nerve inferior, to the superior gemellus muscle. Pokorny et al. (2006) examined 91 cadavers and found an atypical relationship in 19 cases (20.9%).

Natsis et al. (2014) dissected 294 limbs and noted the typical relationship between the common fibular and tibial nerve in 275 (93.6%), demonstrating four additional variations (1.4%) not described in the Beaton and Anson classification. In one of these, the common fibular nerve passed between the superficial and the deep muscle bellies of a doubled piriformis muscle, while the tibial nerve passed below the muscle. In another, the piriformis muscle had three bellies. The common fibular nerve passed between the superficial and intermediate muscle bellies, while the tibial nerve passed through the deep muscle. The other variation presented a bilateral supernumerary muscle located just superior to the piriformis in the suprapiriform foramen. The sciatic nerve ran below the piriformis muscle. Mas et al. (2002) reported a sciatic nerve where the

tibial component traveled inferior to the superior gemellus muscle and the common peroneal part left the pelvis below the piriformis muscle.

The sciatic nerve may innervate the gluteus maximus (Huban et al., 2012).

COMMON FIBULAR NERVE

The common fibular nerve is derived from the dorsal branches of the L4, L5 and S1, S2 ventral rami. It is approximately half the size of the tibial nerve. It descends obliquely along the lateral side of the popliteal fossa to the fibular head, medial to the biceps femoris. It lies between the bicipital tendon and the lateral head of the gastrocnemius. It then passes into the anterolateral compartment of the leg through a tight opening in the thick fascia overlying the tibialis anterior. It curves lateral to the fibular neck, deep to the fibularis longus, and divides into superficial and deep fibular nerves. The course of the common fibular nerve can be indicated by a line drawn from the apex of the popliteal fossa, passing distally, medial to the biceps tendon, to the back of the head of the fibula, where it can be rolled against the bone. In the gluteal region, Santanu et al. (2013) reported the common peroneal part of the sciatic nerve as innervating the gluteus maximus muscle.

It innervates the anterolateral part of the knee joint capsule and the proximal tibiofibular joint via three articular branches. Two of these branches accompany the superior and inferior lateral genicular arteries and can arise together. The third branch is known as the recurrent articular nerve; it arises near the termination of the common fibular nerve. It ascends with the anterior recurrent tibial artery through the tibialis anterior and supplies it. Watt et al. (2014) supported the use of the term "anterior tibial recurrent nerve (ATRN)" for the branch innervating the tibialis anterior and reported four major branching patterns of the common fibular nerve as follows: Type 1, neither the deep fibular nerve nor the ATRN branch before piercing the anterior intermuscular septum; Type 2, the ATRN branches before piercing the anterior intermuscular septum; Type 3, the deep fibular nerve branches before piercing the anterior intermuscular septum; and Type 4, both the deep fibular nerve and the ATRN branch before piercing the anterior intermuscular septum.

The nerve usually gives off two cutaneous branches, the lateral sural and sural communicating nerves. The lateral sural nerve (lateral cutaneous nerve of the calf) supplies the skin on the anterior, posterior, and lateral surfaces of the proximal leg. The sural communicating nerve arises near the head of the fibula and joins the sural nerve crossing over the lateral head of gastrocnemius. It can descend separately as far as the heel (Bergman et al., 1984, 1988; Williams, 2005; Mahadevan, 2008). Occasionally, the sural nerve arises purely from the tibial nerve and, even less commonly, it is purely peroneal (lateral sural cutaneous nerve).

The sciatic usually divides into the common peroneal and tibial nerves at the level of the lower thigh. These two nerves usually arise separately from the sacral plexus. They can be separated in the greater sciatic foramen by the piriformis and pass into the thigh as continuous but separate structures. Huelke (1958) examined 198 adult lower extremities and reported that the peroneal communicating nerve arose directly from the common peroneal nerve in 54.7%, usually as a branch separate from the lateral sural cutaneous nerve (41.5%). The peroneal communicating nerve gave rise to the lateral sural cutaneous branches in 13.2% of sides studied. The peroneal communicating nerve was a terminal branch of the lateral sural cutaneous nerve in one-third of the sides, and arose from a trunk common to it and to the lateral sural cutaneous nerve in 12%. The peroneal communicating nerve was absent in 19.7% of the 198 sides, so no sural nerve was formed in these cases. When this occurs, it is usually the medial sural cutaneous nerve that passes on to the dorsum of the foot as the lateral dorsal cutaneous nerve. Only 58.6% of the cadavers had the same type of origin of the peroneal communicating nerve in both legs. There were no significant differences between the right and left sides, between sexes, or the place where the peroneal communicating or sural nerves arose. The union between the peroneal communicating and medial sural cutaneous nerves was seen on 159 sides (80.3%). This union was more often located in the lower half of the leg (75%) (Bergman et al., 1984, 1988).

DEEP FIBULAR NERVE

This nerve begins at the bifurcation of the common fibular nerve, between the fibula and the proximal part of the fibularis longus. It passes obliquely forward deep to the extensor digitorum longus to the front of the interosseous membrane. Here, it gives muscular branches to the tibialis anterior, extensor hallucis longus, extensor digitorum longus, and fibularis tertius. In the anterior compartment, it accompanies the anterior tibial artery in the proximal third of the leg. It descends with this artery to the ankle, where it divides into lateral and medial terminal branches. As it descends, the nerve is first lateral to the artery, then

anterior, and finally lateral again at the ankle. It is usually divided into medial and lateral branches. It also gives an articular branch to the ankle joint. The lateral terminal branch crosses the ankle deep to the extensor digitorum brevis and supplies that muscle. It also gives three very small interosseous branches, which supply the tarsal and metatarsophalangeal joints of the middle three toes. The medial terminal branch runs distally on the dorsum of the foot lateral to the dorsalis pedis artery and connects with the medial branch of the superficial fibular nerve (SFN) in the first interosseous space. It divides into two dorsal digital nerves, which supply adjacent sides of the great and second toes. Before dividing, it gives off an interosseous branch, which supplies the first metatarsophalangeal joint. The deep fibular nerve can end as three terminal branches instead of two. A number of variations in the digital distribution of the nerve have been reported. It can supply the medial side of the great toe, adjacent sides of the second and third toes, or the lateral three-and-one-half toes. It sometimes has no digital branches at all. Absence of the cutaneous part of the superficial peroneal nerve and the deep peroneal nerve and its branch to the extensor digitorum brevis has been reported. In this case, the nerves were replaced by the saphenous and sural nerves (Bergman et al., 1984, 1988).

SUPERFICIAL FIBULAR NERVE

The SFN begins at the bifurcation of the common fibular nerve. It lies at first deep to the fibularis longus, then passes anteroinferiorly between the fibularis longus and brevis and the extensor digitorum longus and pierces the deep fascia in the distal third of the leg. It divides into a large medial dorsal cutaneous nerve and a smaller, more laterally placed, intermediate dorsal cutaneous nerve, usually after piercing the crural fascia. Sometimes it divides while it is still deep to the fascia. Solomon et al. (2001) reported the SFN to branch into the medial dorsal cutaneous nerve of the foot and the intermediate dorsal cutaneous nerve of the foot before piercing the crural fascia in 24 out of 68 cases (35%). Apaydin et al. (2008a,b) investigated the compartmental anatomy of the SFN and defined three particular types in its course. In 71% of cases, the SFN coursed entirely within the lateral compartment of the leg (Type I). In 23.7%, it penetrated the anterior intermuscular septum, 12.7 cm inferior to the apex of the head of fibula, and coursed in the anterior compartment (Type II). In the remaining 5.3% of the specimens, the SFN had branches in both the anterior and lateral compartments (Type III). Prakash et al. (2010)

examined 60 specimens for the location and course of the SFN and found it was located in the anterior compartment of the leg in 28.3%. In 8.3%, it branched before piercing between the fibularis longus and extensor digitorum longus muscles, whereas in 11.7%, it branched after piercing them. In 41 out of 60 specimens, the sensory division of the superficial peroneal nerve branched into the medial dorsal cutaneous and the intermediate dorsal cutaneous nerve distal to its emergence from the deep fascia.

As the nerve lies between the muscles of the lateral compartment of the leg, it supplies the fibularis longus, fibularis brevis, and the skin of the lower leg. The course, compartmental location, and peripheral digital distribution of the SFN are subject to considerable variation. For example, Browne and Morris (2007) described an adult female cadaver where the SFN bifurcated into two equal-caliber branches 3 cm distal to the fibular head. The two branches remained in the lateral compartment of the leg and passed between the fibularis longus and brevis muscles. The anterior branch pierced the lateral intermuscular septum and then pierced the crural fascia to continue as the medial dorsal cutaneous nerve of the foot. The posterior branch pierced the crural fascia to continue as the intermediate dorsal cutaneous nerve of the foot. Variation in the distribution of the cutaneous nerves of the dorsum of the foot was reported in a series of 229 feet in 1892 by the Committee of Collective Investigation of the Anatomical Society of Great Britain and Ireland: 12 patterns of termination of the dorsal nerves were described, which are known as Kosinski's variants (Kosinski, 1926). Great variability was described in both the deep course (Kosinski, 1926; Von Reinman, 1984; Blair and Botte, 1994; Benjamin et al., 1995) and the peripheral toe distribution (Brodie et al., 1892; Kosinski, 1926) of the sural and superficial fibular nerves. Solomon et al. (2001) described five types additional to Kosinski's variants in their series of 68 feet. Adkinson et al. (1991) reported that 14% of 85 legs had the SFN located in the medial compartment, while in 12% this nerve divided deep to the deep fascia in the lateral compartment and then the medial dorsal cutaneous nerve of the foot passed into the anterior compartment.

Another variant of the SFN with more practical implications in the approach to the lateral malleolus was described by Blair and Botte (1994). These authors reported that in 16% of 25 cases, the nerve branched deep and the medial dorsal cutaneous nerve of the foot pierced the fascia anterior to the lateral malleolus, while the intermediate dorsal cutaneous nerve of the

foot pierced the fascia posterior to the lateral malleolus and then crossed the bone to follow its course toward the dorsum of the foot.

The medial dorsal cutaneous nerve typically passes in front of the ankle joint and divides into two dorsal digital branches, one of which supplies the medial side of the hallux and the other supplies the adjacent side of the second and third toes. It communicates with the saphenous and deep fibular nerves. The intermediate branch traverses the dorsum of the foot laterally. It divides into dorsal digital branches that supply the contiguous sides of the third to fifth toes and the skin of the lateral aspect of the ankle, where it connects with the sural nerve. Some of the lateral branches of the SFN are frequently absent and are replaced by sural branches (Bergman et al., 1984, 1988; Williams, 2005; Mahadevan, 2008).

ACCESSORY FIBULAR NERVES

An accessory SFN and an accessory deep fibular nerve have been described as variant branches of the superficial fibular nerve; both are probably the products of atypical branching of the main nerve deep to the crural fascia. The accessory deep peroneal nerve was reported to be a common variant branch of the superficial peroneal nerve. It participates in the innervation of the extensor digitorum brevis muscle, which can interfere with the differential diagnosis of peroneal nerve lesions (Tzika et al., 2012). Rayegani et al. (2011) found the accessory deep fibular nerve to be present in 28 out of 230 patients (12%). In another study, Prakash et al. (2010) demonstrated the accessory deep peroneal nerve as an additional branch from the sensory division of the SFN in 20 out of 60 specimens. The course of this nerve lay in the anterior compartment of the leg and then passed deep to the extensor retinaculum and supplied the ankle and the dorsum of the foot. Paraskevas et al. (2013) also reported an accessory superficial fibular nerve, which arose from the SFN 0.89 cm proximal to its penetration of the crural fascia.

TIBIAL NERVE

The tibial nerve is the larger component of the sciatic nerve and is derived from the anterior divisions of the L4-L5 and S1-S3 ventral rami. It descends along the back of the thigh and popliteal fossa to the distal border of the popliteus. It then passes anterior to the arch of the soleus with the popliteal artery and continues into the leg. In the thigh, it is overlapped proximally by the hamstring muscles but it becomes more superficial in the popliteal fossa, where it is lateral to the popliteal vessels. At the level of the knee the tibial nerve becomes superficial to the popliteal vessels and crosses to the medial side of the artery. In the distal popliteal fossa, the junction of the two heads of the gastrocnemius overlaps it. In its distal third, it is covered only by skin and fasciae, overlapped sometimes by the flexor hallucis longus. It lies on the tibialis posterior for most of its course except distally, where it adjoins the posterior surface of the tibia.

It gives articular branches to the knee joint forming a plexus with a branch from the obturator nerve. The branches that innervate the gastrocnemius, plantaris, soleus, and popliteus arise proximally either independently or by a common trunk. Apaydin et al. (2008a,b) examined the course and branching pattern of the tibial nerve in the deep posterior compartment of the leg and defined three particular types: Type I (55.6%): separate branches to each of the muscles in the deep posterior compartment of the leg; Type II (30.6%): two main branches of the tibial nerve that provide motor branches; and Type III (13.8%): one main branch, giving rise to separate motor branches to each of the muscles. In 61.1% of their cases, the proximal and distal branches of the tibial nerve innervated the flexor hallucis longus. In 38.9%, this muscle was innervated only by one proximal branch. In all of their cases, the tibialis posterior was innervated by both the proximal and distal branches and the flexor digitorum longus was innervated only distally. The branch to the flexor hallucis longus accompanies the fibular vessels. It has an interosseous branch that descends near the fibula to reach the distal tibiofibular joint. It also gives off the medial calcaneal nerve, which perforates the flexor retinaculum to supply the skin of the heel and medial side of the sole. The medial calcaneal nerve can have two sets of branches, which reunite to form the rest of the nerve (Aasar, 1947).

The tibial nerve ends under the flexor retinaculum by dividing into the medial and lateral plantar nerves. Bareither et al. (1990) dissected 126 human cadaver lower extremities to determine the level of division of the tibial nerve into medial and lateral plantar nerves. They reported a considerable amount of variance in the level of division, documenting a higher incidence of division proximal to the usual description. This is deep to the flexor retinaculum between the calcaneus and medial malleolus.

The medial plantar nerve is the larger terminal division of the tibial nerve. The medial plantar artery accompanies it laterally. It originates under the flexor retinaculum and passes deep to the abductor hallucis.

Between the abductor hallucis and flexor digitorum brevis, it gives off a medial proper digital nerve to the hallux and divides near the metatarsal bases into three common plantar digital nerves. Its cutaneous branches pierce the plantar aponeurosis between the abductor hallucis and flexor digitorum brevis to supply the skin of the sole of the foot.

Muscular branches supply the abductor hallucis, flexor digitorum brevis, flexor hallucis brevis, and the first lumbrical. The former two arise near the origin of the nerve and enter the deep surfaces of the muscles. The branch to the flexor hallucis brevis is from the medial digital nerve of the great toe, and that to the first lumbrical from the first common plantar digital nerve. Articular branches supply the joints of the tarsus and metatarsus. Three common plantar digital nerves pass between the slips of the plantar aponeurosis, each dividing into two proper digital branches. The first supplies adjacent sides of the hallux and second toe; the second supplies adjacent sides of the second and third toes; the third supplies adjacent sides of the third and fourth toes, and also connects with the lateral plantar nerve. The first gives a branch to the first lumbrical. Each proper digital nerve has cutaneous and articular branches: near the distal phalanges a dorsal branch supplies structures around the nail, and the termination of each nerve supplies the ball of the toe.

The lateral plantar nerve supplies the skin of the fifth toe, the lateral half of the fourth toe, and most of the deep muscles of the foot. It has superficial and deep branches. Before division, it supplies the flexor digitorum accessorius and abductor digiti minimi and gives rise to small branches that pierce the plantar fascia to supply the skin of the lateral part of the sole. The superficial branch splits into two common plantar digital nerves: the lateral supplies the lateral side of the fifth toe, the flexor digiti minimi brevis, and the two interossei in the fourth intermetatarsal space; the medial connects with the third common plantar digital branch of the medial plantar nerve and divides into two to supply the adjoining sides of the fourth and fifth toes. The deep branch accompanies the lateral plantar artery deep to the flexor tendons and adductor hallucis and supplies the second to fourth lumbricals, adductor hallucis, and all the interossei (except those of the fourth intermetatarsal space). Branches to the second and third lumbricals pass distally deep to the transverse head of the adductor hallucis and curl round its distal border to reach them. The first and second lumbricals can receive branches from both the lateral and medial plantars. The branch of the lateral nerve to the second lumbrical courses forward beneath the transversus (adductor hallucis), then turns backward over the transversus to reach the lumbrical muscle. Cruveilhier (1844) described a branch of the lateral plantar that pierced the transversus to reach the third lumbrical. The lateral nerve rarely provides a branch to the lateral head of the flexor hallucis brevis (Bergman et al., 1984, 1988).

Hallopeau's nerve is a branch of the lateral plantar nerve that supplies the flexor hallucis brevis muscle while also forming an anastomosis with the medial plantar nerve. In a study by Chou et al. (2008), this neural anastomosis was found in 4 out of 26 specimens.

SURAL NERVE

The sural nerve is typically formed by the union of the lateral and medial sural communicating nerves, which originate from the common fibular and tibial nerves. After its formation, the sural nerve descends between the heads of the gastrocnemius, piercing the deep fascia proximally in the leg. It is not uncommon for the medial sural communicating branch to be joined at a variable level by the lateral sural communicating branch of the common fibular nerve after piercing the deep fascia. The sural nerve descends lateral to the calcaneal tendon, near the short saphenous vein, to the region between the lateral malleolus and the calcaneus, and supplies the posterior and lateral skin of the distal third of the leg. It then passes distal to the lateral malleolus along the lateral side of the foot and little toe, supplying the overlying skin. It connects with the posterior femoral cutaneous nerve in the leg and with the SFN on the dorsum of the foot. The surface marking at the ankle is a line parallel to the calcaneal tendon halfway between the tendon and the lateral malleolus. Its position is variable, however (Webb et al., 2000). Apaydin et al. (2009a,b) demonstrated that in 95.5% of their specimens the sural nerve was initially medial to the lateral border of the CT proximally and intersected with the lateral border of the CT at 55% of the mid-tendon line.

Several variations have been reported in the formation and distribution of branches of these nerves. The point of union of the two branches of the sural nerve is subject to wide variation. It can be high in the popliteal space or sometimes there is no union at all. The union can occur 3 cm below the origin of the peroneal communicating nerve. The two branches of the sural nerve can arise 3 cm apart about 10 cm above the knee and pierce the medial head of the gastrocnemius muscle before joining the peroneal communicating nerve. In some cases the two branches do not rejoin.

The sural nerve sometimes supplies the dorsal cutaneous area of the lateral two-and-one-half toes. It can terminate at the lateral border of the foot without providing any digital branches. When the medial sural cutaneous nerve is joined by the peroneal communicating nerve, the combined nerve is termed the sural nerve (Bergman et al., 1984, 1988).

Eid and Hegazy (2011) examined 24 specimens and noted a sural communicating nerve connected with the sural nerve in 87.5%. In 62%, the predominant site of union between these two nerves was in the lower one-third of the leg and ankle region. There were four types of pattern of innervation of the toes by the sural nerve. The predominant pattern was type I (45.8%), where the lateral side of the little toe was supplied by the sural nerve alone. The second most common pattern was type IV (29.2%), where the lateral two-and-a-half toes were supplied by the sural nerve alone (Eid and Hegazy, 2011). Madhavi et al. (2005) determined the cutaneous pattern of distribution of the sural nerve on the dorsum of the foot in 260 Indian feet and demonstrated 6 patterns of innervation of the toes. The reported types did not differ from those reported by Kosinski in 1926. There was no association between the innervation pattern and side or sex. Two cases of anomalous innervation of the abductor digiti quinti muscle of the foot via the sural nerve have been described (Ragno and Santoro, 1995). Amoiridis et al. (1997) reported motor fibers from the sural nerve innervating the abductor digiti minimi in 13 out of 207 individuals. The sural nerve may have an intramuscular course through the gastrocnemius muscle (Shankar and Veeramani, 2008).

PUDENDAL NERVE

The pudendal nerve arises from the ventral rami of the S2-S4 ventral rami and is formed just above the superior border of the sacrotuberous ligament and the upper fibers of the coccygeus. It leaves the pelvis via the greater sciatic foramen between the piriformis and coccygeus. It enters the gluteal region and crosses the sacrospinous ligament close to its attachment to the ischial spine, medial to the internal pudendal vessels. It accompanies the internal pudendal artery through the lesser sciatic foramen into the pudendal (Alcock's) canal on the lateral wall of the ischioanal fossa. It travels ventrally through the pudendal canal, and in the posterior part of the canal it gives rise to their main branches: the inferior rectal nerve, the perineal nerve, and the dorsal nerve of the penis or clitoris. The inferior rectal nerve was previously known as the hemorrhoidal nerve. It arises from

S3, S4, and occasionally S2. It can arise from the sacral plexus directly rather than being one of the aforementioned three terminal branches of the pudendal nerve (Aasar, 1947; Hollinshead, 1956; Bergman et al., 1984, 1988). Mahakkanukrauh et al. (2005) reported that 15 inferior rectal nerves out of 73 specimens originated independently from S4.

Several variations have been reported in the formation of the pudendal nerve and the course of its branches. Its roots can arise from both the S4 and S5 spinal nerves. Piersol (1918) reported a possible contribution from either the L5 or S1 spinal nerves. The inferior rectal branch can pierce the sacrospinous ligament on its course to the perineum. The lateral superficial perineal branch of the pudendal sometimes pierces the sacrotuberous ligament (Aasar, 1947; Bergman et al., 1984, 1988). Yi and Itoh (2010) reported an "accessory pudendal nerve" that originates primarily from the rami of S2, receiving contributions from the adjacent roots of S1 and S3. The accessory nerve had two branches: the main branch supplied the dorsum of the clitoris, and another thin branch joined to supply the area of the posterior femoral cutaneous nerve. Mahakkanukrauh et al. (2005) investigated the branching of the pudendal nerve in relation to the sacrospinous ligament in 73 sides of 37 cadavers and grouped the branching patterns as follows: Type I: one trunk (56.2%); Type II: two trunks (11%); Type III: two trunks, one being an inferior rectal nerve piercing through the sacrospinous ligament (11%); Type IV: two trunks, one being inferior rectal nerve not piercing through the sacrospinous ligament (9.5%); and Type V: three trunks (12.3%).

SACRAL MUSCULAR BRANCHES

Several muscular branches arise from the S4 ventral ramus to supply the superior surface of the levator ani and the upper part of the external anal sphincter. The levator ani can be supplied by S2, S3, or S4 ventral rami. The branches to the levator ani enter the pelvic surface of the muscle while the branch to the external anal sphincter (perineal branch of the S4) reaches the ischioanal fossa by running either through the ischiococcygeus or between the ischiococcygeus and iliococcygeus. It supplies the skin between the anus and coccyx via its cutaneous branches. The nerve to the external sphincter ani can pass between the coccygeus and levator ani instead of piercing the coccygeus (Bergman et al., 1984, 1988; Williams, 2005; Mahadevan, 2008).

REFERENCES

Aasar, Y.H., 1947. Anatomical Anomalies. Fouad I University Press, Cairo, pp. 92–101.

Adkinson, D.P., Bosse, M.J., Gaccione, D.R., Gabriel, K.R., 1991. Anatomical variations in the course of the superficial peroneal nerve. J. Bone Jt. Surg. 73A, 112–114.

Amoiridis, G., Schols, L., Ameridis, N., Przuntek, H., 1997. Motor fibers in the sural nerve of humans. Neurology 49, 1725–1728.

Apaydin, N., Basarir, K., Loukas, M., Tubbs, R.S., Uz, A., Kinik, H., 2008a. Compartmental anatomy of the superficial fibular nerve with an emphasis on fascial release operations of the leg. Surg. Radiol. Anat. 30 (1), 47–52.

Apaydin, N., Loukas, M., Kendir, S., Tubbs, R.S., Jordan, R., Tekdemir, I., Elhan, A., 2008b. The precise localization of distal motor branches of the tibial nerve in the deep posterior compartment of the leg. Surg. Radiol. Anat. 30 (4), 291–295.

Apaydin, N., Bozkurt, M., Loukas, M., Tubbs, R.S., Esmer, A.F., 2009a. The course of the inferior gluteal nerve and surgical landmarks for its localization during posterior approaches to hip. Surg. Radiol. Anat. 31 (6), 415–418.

Apaydin, N., Bozkurt, M., Loukas, M., Vefali, H., Tubbs, R.S., Esmer, A.F., 2009b. Relationships of the sural nerve with the calcaneal tendon: an anatomical study with surgical and clinical implications. Surg. Radiol. Anat. 1 (10), 775–780.

Apaydin, N., Kendir, S., Loukas, M., Tubbs, R.S., Bozkurt, M., 2013. Surgical anatomy of the superior gluteal nerve and landmarks for its localization during minimally invasive approaches to the hip. Clin. Anat. 26 (5), 614–620.

Arifoglu, Y., Sürücü, H.S., Sargon, M.F., Tanyeli, E., Yazar, F., 1997. Double superior gemellus together with double piriformis and high division of the sciatic nerve. Surg. Radiol. Anat. 19 (6), 407–408.

Aung, H.H., Sakamoto, H., Akita, K., Sato, T., 2001. Anatomical study of the obturator internus, gemelli and quadratus femoris muscles with special reference to their innervation. Anat. Rec. 263 (1), 41–52.

Babinski, M.A., Machado, F.A., Costa, W.S., 2003. A rare variation in the high division of the sciatic nerve surrounding the superior gemellus muscle. Eur. J. Morphol. 41 (1), 41–42.

Bardeen, C.R., Elting, A.W., 1901. A statistical study of the variations in the formation and position of the lumbosacral plexus in man. Anat. Anzeiger 19, 124–128 and 209–232.

Bareither, D.J., Genau, J.M., Massaro, J.C., 1990. Variation in the division of the tibial nerve: application to nerve blocks. J. Foot. Surg. 29 (6), 581–583.

Benjamin, A.C., Tuma Jr., P., Grillo, M.A., Ferreira, M.C., 1995. Surgical anatomy of the sural nerve. Rev. Hosp. Clin. Fac. Med. Sao Paulo 50, 25–29.

Bergman, R.A., Thompson, S.A., Afifi, A.K., 1984. Catalogue of Human Variations. Urban & Schwarzenberg, Baltimore and Munich, pp. 158–161.

Bergman, R.A., Thompson, S.A., Aww, A.K., Saddeh, F.A., 1988. Compendium of Human Anatomical Variations. Urban and Schwarzenburg, Baltimore, pp. 143–148.

Blair, J.M., Botte, M.J., 1994. Surgical anatomy of the superficial peroneal nerve in the ankle and foot. Clin. Orthop. Relat. Res. 305, 229–238.

Brodie, G., Shaw, E.H., Macload, P., Harris, W.A., Fawcett, E., 1892. Collective investigation on the distribution of cutaneous nerve of the dorsum of the foot. J. Anat. Physiol. 26, 89–90.

Browne, J.A., Morris, M.J., 2007. Variant superficial fibular (peroneal) nerve anatomy in the middle third of the lateral leg. Clin. Anat. 20, 996–997.

Carare, R.O., Goodwin, M., 2008. A unique variation of the sciatic nerve. Clin. Anat. 21 (8), 800–801.

Chou, L.B., Choi, L.E., Ramachandra, T., Ma, G., 2008. Variation of nerve to flexor hallucis brevis. Foot Ankle. Int. 29 (10), 1042–1044.

Cruveilhier, J., 1844. The Anatomy of the Human Body. Harper & Brothers, New York.

Eid, E.M., Hegazy, A.M., 2011. Anatomical variations of the human sural nerve and its role in clinical and surgical procedures. Clin. Anat. 24 (2), 237–245.

Eisler, P., 1892. Der Plexus lumbosacralis des Menschen. Halle.

Hollinshead, W.H., 1956. Anatomy for Surgeons. Volume 2. The Thorax, Abdomen and Pelvis. Cassell & Co. Ltd., London, pp. 636–638.

Honma, S., Jun, Y., Horiguchi, M., 1998. The human gemelli muscles and their nerve supplies. Kaibogaku Zasshi 73, 329–335.

Huban, T.R., Nayak, V.S., D'Souza, A.S., 2012. A rare variation in the innervation of the gluteus maximus muscle. A case report. Proceed. Anat. Assoc. Thai 1 (12).

Huelke, D.F., 1958. Origin of the peroneal communicating nerve in adult man. Anat. Rec. 132, 81–92.

Jacobs, L.G.H., Buxton, R.A., 1989. The course of the SGN in the lateral approach to the hip. J. Bone. Jt. Surg. 71A, 1239–1243.

Kikuchi, T., 1987. A macroscopical observation of the nerves to the pelvic floor muscles, the obturator internus, the quadratus femoris and the gemelli (in Japanese with English abstract). Sapporo. Med. J. 56, 319–332.

Kosinski, C., 1926. The course, mutual relations and distribution of the cutaneous nerves of the metazonal region of the leg and foot. J. Anat. Physiol. 60, 274–297.

Madhavi, C., Isaac, B., Antoniswamy, B., Holla, S.J., 2005. Anatomical variations of the cutaneous innervation patterns of the sural nerve on the dorsum of the foot. Clin. Anat. 18 (3), 206–209.

Mahadevan, V., 2008. Pelvic girdle and lower limb. In: Standring, S. (Ed.), Gray's Anatomy, fortyth ed. Elsevier, New York, pp. 1327–1429.

Mahakkanukrauh, P., Surin, P., Vaidhayakarn, P., 2005. Anatomical study of the pudendal nerve adjacent to the sacrospinous ligament. Clin. Anat. 18, 200–205.

Mas, N., Ozeksi, P., Ozdemir, B., Kapakin, S., Sargon, M.F., Celik, H.H., Yener, N., 2002. A case of bilateral high division of the sciatic nerves, together with a unilateral unusual course of the tibial nerve. Neuroanatomy 2, 13–15.

Natsis, K., Totlis, T., Konstantinidis, G.A., Paraskevas, G., Piagkou, M., Koebke, J., 2014. Anatomical variations between the sciatic nerve and the piriformis muscle: a contribution to surgical anatomy in piriformis syndrome. Surg. Radiol. Anat. 36 (3), 273–280.

Paraskevas, G.K., Natsis, K., Tzika, M., Ioannidis, O., 2013. Potential entrapment of an accessory superficial peroneal sensory nerve at the lateral malleolar area: a cadaveric case report and review of the literature. J. Foot Ankle Surg. 52, 92–95.

Patel, S., Shah, M., Vora, R., Zalawida, A., Rathod, S.P., 2011. A variation in the high division of the sciatic nerve and its relation with piriformis syndrome. Natl. J. Med. Res. 1 (2), 27–30.

Piersol, G.A., 1918. Human Anatomy. JB Lippincott, Philadelphia.

Pokorny, D., Jahoda, D., Veigl, D., Pinskerova, V., Sonsa, A., 2006. Topographic variations of the relationship of the sciatic nerve and the piriformis muscle and its relevance to palsy after total hip arthroplasty. Surg. Radiol. Anat. 28, 88–91.

Prakash, Bhardwaj, A.K., Singh, D.K., Rajini, T., Jayanthi, V., Singh, G., 2010. Anatomic variations of superficial peroneal nerve: clinical implications of a cadaver study. Ital. J. Anat. Embryol. 115 (3), 223–228.

Ragno, M., Santoro, L., 1995. Motor fibers in human sural nerve. Electromyogr. Clin. Neurophysiol. 35 (1), 61–63.

Rayegani, S.M., Daneshtalab, E., Bahrami, M.H., Eliaspour, D., Raeissadat, S.A., Rezaei, S., Babaee, M., 2011. Prevalence of accessory deep peroneal nerve in referred patients to an electrodiagnostic medicine clinic. J. Brachial Plexus Peripher. Nerve Inj. 6 (1), 3.

Santanu, B., Pitbaran, C., Sudeshna, M., Hasi, D., 2013. Different neuromuscular variations in the gluteal region. IJAV 6, 136–139.

Shankar, N., Veeramani, R., 2008. An unusual origin and intramuscular course of the sural nerve: a case report. Neuroanatomy 7, 79–82.

Solomon, L.B., Ferris, L., Tedman, R., Henneberg, M., 2001. Surgical anatomy of the sural and superficial fibular nerves with an emphasis on the approach to the lateral malleolus. J. Anat. 199 (6), 717–723.

Tubbs, R.S., Miller, J., Loukas, M., Shoja, M.M., Shokouhi, G., Cohen-Gadol, A.A., 2009. Surgical and anatomical landmarks for the perineal branch of the posterior femoral cutaneous nerve: implications in perineal pain syndromes. Laboratory investigation. J. Neurosurg. 111 (2), 332–335.

Tunali, S., Cankara, N., Albay, S., 2011. A rare case of communicating branch between the posterior femoral cutaneous and the sciatic nerves. Rom. J. Morphol. Embryol. 52 (1), 203–205.

Tzika, M., Paraskevas, G.K., Kitsoulis, P., 2012. The accessory deep peroneal nerve: a review of the literature. Foot 22 (3), 232–234.

von Lanz, B., Wachsmuth, W., 2004. Praktische Anatomie. Springer-Verlag, Berlin.

Von Reinman, R., 1984. Uberzählige nervi peronei beim menschen. Accessory peroneal nerves in the human. Anat. Anzeiger 155, 257−267.

Watt, T., Hariharan, A.R., Brzezinski, D.W., Caird, M.S., Zeller, J.L., 2014. Branching patterns and localization of the common fibular (peroneal) nerve: an anatomical basis for planning safe surgical approaches. Surg. Radiol. Anat. 36 (8), 821−828.

Webb, J., Moorjani, N., Radford, M., 2000. Anatomy of the sural nerve and its relation to the Achilles tendon. Foot Ankle. Int. 21, 475−477.

Williams, A., 2005. Pelvic girdle and lower limb. In: Standring, S. (Ed.), Gray's Anatomy, thirtyninth ed. Elsevier, New York, pp. 1456−1499.

Wilson, J.T., 1889. Abnormal distribution of the nerve to the quadratus femoris in man, with remarks on its significance. J. Anat. Physiol. 23 (3), 354−357.

Yi, S.Q., Itoh, M., 2010. A unique variation of the pudendal nerve. Clin. Anat. 23 (8), 907−908.

CHAPTER 17

Microanatomy of the Sacral Plexus Roots

ANNA CARRERA • FRANCISCO REINA • JAVIER MORATINOS-DELGADO •
VIRGINIA GARCÍA-GARCÍA • ANDRÉ P. BOEZAART • MIGUEL A. REINA

The sacral plexus is formed by the lumbosacral trunk, which includes the anterior branch from the fifth lumbar nerve root, a branch from the anterior fourth lumbar nerve root, and the anterior branches of the first, second, and third sacral nerve roots, as well as a part of the anterior fourth sacral nerve root. The remaining sacral nerve roots join to form a coccygeal plexus. The inferior part of the sacral plexus is small and plexiform and is formed mainly from the third sacral nerve root joined to a part of the fourth sacral nerve root and a small nerve anastomosis from the second sacral nerve root (Fig. 17.1).

Our group examined the motor, sensory, and sympathetic nerves from their origins after they entered or exited the subarachnoid spaces within the nerve root cuffs to the epidural space level and where they entered or exited through the intervertebral canals. Cross sections were obtained at each level:

1. The first cross section was a full transverse cross section of the nerve root cuff between its entry (afferent sensory nerves) or exit (efferent motor nerves) into or from the dural sac and the dorsal root ganglion (DRG). This cross section was obtained perpendicular to the longitudinal axis of the nerve root cuff.
2. The second transverse cross section was a full cross section perpendicular to the longitudinal axis of the nerve root cuff at the level of the DRG, including the anterior efferent motor nerve roots at that level.
3. The third transverse cross section consisted of a complete transverse cross section perpendicular to the longitudinal axis of the nerve root cuff, immediately peripheral to the DRG.
4. A final cross section was obtained 2 mm more peripheral to the third cut.

The term "nerve root" may be confusing if it is used to refer to structures found at different levels, as they may not share similar morphology. Nerve rootlets leave and enter the spinal cord at the ventrolateral and dorsolateral sulci, respectively. Anterior rootlets contain predominately efferent fibers from the ventral horn and carry motor signals to voluntary muscles. In the thoracic and upper lumbar regions, they also carry preganglionic sympathetic fibers from the lateral horns. It may, however, be questioned whether the anterior nerve roots in the cauda equina should be called rootlets or nerve roots; the term subarachnoid nerve root may be more appropriate. Subarachnoid nerve roots joined the spinal cord centrally in one to two anterior nerve roots and two to five posterior nerve roots to exit (anterior roots) or enter (posterior roots) through the anterolateral subarachnoid space toward the nerve root cuffs. Inside the nerve root cuffs, these nerves are referred to as anterior (efferent motor) and posterior (afferent sensory) nerve roots, respectively.

At the level of the DRG, the bodies of pseudounipolar nerve cells and their sensory axons were present (Figs. 17.3, 17.7, 17.11, 17.15, 17.24–17.32). At similar cross-sectional levels where the DRGs were found, anterior motor nerve roots were present inside the neural foramina or vertebral canal (Figs. 17.33–17.38).

The external parts of nerve root cuffs were enveloped in transitional tissue, similar in appearance to the network of interlacing collagen fibers found in the epineurium of peripheral nerves and dura mater of the dural sac (Figs. 17.2, 17.6, 17.10, 17.14). All structures that look like fascicles (pseudo-fascicles) found in the neural foramina (intervertebral canals) and the anterior and posterior nerve roots were surrounded by a transitional arachnoid layer with different properties from the arachnoid layer inside the dural sac (Figs. 17.2, 17.6, 17.10, 17.14).

Surgical Anatomy of the Sacral Plexus and Its Branches. https://doi.org/10.1016/B978-0-323-77602-8.00017-9

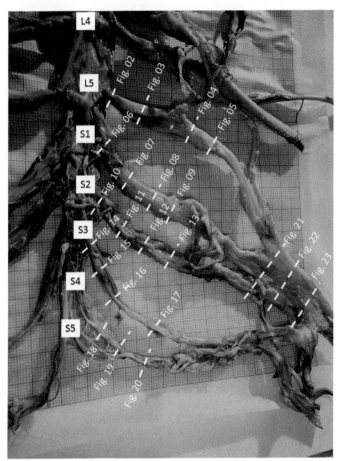

FIG. 17.1 Human dural sac, nerve root cuffs, and roots of the lumbar-sacral plexus. The positions of the cuts made for the subsequent figures are shown. The dural sac appears flattened due to the absence of cerebrospinal fluid after the dissection.

At the level of the DRG, cross-sectional images demonstrated that the transitional arachnoid layer was replaced by a membrane that resembled the perineurium of peripheral nerves, with multiple layers of perineurial cells (Figs. 17.24–17.26, 17.31–17.34, 17.36-17.38).

The true perineuriums were seen only immediately peripheral to the DRG, at the levels of the microscopic origins of peripheral nerves (Figs. 17.4, 17.5, 17.8, 17.9, 17.12, 17.13, 17.16–17.19).

The macroscopic origin of peripheral nerves outside the neuroforamens is an arbitrary description from gross anatomy and did not correspond with microscopic findings. The DRGs occupied different positions inside the neural foramina (or vertebral canals) at the different vertebral levels. At some vertebral levels, the true origins of peripheral nerves were found within the intervertebral canal, whereas at other levels, this was not the case.

Intraneural plexuses of fascicles have been described in peripheral nerves. The question is where these intraneural plexuses start.

The cross sections performed centrally to the nerve root cuff and perpendicular to the longitudinal axis of the nerve root cuff showed the first and most proximal fascicular interconnections. In peripheral nerves, however, these fascicular interconnections start immediately peripheral to the DRG. This finding was not identical for each vertebral level we studied.

Details of the microanatomy of the sciatic nerve at its origin are included. The microanatomy of sympathetic trunks at the lumbar level was also studied and showed the differences between the histology of somatic nerve root ganglia and sympathetic ganglia.

Fig. 17.1 shows the gross anatomy of a dissected human sacral plexus from which our group obtained the samples shown in the cross sections (Figs. 17.2–17.47).

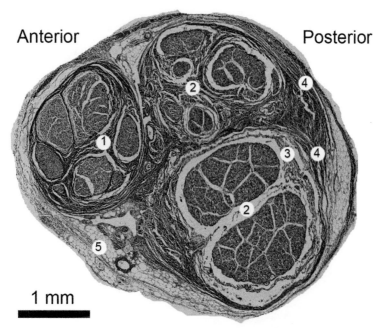

FIG. 17.2 Transverse cross section of the fifth lumbar vertebral nerve root cuff between the dural sac and the dorsal root ganglion. The image shows the anterior and posterior nerve roots separately enveloped by a transitional arachnoid layer and dura mater on the outer aspect. In the area of the dural cuffs, adipose tissue appears scarcely distributed among the dural layers. The dura mater at this level appears thinner than in the dural sac, although the overall thickness of the dura that covered nerve roots was greater. 1 = anterior nerve root, 2 = posterior nerve root, 3 = arachnoid layer, 4 = dura mater, 5 = adipose tissue. Stained with hematoxylin and eosin. Magnification ×40. Bar = 1 mm.

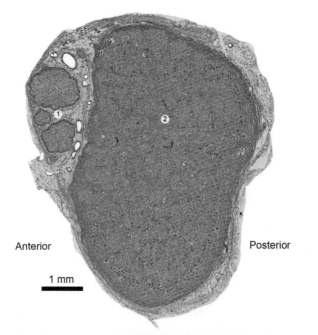

FIG. 17.3 Transverse cross section of a nerve root cuff at the level of the fifth lumbar dorsal root ganglion (DRG). The image includes the anterior nerve root at the same level. Three anterior nerve roots were found. 1 = anterior nerve roots. 2 = DRG. Stained with hematoxylin and eosin. Magnification ×40. Bar = 1 mm.

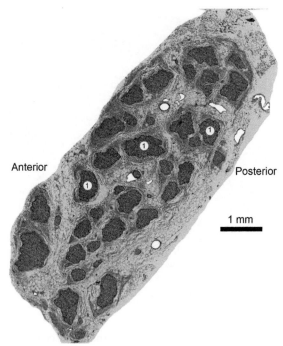

Anterior

Posterior

1 mm

FIG. 17.4 Transverse cross section of the fifth lumbar nerve root located immediately distal (peripheral) to the dorsal root ganglion. Origin of a peripheral nerve. 1 = fascicle. Stained with hematoxylin and eosin. Magnification ×40. Bar = 1 mm.

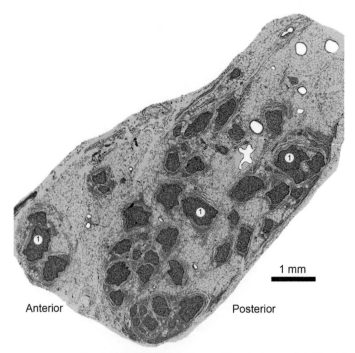

1 mm

Anterior

Posterior

FIG. 17.5 Transverse cross section of the fifth lumbar nerve root located more distal (peripheral) to the dorsal root ganglion. Peripheral nerve. 1 = fascicle. Stained with hematoxylin and eosin. Magnification ×40. Bar = 1 mm.

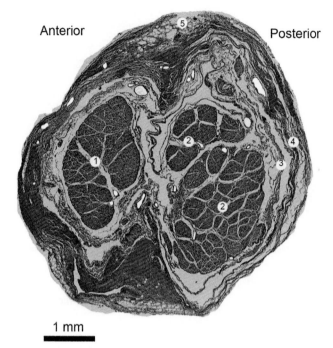

Anterior Posterior

1 mm

FIG. 17.6 Transverse cross section of the nerve root cuff between dural sac and dorsal root ganglion at first sacral vertebral level. The image shows the anterior and posterior nerve roots, each enveloped by a transitional arachnoid layer and outside by dura mater. 1 = anterior nerve root, 2 = posterior nerve root, 3 = arachnoid layer, 4 = dura mater, 5 = adipose tissue. Stained with hematoxylin and eosin. Magnification ×40. Bar = 1 mm.

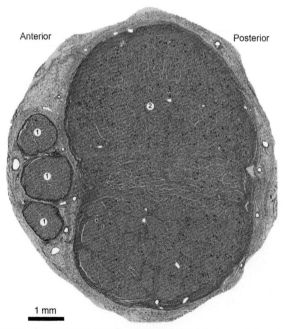

Anterior Posterior

1 mm

FIG. 17.7 Transverse cross section of the nerve root cuff at the level of the first sacral dorsal root ganglion (DRG) (2), showing the anterior nerve root (1) at the same level. Three anterior nerve roots were found. 1 = anterior nerve root, 2 = DRG. Stained with hematoxylin and eosin. Magnification ×40. Bar = 1 mm.

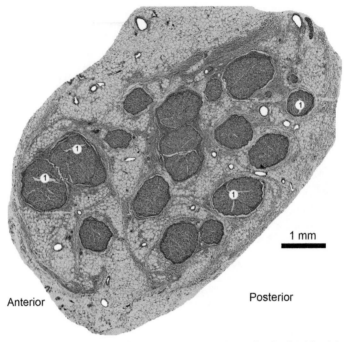

FIG. 17.8 Transverse cross section of the first sacral nerve root immediately distal (peripheral) to the dorsal root ganglion. Origin of a peripheral nerve. 1 = fascicle. Stained with hematoxylin and eosin. Magnification ×40. Bar = 1 mm.

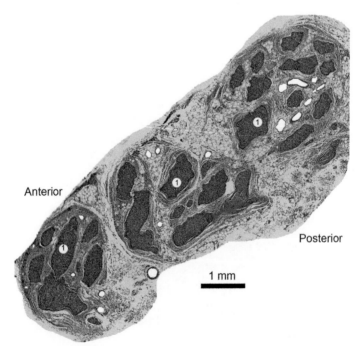

FIG. 17.9 Transverse cross section of the first sacral motor nerve root more distal (peripheral) to the dorsal root ganglion. Peripheral nerve. 1 = fascicle. Stained with hematoxylin and eosin. Magnification ×40. Bar = 1 mm.

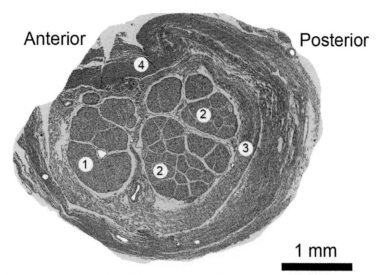

FIG. 17.10 Transverse cross section of the nerve root cuff between the dural sac and dorsal root ganglion (DRG) at the second sacral vertebral level. The image shows the anterior and posterior nerve roots each enveloped by a transitional arachnoid layer and dura mater. This cross section was obtained near and proximal (central) to the DRG. The axons seen within the pseudo-fascicles of the posterior nerve root are the same axons located within the DRG in Fig. 17.15. 1 = anterior nerve root, 2 = posterior nerve root, 3 = arachnoid layer, 4 = dura mater. Stained with hematoxylin and eosin. Magnification ×40. Bar = 1 mm.

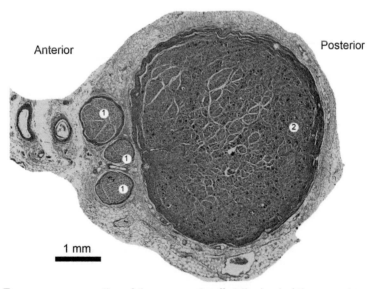

FIG. 17.11 Transverse cross section of the nerve root cuff at the level of the second sacral dorsal root ganglion (DRG) including the anterior nerve root (1) at the same level. Three anterior nerve roots were found. 1 = anterior nerve root. 2 = DRG. Stained with hematoxylin and eosin. Magnification ×40. Bar = 1 mm.

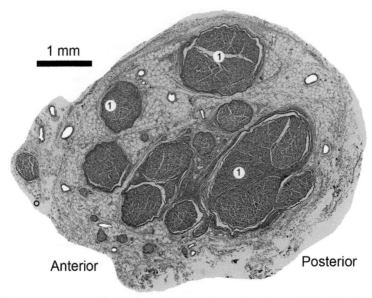

FIG. 17.12 Transverse cross section of the second sacral nerve root immediately distal (peripheral) to the dorsal root ganglion. Origin of peripheral nerve. 1 = fascicle. Stained with hematoxylin and eosin. Magnification ×40. Bar = 1 mm.

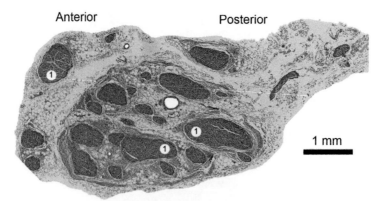

FIG. 17.13 Transverse cross section of the second sacral nerve root more distal (peripheral) to the dorsal root ganglion. Peripheral nerve. 1 = fascicle. Stained with hematoxylin and eosin. Magnification ×40. Bar = 1 mm.

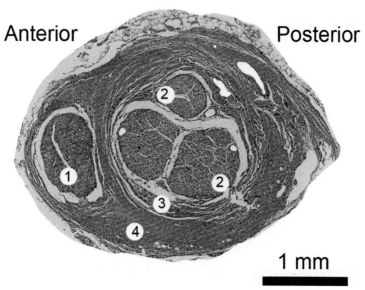

FIG. 17.14 Transverse cross section of the nerve root cuff between the dural sac and the dorsal root ganglion at the third sacral vertebral level. The image shows the anterior and posterior nerve roots each enveloped by a transitional arachnoid layer and dura mater. 1 = anterior nerve root, 2 = posterior nerve root, 3 = arachnoid layer, 4 = dura mater. Stained with hematoxylin and eosin. Magnification ×40. Bar = 1 mm.

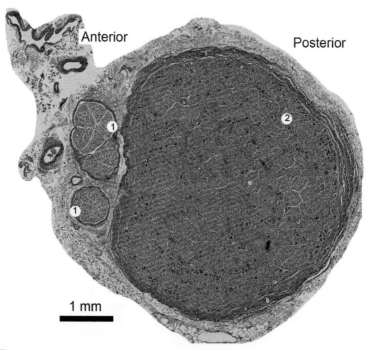

FIG. 17.15 Transverse cross section of the nerve root cuff at the third sacral dorsal root ganglion (DRG) including the anterior nerve root at the same level. Two anterior nerve roots were found. 1 = anterior nerve root, 2 = DRG. Stained with hematoxylin and eosin. Magnification ×40. Bar = 1 mm.

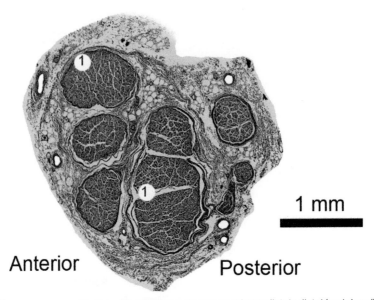

FIG. 17.16 Transverse cross section of the third sacral nerve root immediately distal (peripheral) to the dorsal root ganglion. Origin of a peripheral nerve. 1 = fascicle. Stained with hematoxylin and eosin. Magnification ×40. Bar = 1 mm.

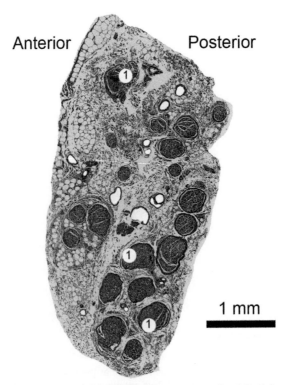

FIG. 17.17 Transverse cross section of the third sacral nerve root more distal (peripheral) to the dorsal root ganglion. Peripheral nerve. 1 = fascicle. Stained with hematoxylin and eosin. Magnification ×40. Bar = 1 mm.

Anterior   Posterior

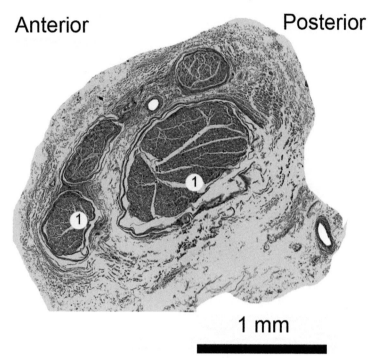

1 mm

FIG. 17.18 Transverse cross section of the fourth lumbar nerve root immediately distal (peripheral) to the dorsal root ganglion. Origin of a peripheral nerve. 1 = fascicle. Stained with hematoxylin and eosin. Magnification ×40. Bar = 1 mm.

Anterior   Posterior

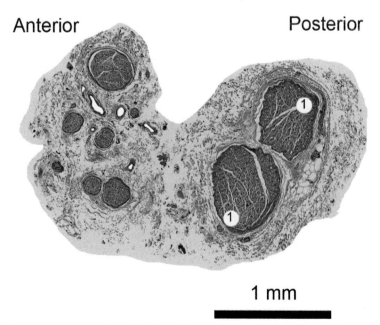

1 mm

FIG. 17.19 Transverse cross section of the fourth lumbar motor nerve root more distal (peripheral) to the dorsal root ganglion. Peripheral nerve. 1 = fascicle. Stained with hematoxylin and eosin. Magnification ×60. Bar = 1 mm.

Anterior   Posterior

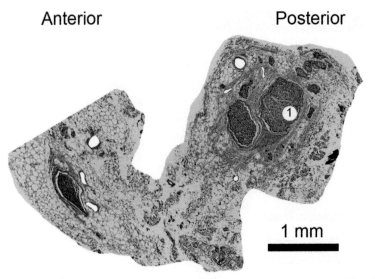

1 mm

FIG. 17.20 Transverse cross section of the fourth and fifth sacral nerve roots more peripheral to the cross section from Fig. 17.19. 1 = fascicle. Stained with hematoxylin and eosin. Magnification ×40. Bar = 1 mm.

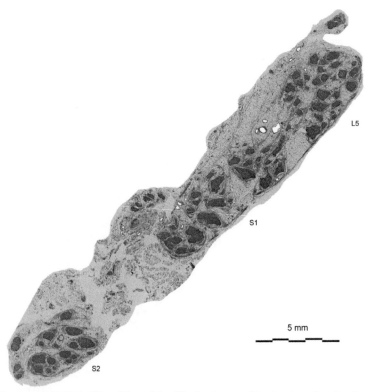

L5

S1

5 mm

S2

FIG. 17.21 Transverse cross section of the origin of the lumbosacral trunk, where the structures from L5, S1, and S2 nerve roots converge. Cross section obtained more peripheral to the cross sections of Figs. 17.5, 17.9, and 17.13. Stained with hematoxylin and eosin. Magnification ×40. Bar = 5 mm.

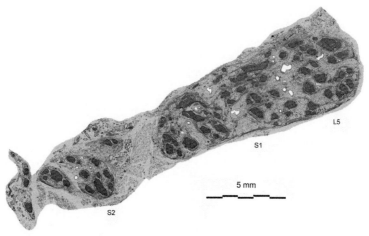

FIG. 17.22 Transverse cross section of the lumbosacral trunk, where the structures from L5, S1, and S2 nerve roots can be seen. Cross section obtained more peripheral to the cross section of Fig. 17.21. Stained with hematoxylin and eosin. Magnification ×40. Bar = 5 mm.

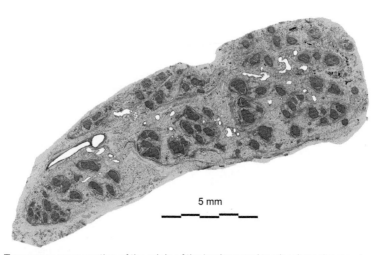

FIG. 17.23 Transverse cross section of the origin of the lumbosacral trunk, where the structures from L5, S1, and S2 nerve roots can be seen. Cross section obtained distal to the cross section of Fig. 17.22. Stained with hematoxylin and eosin. Magnification ×40. Bar = 5 mm.

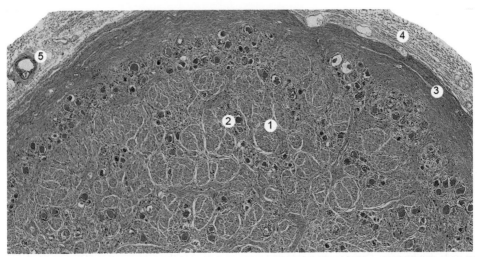

FIG. 17.24 Transverse cross section of the nerve root cuff at the level of the first sacral dorsal root ganglion, showing the details of Fig. 17.7 at a greater level of magnification. 1 = axons of sensory neurons, 2 = cell bodies of the sensory neurons, 3 = perineurium-like, 4 = dura mater—like, 5 = vessel. Stained with hematoxylin and eosin. Magnification ×80.

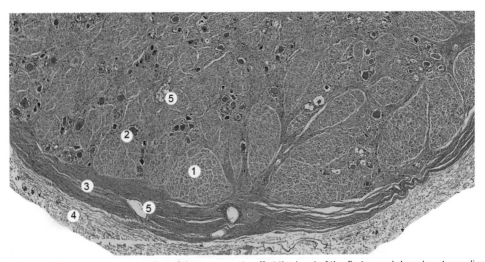

FIG. 17.25 Transverse cross section of the nerve root cuff at the level of the first sacral dorsal root ganglion, showing the details of Fig. 17.7 at higher magnification. 1 = axons of sensory neurons, 2 = cell bodies of the sensory neurons, 3 = perineurium-like, 4 = dura mater—like, 5 = vessel. Stained with hematoxylin and eosin. Magnification ×80.

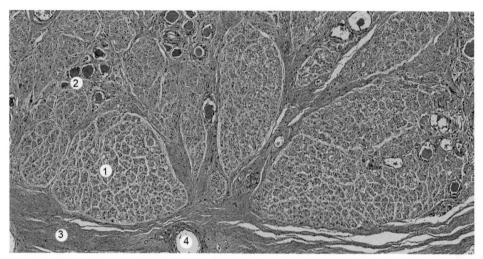

FIG. 17.26 Transverse cross section of the nerve root cuff at the level of the first sacral dorsal root ganglion, showing the details of Fig. 17.7 at higher magnification. 1 = axons of sensory neurons, 2 = cell bodies of the sensory neurons, 3 = perineurium-like, 4 = vessel. Stained with hematoxylin and eosin. Magnification ×160.

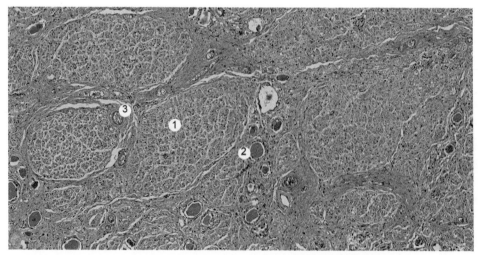

FIG. 17.27 Transverse cross section of the nerve root cuff at the level of the first sacral dorsal root ganglion, showing the details of Fig. 17.7 at higher magnification. 1 = axons of sensory neurons, 2 = cell bodies of the sensory neurons, 3 = vessel. Stained with hematoxylin and eosin. Magnification ×160.

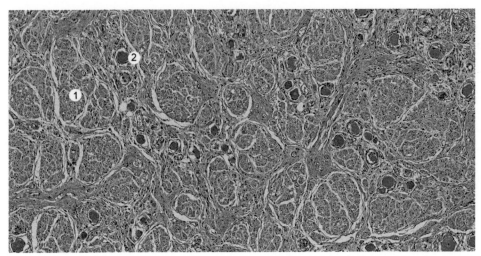

FIG. 17.28 Transverse cross section of the nerve root cuff at the level of the first sacral dorsal root ganglion, showing the details of Fig. 17.7 at higher magnification. 1 = axons of sensory neurons, 2 = cell body of the sensory neurons. Stained with hematoxylin and eosin. Magnification ×160.

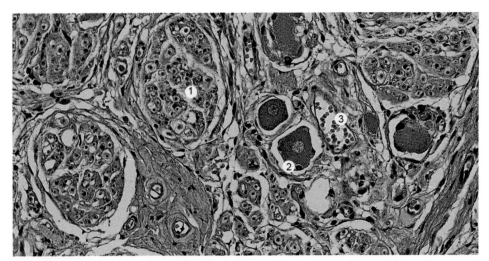

FIG. 17.29 Transverse cross section of the nerve root cuff at the level of the first sacral dorsal root ganglion, showing the details of Fig. 17.7 at higher magnification. 1 = axons of sensory neurons, 2 = cell bodies of the sensory neurons, 3 = vessel. Stained with hematoxylin and eosin. Magnification ×600.

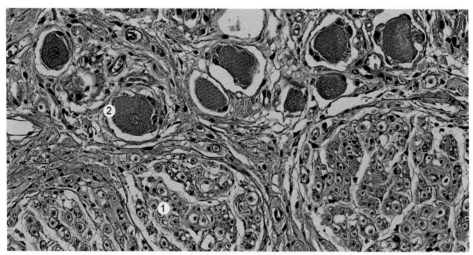

FIG. 17.30 Transverse cross section of the nerve root cuff at the level of the first sacral dorsal root ganglion, showing the details of Fig. 17.7 at higher magnification. 1 = axons of sensory neurons, 2 = cell bodies of the sensory neurons. Stained with hematoxylin and eosin. Magnification ×600.

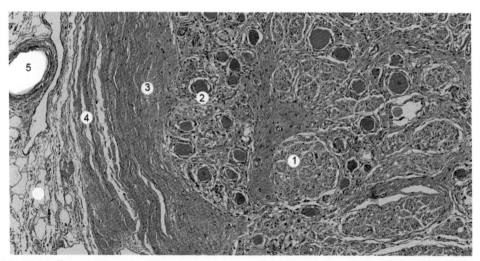

FIG. 17.31 Transverse cross section of the nerve root cuff at the level of the first sacral dorsal root ganglion, showing the details of Fig. 17.7 at higher magnification. 1 = axons of sensory neurons, 2 = cell bodies of the sensory neurons, 3 = perineurium-like, 4 = dura mater–like, 5 = vessel. Stained with hematoxylin and eosin. Magnification ×200.

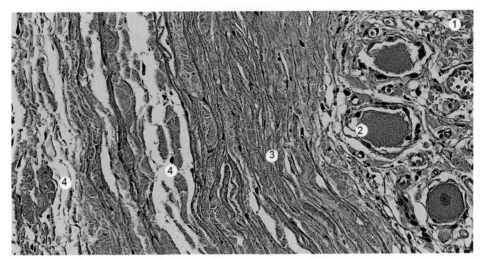

FIG. 17.32 Transverse cross section of the nerve root cuff at the level of the first sacral dorsal root ganglion, showing the details of Fig. 17.7 at higher magnification. 1 = axons of motor neurons, 2 = cell body of the sensory neurons, 3 = perineurium-like, 4 = dura mater–like. Stained with hematoxylin and eosin. Magnification ×600.

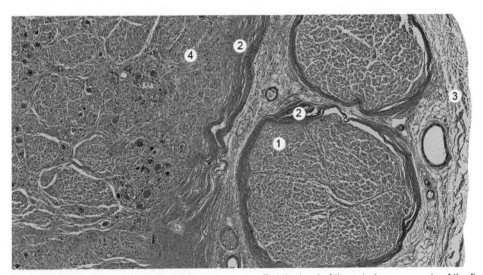

FIG. 17.33 Transverse cross section of the nerve root cuff at the level of the anterior nerve roots of the first sacral nerve root cuff, showing the details of Fig. 17.7 at higher magnification. 1 = axons of motor neurons, 2 = perineurium-like, 3 = dura mater–like, 4 = axons of sensory neurons. Stained with hematoxylin and eosin. Magnification ×80.

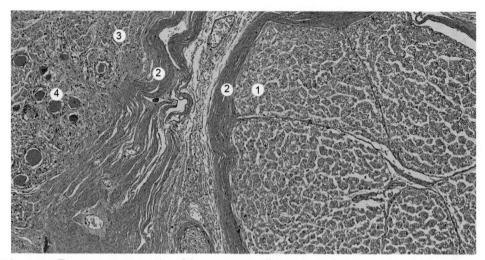

FIG. 17.34 Transverse cross section of the nerve root cuff at the level of the anterior nerve roots of the first sacral nerve root cuff, showing the details of Fig. 17.7 at higher magnification. 1 = axons of motor neurons, 2 = perineurium-like, 3 = axons of sensory neurons, 4 = cell bodies of the sensory neurons. Stained with hematoxylin and eosin. Magnification ×160.

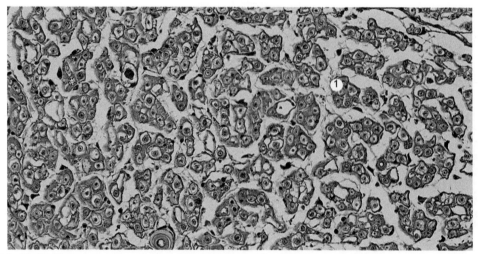

FIG. 17.35 Transverse cross section of the nerve root cuff at the level of the anterior nerve roots of the first sacral nerve root cuff, showing the details of Fig. 17.7 at higher magnification. 1 = axons of motor neurons. Stained with hematoxylin and eosin. Magnification ×600.

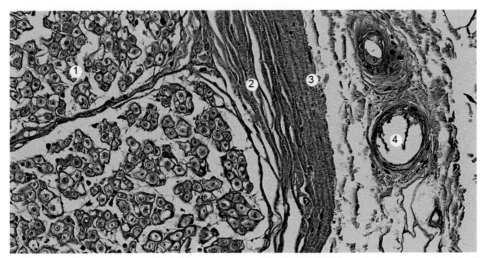

FIG. 17.36 Transverse cross section of the nerve root cuff at the level of the anterior nerve roots of the first sacral nerve root cuff, showing the details of Fig. 17.7 at higher magnification. 1 = axons of motor neurons, 2 = perineurium-like, 3 = dura mater–like. Stained with hematoxylin and eosin. Magnification ×600.

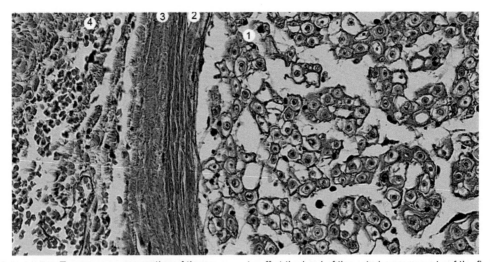

FIG. 17.37 Transverse cross section of the nerve root cuff at the level of the anterior nerve roots of the first sacral nerve root cuff, showing the details of Fig. 17.7 at higher magnification. 1 = axons of motor neurons, 2 = perineurium-like, 3 = collagen fiber layer close to perineurium-like layer, 4 = dura mater–like. Stained with hematoxylin and eosin. Magnification ×800.

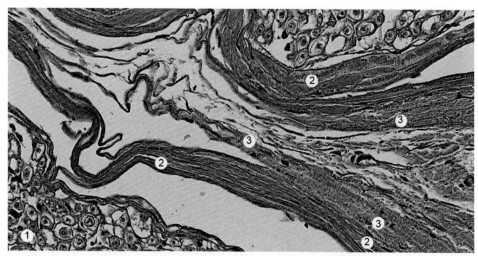

FIG. 17.38 Transverse cross section of the nerve root cuff at the level of the anterior nerve roots of the first sacral nerve root cuff, showing the details of Fig. 17.7 at higher magnification. 1 = axons of motor neurons, 2 = perineurium-like, 3 = collagen fibers between two anterior nerve roots. Stained with hematoxylin and eosin. Magnification ×800.

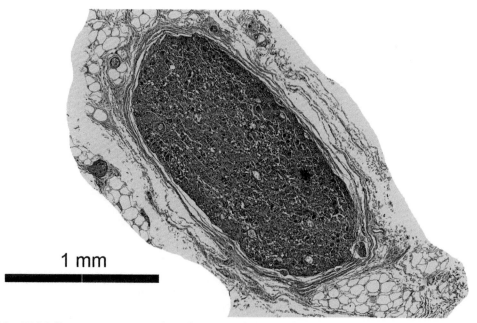

FIG. 17.39 Transverse cross section of a sympathetic ganglion in the lumbar region. Stained with hematoxylin and eosin. Magnification ×80.

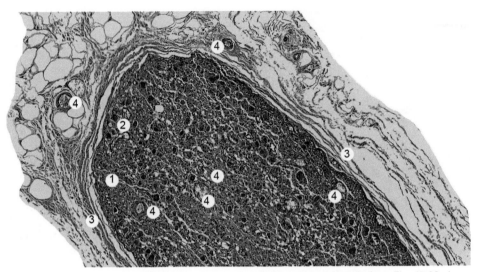

FIG. 17.40 Details of the sympathetic axons and sympathetic body nerve cells from Fig. 17.39 shown at higher magnification. 1 = axons of sympathetic neurons, 2 = cell bodies of the sympathetic neurons, 3 = collagen fiber layers, 4 = vessel. Stained with hematoxylin and eosin. Magnification ×160.

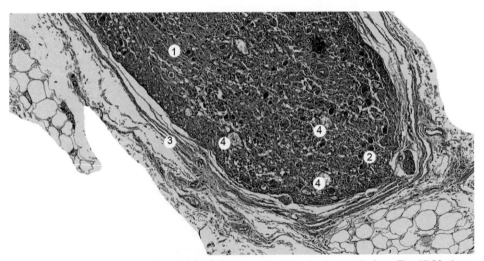

FIG. 17.41 Details of the sympathetic axons and sympathetic body nerve cells from Fig. 17.39 shown at higher magnification. 1 = axons of sympathetic neurons, 2 = cell bodies of the sympathetic neurons, 3 = collagen fiber layers, 4 = vessel. Stained with hematoxylin and eosin. Magnification ×160.

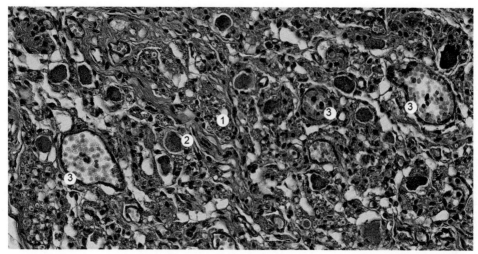

FIG. 17.42 Details of the sympathetic axons and sympathetic body nerve cells from Fig. 17.39 shown at higher magnification. 1 = axons of sympathetic neurons, 2 = cell bodies of the sympathetic neurons, 3 = vessel. Stained with hematoxylin and eosin. Magnification ×600.

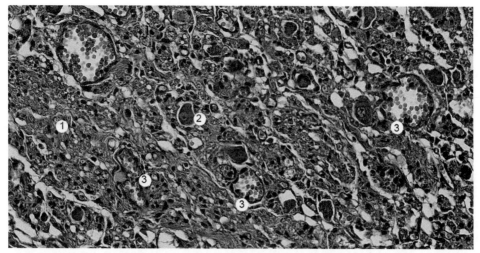

FIG. 17.43 Details of the sympathetic axons and sympathetic body nerve cells from Fig. 17.39 shown at higher magnification. 1 = axons of sympathetic neurons, 2 = cell bodies of the sympathetic neurons, 3 = vessel. Stained with hematoxylin and eosin. Magnification ×600.

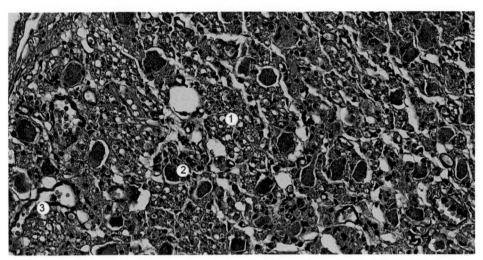

FIG. 17.44 Details of the sympathetic axons and sympathetic body nerve cells from Fig. 17.39 shown at higher magnification. 1 = axons of sympathetic neurons, 2 = cell bodies of the sympathetic neurons, 3 = vessel. Stained with hematoxylin and eosin. Magnification ×600.

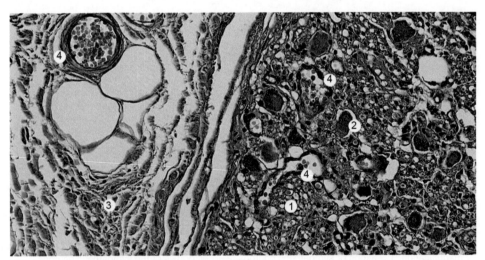

FIG. 17.45 Details of the sympathetic axons and sympathetic body nerve cells from Fig. 17.39 shown at higher magnification. 1 = axons of sympathetic neurons, 2 = cell bodies of the sympathetic neurons, 3 = collagen fiber layers, 4 = vessel. Stained with hematoxylin and eosin. Magnification ×600.

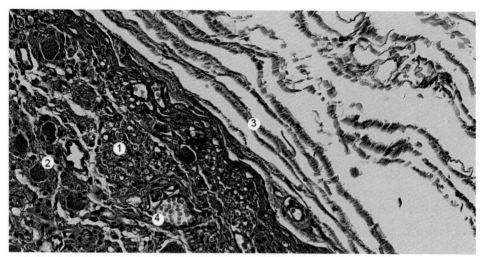

FIG. 17.46 Details of the sympathetic axons and sympathetic body nerve cells from Fig. 17.39 shown at higher magnification. 1 = axons of sympathetic neurons, 2 = cell bodies of the sympathetic neurons, 3 = collagen fiber layers, 4 = vessel. Stained with hematoxylin and eosin. Magnification ×600.

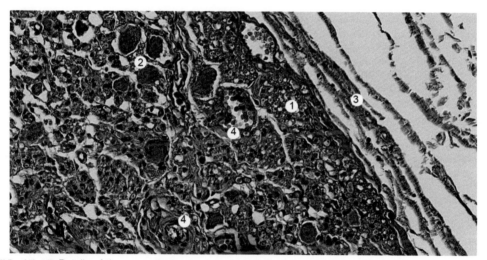

FIG. 17.47 Details of the sympathetic axons and sympathetic body nerve cells from Fig. 17.39 shown at higher magnification. 1 = axons of sympathetic neurons, 2 = cell bodies of the sympathetic neurons, 3 = collagen fiber layers, 4 = vessel. Stained with hematoxylin and eosin. Magnification ×600.

FURTHER READING

Reina, M.A., 2015. Atlas of Functional Anatomy for Regional Anesthesia and Pain Medicine. Human Structure, Ultra-structure, and 3D Reconstruction Images. Springer, New York, 1–935.

FIG. 17.24

CHAPTER 18

Axial Sections of the Nerves of the Lower Limb. Anatomy and Microanatomy

FRANCISCO REINA • MIGUEL A. REINA • PALOMA FERNÁNDEZ •
XAVIER SALA-BLANCH • ANDRÉ P. BOEZAART • ANNA CARRERA

INTRODUCTION

The lower limb nerves originate from the lumbar and sacral plexuses. Each one has specific muscle group and cutaneous innervations. Herein, muscles, vessels, and nerves are shown in cross-sections. Twenty axial sections (Figs. 18.1–18.20) from a total of 91 (thickness slice = 1 cm) human cadaveric lower limbs were analyzed in this chapter.

The **femoral nerve** originates from the lumbar plexus from the dorsal divisions of the second to fourth lumbar ventral rami. It is initially located in the iliac fossa at the sulcus formed between the iliacus muscle and the lateral edge of the psoas major muscle (Fig. 18.1, *axial* section 5). The femoral nerve accompanies the iliopsoas muscle and is in the same fascial compartment as this muscle. It then enters the anterior surface of the lower limb by passing through the femoral ring under the inguinal ligament. At this point, the femoral nerve has a bandlike appearance, and the iliopsoas fascia covers it and forms the iliopectineal arch (Figs. 18.2 and 18.3, *axial* sections 8 and 10). This arch separates the femoral nerve from the femoral artery, which runs medial to it. The femoral vein, in turn, is situated medial to the artery. Once the femoral nerve reaches the femoral triangle, the nerve is divided into several terminal branches that are distributed to the anterior aspect of the thigh. The deep terminal branches are responsible for the motor innervation of the muscle group of the anterior of thigh—the quadriceps femoris and sartorius muscles—and also provide partial motor innervation to the pectineus and adductor magnus muscles. The

superficial terminal branches are cutaneous and are distributed along the anterior subcutaneous surface of the thigh (Fig. 18.4, *axial* section 16). One of these cutaneous branches, the **saphenous nerve**, descends with the femoral vessels through the femoral triangle and the adductor canal (Fig. 18.5, *axial* section 19). Here, it is initially located lateral to the femoral artery and, progressively along the adductor canal, it moves anterior to it (Figs. 18.6 and 18.7, *axial* sections 25 and 31). Upon reaching the knee, at the distal opening of the adductor canal, it becomes superficial by crossing the vastoadductor membrane and, occasionally, the belly of the sartorius muscle (Figs. 18.8 and 18.9, *axial* sections 37 and 40). From here, it continues distally at the medial aspect of the leg to reach the medial malleolus. It is often thought of as a purely cutaneous nerve here, but Sarrafian has clearly demonstrated that it also innervates the medial aspects of the ankle joint. At the medial aspect of the leg below the knee and at the ankle joint, it is closely related to the great saphenous vein (Fig. 18.15, *axial* section 61).

The anterolateral cutaneous region of the thigh is innervated by the **lateral femoral cutaneous nerve**. This nerve emerges from dorsal divisions of the lumbar plexus and is located on the lateral border of the psoas major muscle. It crosses transversally on the surface of the iliacus muscle to reach the anterior superior iliac spine (Figs. 18.1 and 18.2, *axial* sections 5 and 8). At this point it becomes superficial and passes medial to the sartorius muscle's insertion point where it ends up as two or three cutaneous

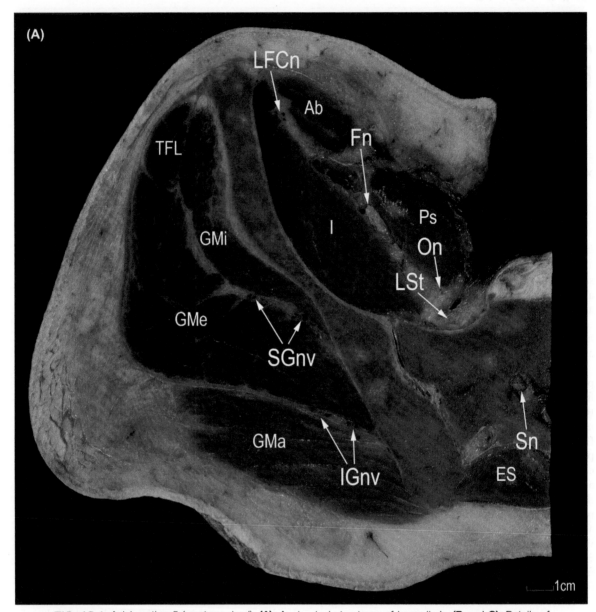

FIG. 18.1 Axial section 5 (most proximal). **(A)**: Anatomical structures of lower limb. **(B** and **C)**: Details of microanatomy. Studied area within the axial section in Fig. 18.25. *Ab*, anterolateral abdominal wall; *ES*, erector spinae; *Fn*, femoral nerve; *Gmi*, gluteus minimus; *Gme*, gluteus medius; *Gma*, gluteus maximus; *I*, iliacus; *Ignv*, inferior gluteal; *LCFn*, lateral femoral cutaneous nerve; *LSt*, lumbosacral trunk; *On*, obturator nerve; *Ps*, psoas major; *Sn*, sacral nerve; *SGnv*, superior gluteal nerve and vessels; *TFL*, tensor fasciae latae; nerve and vessels.

branches on the anterolateral region of the thigh (Fig. 18.3, *axial* section 10).

The **obturator nerve** originates from the anterior divisions of the lumbar plexus and emerges at the medial edge of the psoas major muscle (Fig. 18.1, *axial* section 5). It initially descends anterior to the sacroiliac joint and deep to the external iliac vessels. At this level it is located medial to the external iliac vein

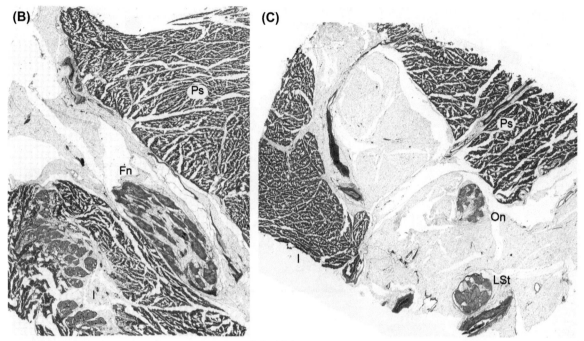

FIG. 18.1   cont'd.

(Fig. 18.2, *axial* section 8). Following an anterior and caudal direction at the level of the lesser pelvis, it reaches the obturator canal, in the superior part of the obturator foramen, under the superior pubic ramus (Fig. 18.3, *axial* section 10). In this canal, it is accompanied by the obturator artery and vein, and then crosses the superior edge of the obturator internus muscle, the obturator membrane and the obturator externus muscle, innervating this latter muscle. Generally, before exiting the obturator canal, it divides into anterior and posterior branches that supply motor innervation to the muscles of the adductor group of the thigh. The **anterior branch** is located superficial to the adductor brevis muscle and deep to the pectineus and adductor longus muscles (Figs. 18.4 and 18.5, *axial* sections 16 and 19). From this branch generally emerges a cutaneous branch that reaches and provides sensory innervation to a variable portion of skin at the medial surface of the lower third of the thigh and the knee. The **posterior branch** is located between the adductor brevis and adductor magnus muscles (Figs. 18.4 and 18.5, *axial* sections 16 and 19). This branch innervates the adductor magnus muscle and also the obturator externus muscle

partially. Furthermore, some articular branches reach the popliteal fossa, passing through the adductor magnus in the adductor canal, to form part of the posterior genicular nervous plexus that innervate the posterior knee capsule.

The **sciatic nerve** originates as the terminal branch of the sacral plexus (from the anterior and posterior divisions of the fourth–fifth lumbar to the 3rd sacral ventral rami) and is formed by the **tibial** and **common peroneal** nerves. It forms in the posterior wall of the lesser pelvis and is placed on the anterior surface of the piriformis muscle (Fig. 18.3, *axial* section 10). It leaves the pelvis by passing through the infrapiriform space of the greater sciatic foramen and reaches the gluteal region where the nerve is deep to the gluteus maximus muscle. It travels distally by crossing the superior and inferior gemellus, which cover the tendon of the internal obturator muscle, and then crosses over the quadratus femoris muscle. At this point, the sciatic nerve is located between the ischial tuberosity and the greater trochanter (Fig. 18.4, *axial* section 16). The sciatic nerve then follows its descending course in the posterior compartment of the thigh lateral to the hamstring muscles (semitendinosus,

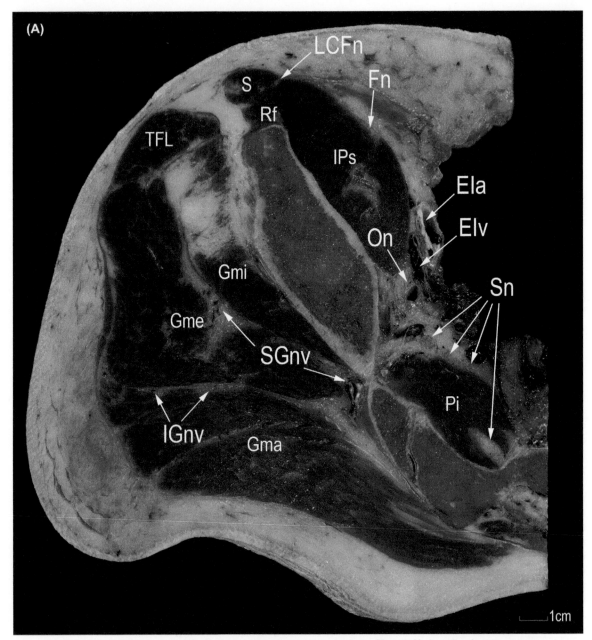

FIG. 18.2 Axial section 8. **(A)**: Anatomical structures of lower limb. **(B and C)**: Details of microanatomy. Studied area within the axial section in Fig. 18.25. *Elv*, external iliac vein; *Eia*, external iliac artery; *Fn*, femoral nerve; *Gmi*, gluteus minimus; *Gme*, gluteus medius; *Gma*, gluteus maximus; *IPs*, iliopsoas; *IGnv*, inferior gluteal nerves and vessels; *LCFn*, lateral femoral cutaneous nerve; *Pi*, piriformis; *Rf*, rectus femoris; *Sn*, sacral nerve; *SGnv*, superior gluteal nerve and vessels; *S*, sartorius; *TFL*, tensor fasciae latae.

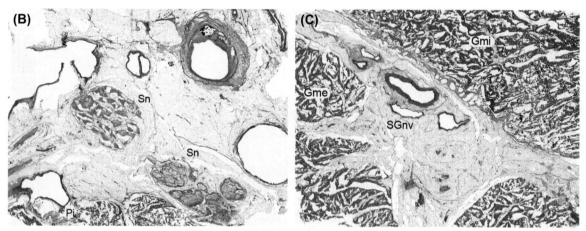

FIG. 18.2 **cont'd.**

semimembranosus, and long head of biceps femoris muscles) (Fig. 18.5, *axial* section 19). Further distal in its course, the sciatic nerve overlies the posterior surface of the adductor magnus muscle and is crossed by the long head of the biceps femoris muscle, which moves laterally to its insertion point on the head of the fibula superficially (Figs. 18.6, 18.7 and 18.8, *axial* sections 25, 31, 37). On the posterior surface of the thigh, the sciatic nerve supplied motor innervation to the hamstring muscles and the extensor part of the adductor magnus muscle through the tibial component of the nerve and the short head of the biceps femoris muscle through the common peroneal part of the nerve. When it reaches the apex of the popliteal fossa, where the sciatic nerve is located in the midline and immediately deep to the fascia, it divides into the tibial and the common peroneal nerves (Fig. 18.9, *axial* section 40).

The **tibial nerve** continues distally in the middle of the popliteal fossa and is accompanied by the popliteal vessels. Here the vein and artery are deeper and medial to the nerve (Fig. 18.10, *axial* section 43). With these vessels, the tibial nerve courses in the posterior aspect of the lower leg; passing between the two heads of the gastrocnemius muscle and then positioned on the surface of the popliteus muscle (Figs. 18.11 and 18.12, *axial* sections 47 and 50). Thereafter, still accompanied by the posterior tibial blood vessels, it courses through the tendinous arch of the soleus muscle and is now located in the plane between the triceps surae superficially and the tibialis

posterior, flexor hallucis longus, and flexor digitorum longus muscles (Figs. 18.13 and 18.14, *axial* sections 53 and 56). The tibial nerve and the posterior tibial vessels now course medially toward the posterior surface of the medial malleolus (Figs. 18.13–18.18, *axial* sections 53, 56, 61, 69, 73, and 76). The entire muscular compartment of the posterior aspect of the leg receives its motor innervation from the tibial nerve en route through this region. After passing the medial malleolus, the tibial nerve and its accompanying vessels pass through the tarsal tunnel underneath the flexor retinaculum to enter the plantar aspect of the foot (Fig. 18.19, *axial* section 79). In the tarsal canal, the nerve divides into the **lateral** and **medial plantar nerves**, both supplying motor innervation to the muscles of the plantar region of the foot (Figs. 18.19 and 18.20, *axial* sections 79 and 86).

The **common peroneal nerve** in the popliteal fossa takes an oblique route caudally and laterally following the posteromedial border of the biceps femoris muscle (Figs. 18.10 and 18.11, *axial* sections 43 and 47) to reach the proximal end of the fibula where it encircles the fibular neck and enters the lateral compartment of the leg, into the peroneus longus muscle (Fig. 18.12, *axial* section 50). Here, it divides into the superficial and the deep peroneal nerves (Fig. 18.13, *axial* section 53).

The **superficial peroneal nerve** descends in the lateral compartment of the leg where it innervates the peroneus muscles (Fig. 18.14, *axial* section 56). In the lower third of the leg, it is in the intermuscular

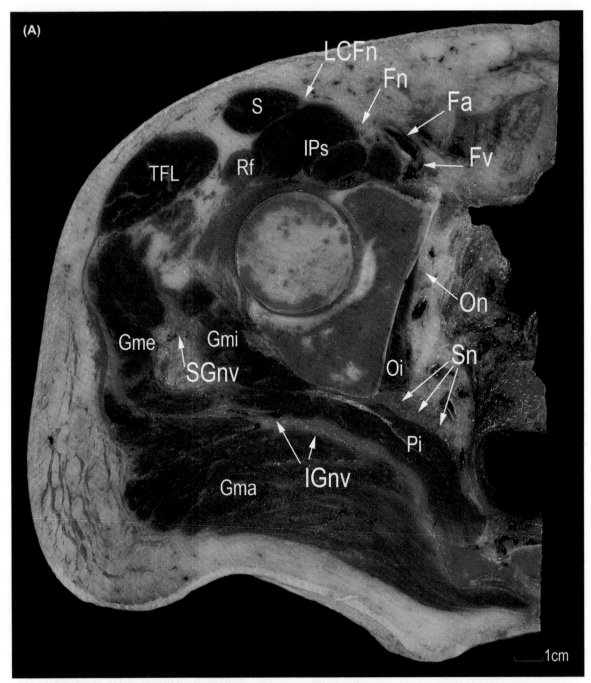

FIG. 18.3 Axial section 10. **(A)**: Anatomical structures of lower limb. **(B** and **C)**: Details of microanatomy. Studied area within the axial section in Fig. 18.25. *Fn*, femoral nerve; *Fa*, femoral artery; *Fv*, femoral vein; *Gmi*, gluteus minimus; *Gme*, gluteus medius; *Gma*, gluteus maximus; *LCFn*, lateral cutaneous femoral nerve; *IPs*, iliopsoas; *IGnv*, inferior gluteal nerves and vessels; *Oi*, obturator internus; *Oi*, obturator internus; *Oi*, obturator internus; *Pi*, piriformis; *Pit/Gm*, *Rf*, rectus femoris; *S*, sartorius; *Sn*, sacral nerve; *SGnv*, superior gluteal nerves and vessels; *TFL*, tensor fasciae latae; piriformis tendon with gemellus.

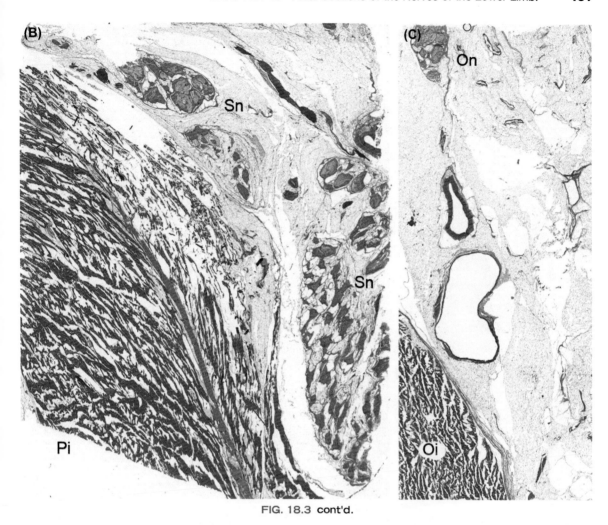

FIG. 18.3 cont'd.

septum between the peronei and the extensor digitorum longus muscles where it perforates the deep fascia (Figs. 18.15 and 18.16, *axial* sections 61 and 69). Now in a subcutaneous position, it branches out and supplies sensory innervation to the skin of the anterolateral distal third of the leg and the dorsum of the foot except for the first interdigital space, which receives its sensory innervation from the deep peroneal nerve.

The **deep peroneal nerve**, after encircling the neck of the fibula, pierces the anterior intermuscular septum to enter the anterior compartment of the leg where it innervates all of its muscles (Figs. 18.13 and 18.14, *axial* sections 53 and 56). It descends on the interosseous membrane where it travels with the anterior tibial vessels (Fig. 18.15, *axial* section 61). Initially it is located between the tibialis anterior and the extensor digitorum longus muscles (Figs. 18.15 and 18.16, *axial* sections 61 and 69), and more distally between the tibialis anterior and the extensor hallucis longus muscle tendons (Figs. 18.17 and 18.18 and 18.19, *axial* sections 73, 76, and 79). In the lower third of the leg, the tendon of the extensor hallucis longus muscle moves medially and crosses over the nerve so that, in the anterior part of the ankle and dorsum of the foot, the deep peroneal nerve is located laterally to the extensor hallucis longus tendon (Fig. 18.20, *axial* section 86).

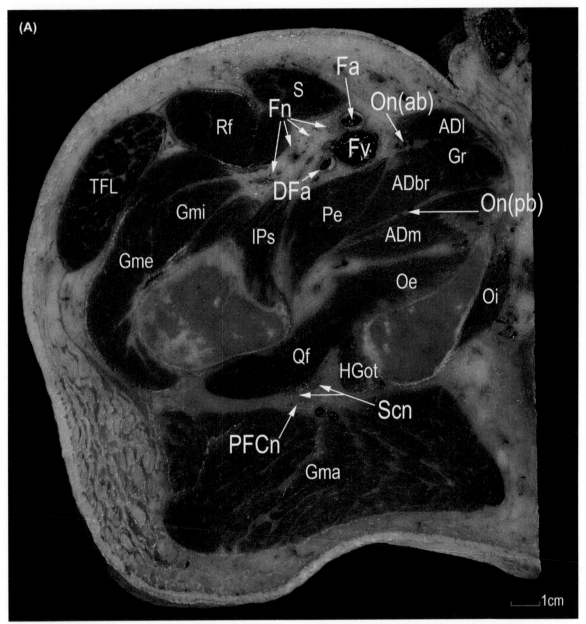

FIG. 18.4 Axial section 5. **(A)**: Anatomical structures of lower limb. **(B** and **C)**: Details of microanatomy. Studied area within the axial section in Fig. 18.25. *ADl*, adductor longus; *ADbr*, adductor brevis; *ADm*, adductor magnus; *DFa*, deep femoral artery; *Fn*, femoral nerve; *Fa*, femoral artery; *Fv*, femoral vein; *Gmi*, gluteus minimus; *Gme*, gluteus medius; *Gma*, gluteus maximus; *Gr*, gracilis; *Hgot*, hamstring group origin tendon; *IPs*, iliopsoas; *Isch*, insertion of ischial muscles; *Oi*, obturator internus; *Oe*, obturator externus; *On(ab)*, obturator nerve anterior branch; *On(pb)*, obturator nerve posterior branch; *Pe*, pectineus; *Qf*, quadratus femoris; *Rf*, rectus femoris; *S*, sartorius; *Scn*, sciatic nerve; *TFL*, tensor fasciae latae.

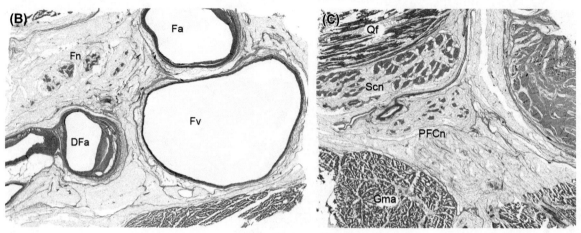

FIG. 18.4 cont'd.

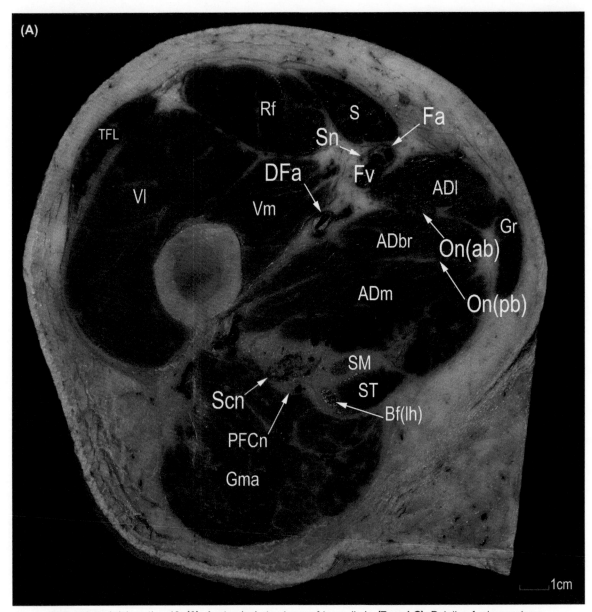

FIG. 18.5 Axial section 19. **(A)**: Anatomical structures of lower limb. **(B and C)**: Details of microanatomy. Studied area within the axial section in Fig. 18.25. *ADbr*, adductor brevis; *ADl*, adductor longus; *ADm*, adductor magnus; *Bf (lh)*, long head of biceps femoris; *DFa*, deep femoral artery; *Fa*, femoral artery; *Fv*, femoral vein; *Gma*, gluteus maximus; *Gr*, gracilis; *On(ab)*, obturator nerve anterior branch; *On(pb)*, obturator nerve posterior branch; *Rf*, rectus femoris; *S*, sartorius; *Scn*, sciatic nerve; *Sn*, saphenous nerve; *SM*, semimembranosus; *ST*, semitendinosus; *TFL*, tensor fasciae latae; *Vl*, vastus lateralis; *Vm*, vastus medialis.

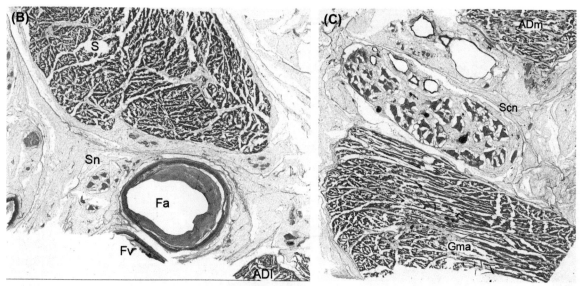

FIG. 18.5 cont'd.

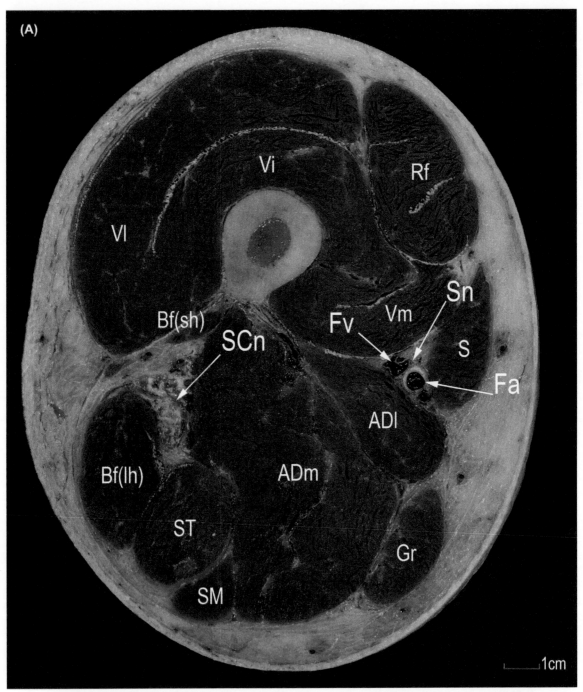

FIG. 18.6 Axial section 25. **(A)**: Anatomical structures of lower limb. **(B and C)**: Details of microanatomy. Studied area within the axial section in Fig. 18.25. *ADl*, adductor longus; *ADm*, adductor magnus; *Bf (lh)*, long head of biceps femoris; *Fa*, femoral artery; *Fv*, femoral vein; *Gr*, gracilis; *Rf*, rectus femoris; *S*, sartorius; *Scn*, sciatic nerve; *SM*, semimembranosus; *Sn*, saphenous nerve; *ST*, semitendinosus; *Vi*, vastus intermedius; *Vl*, vastus lateralis; *Vm*, vastus medialis.

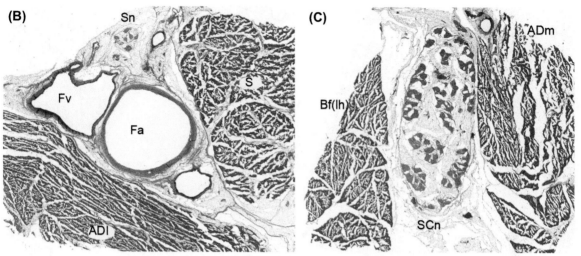

FIG. 18.6 cont'd.

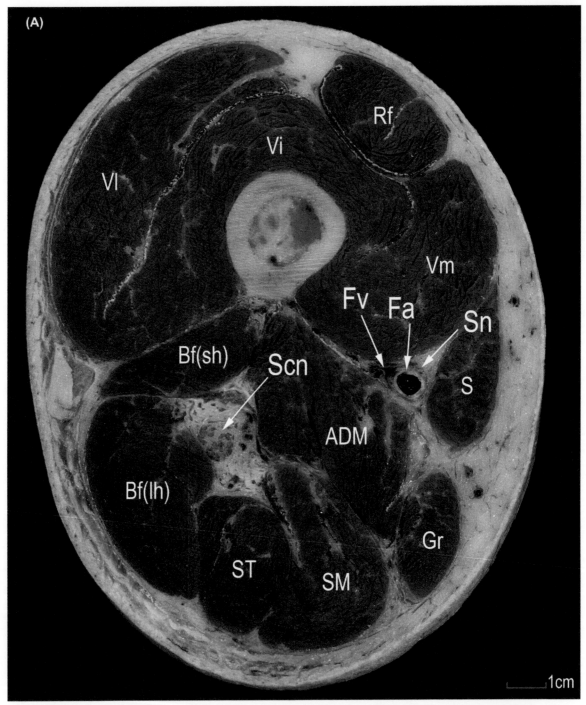

FIG. 18.7 Axial section 31. **(A)**: Anatomical structures of lower limb. **(B** and **C)**: Details of microanatomy. Studied area within the axial section in Fig. 18.25. *ADm*, adductor magnus; *Bf (lh)*, long head of biceps femoris; *BF(sh)*, short head of biceps femoris; *Fa*, femoral artery; *Fv*, femoral vein; *Gr*, gracilis; *Rf*, rectus femoris; *S*, sartorius; *Scn*, sciatic nerve; *SM*, semimembranosus; *Sn*, saphenous nerve; *ST*, semitendinosus; *Vi*, vastus intermedius; *Vl*, vastus lateralis; *Vm*, vastus medialis.

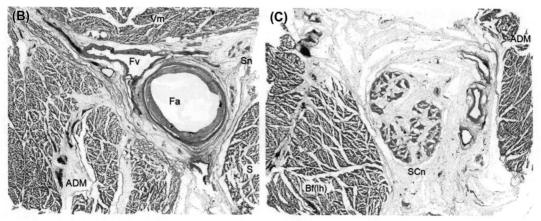

FIG. 18.7 cont'd.

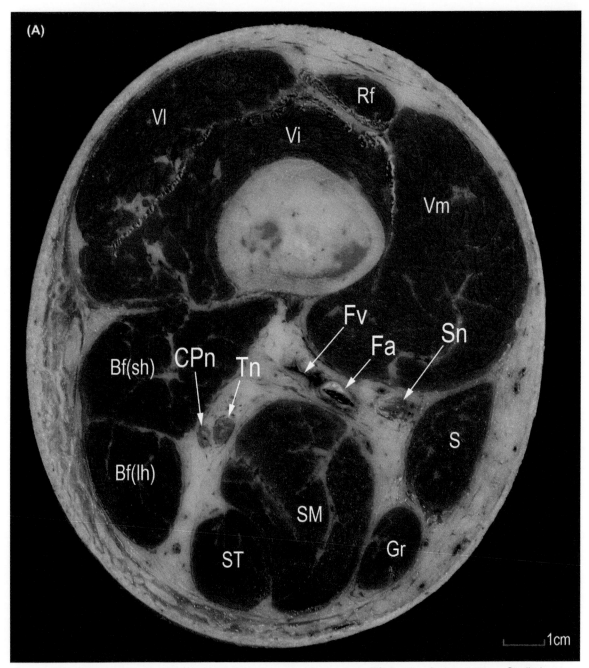

FIG. 18.8 Axial section 37. **(A)**: Anatomical structures of lower limb. **(B)**: Details of microanatomy. Studied area within the axial section in Fig. 18.25. *Bf (lh)*, long head of biceps femoris; *BF(sh)*, short head of biceps femoris; *CPn*, common peroneal nerve; *Fa*, femoral artery; *Fv*, femoral vein; *Gr*, gracilis; *Rf*, rectus femoris; *S*, sartorius; *SM*, semimembranosus; *Sn*, saphenous nerve; *ST*, semitendinosus; *Tn*, tibial nerve; *Vi*, vastus intermedius; *Vl*, vastus lateralis; *Vm*, vastus medialis.

(B)

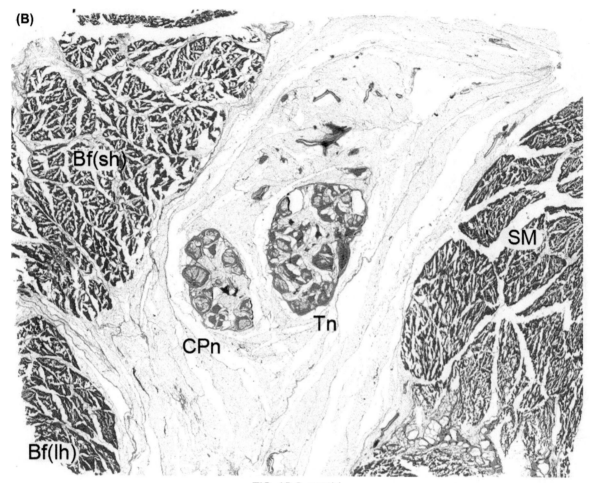

FIG. 18.8 cont'd.

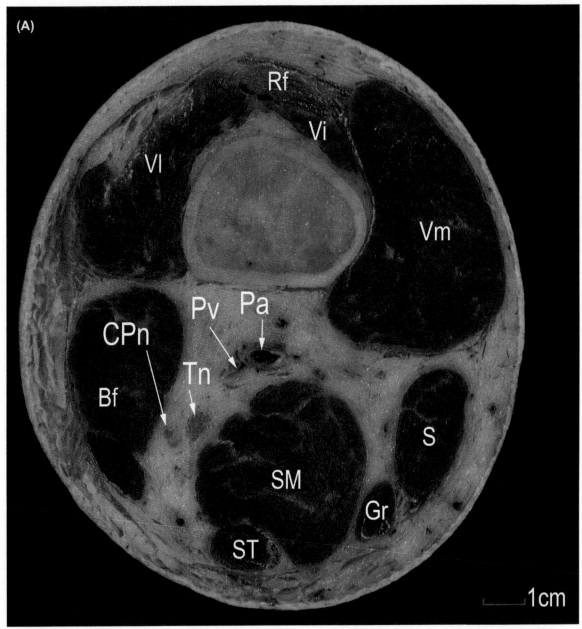

FIG. 18.9 Axial section 40. **(A)**: Anatomical structures of lower limb. **(B)**: Details of microanatomy. Studied area within the axial section in Fig. 18.25. *Bf*, biceps femoris; *CPn*, common peroneal nerve; *Gr*, gracilis; *Pa*, popliteal artery; *Pv*, popliteal vein; *Rf*, rectus femoris; *S*, sartorius; *SM*, semimembranosus; *ST*, semitendinosus; *Tn*, tibial nerve; *Vl*, vastus lateralis; *Vi*, vastus intermedius; *Vm*, vastus medialis.

(B)

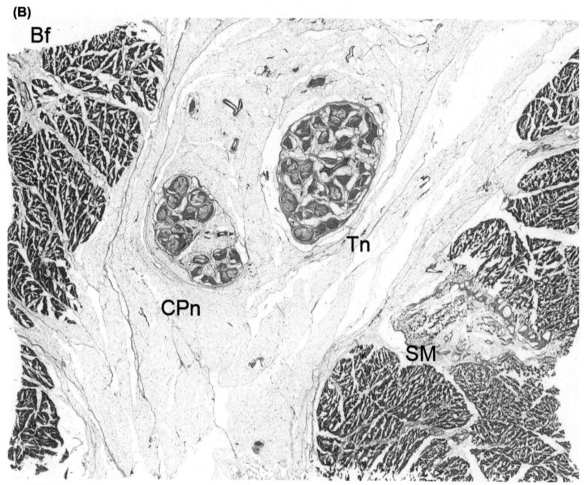

FIG. 18.9 cont'd.

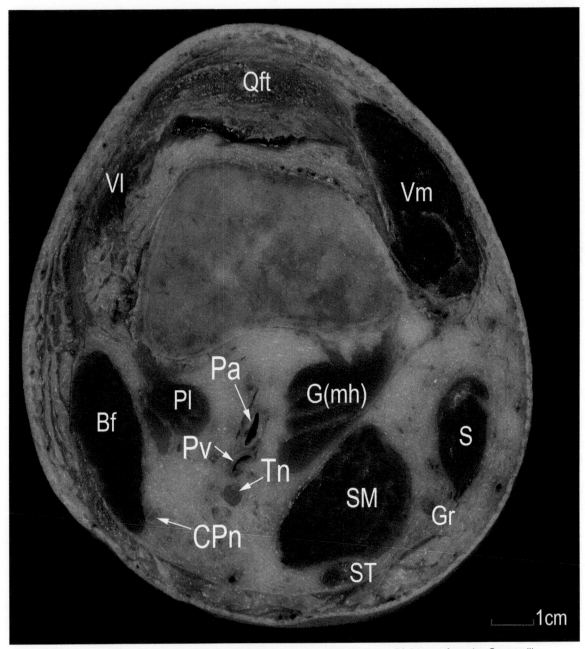

FIG. 18.10 Axial section 43. **(A):** Anatomical structures of lower limb. *Bf,* biceps femoris; *Gr,* gracilis; *G(mh),* gastrocnemius medial head; *Pa,* popliteal artery; *Pl,* plantaris; *Pv,* popliteal vein; *Qft,* quadriceps femoris tendon; *S,* sartorius; *SM,* semimembranosus; *ST,* semitendinosus; *Tn,* tibial nerve; *Vl,* vastus lateralis; *Vm,* vastus medialis.

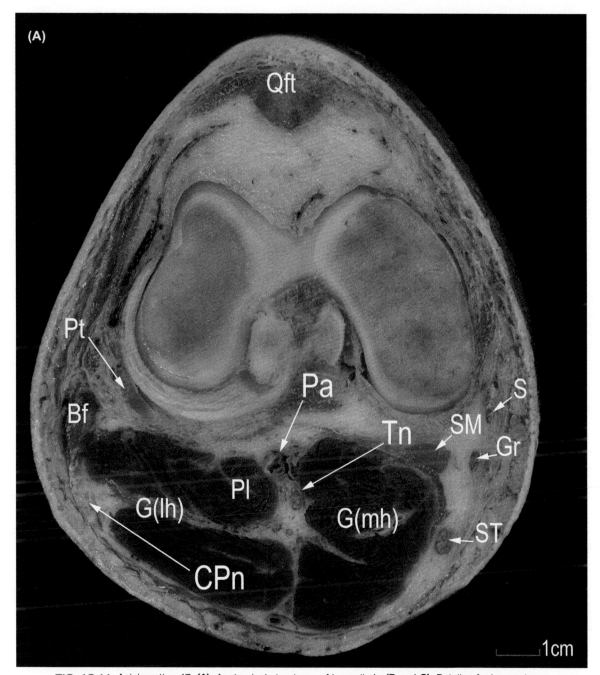

FIG. 18.11 Axial section 47. **(A)**: Anatomical structures of lower limb. **(B and C)**: Details of microanatomy. Studied area within the axial section in Fig. 18.25. *Bf*, biceps femoris; *CPn*, common peroneal nerve; *G(lh)*, gastrocnemius lateral head; *G(mh)*, gastrocnemius medial head; *Gr*, gracilis; *Pa*, popliteal artery; *Pl*, plantaris; *Pt*, popliteus tendon; *Pv*, popliteal vein; *Qft*, quadriceps femoris tendon; *S*, sartorius; *SM*, semimembranosus; *ST*, semitendinosus; *Tn*, tibial nerve.

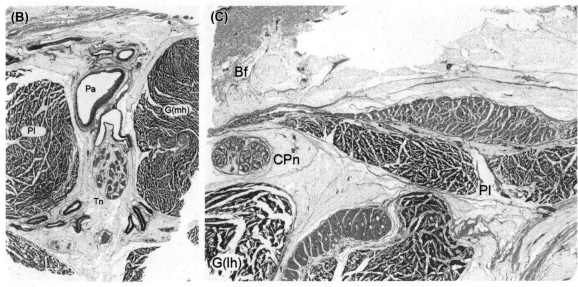

FIG. 18.11 cont'd.

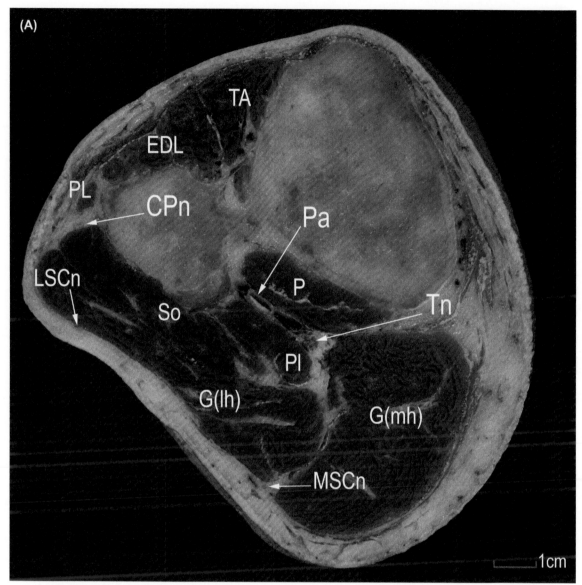

FIG. 18.12 Axial section 50. **(A)**: Anatomical structures of lower limb. **(B)**: Details of microanatomy. Studied area within the axial section in Fig. 18.25. *CPn*, common peroneal nerve; *EDL*, extensor digitorum longus; *G(lh)*, gastrocnemius lateral head; *G(mh)*, gastrocnemius medial head; *LSCn*, lateral sural cutaneous nerve; *MSCn*, medial sural cutaneous nerve; *P*, popliteus; *Pa*, popliteal artery; *Pl*, plantaris; *PL*, peroneus longus; *So*, soleus; *TA*, tibialis anterior; *Tn*, tibial nerve.

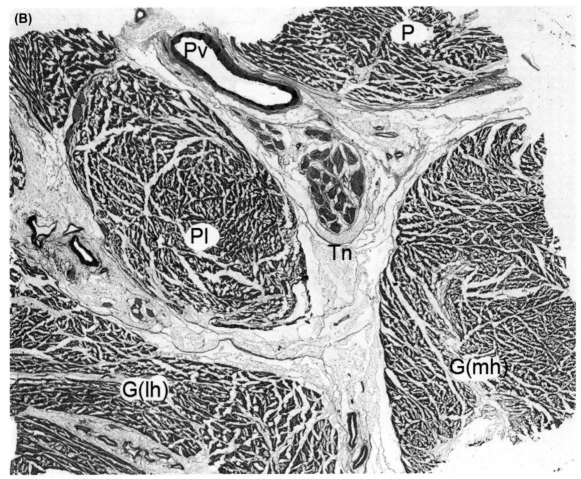

FIG. 18.12 cont'd.

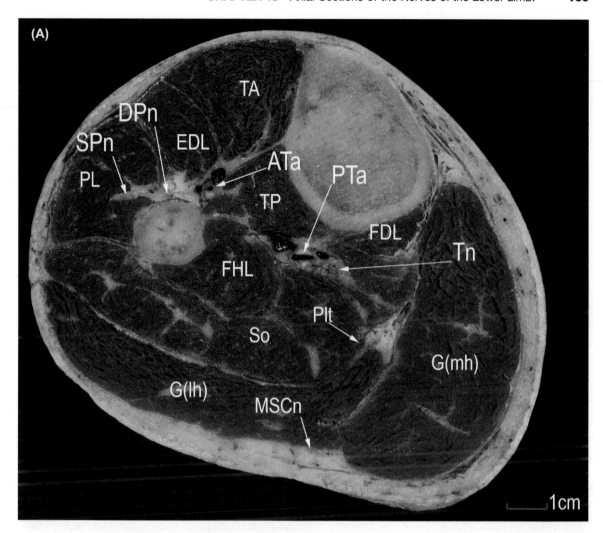

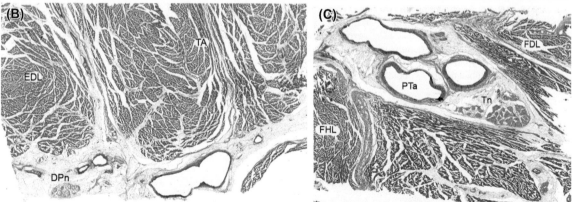

FIG. 18.13 Axial section 53. **(A):** Anatomical structures of lower limb. **(B** and **C):** Details of microanatomy. Studied area within the axial section in Fig. 18.25. *Ata,* anterior tibial artery; *DPn,* deep peroneal nerve; *EDL,* extensor digitorum longus; *FDL,* flexor digitorum longus; *FHL,* flexor hallucis longus; *G(lh),* gastrocnemius lateral head; *G(mh),* gastrocnemius medial head; *PTa,* posterior tibial artery; *PL,* peroneus longus; *Plt,* plantaris tendon; *So,* soleus; *SPn,* superficial peroneal nerve; *TA,* tibialis anterior; *Tn,* tibial nerve; *TP,* tibialis posterior.

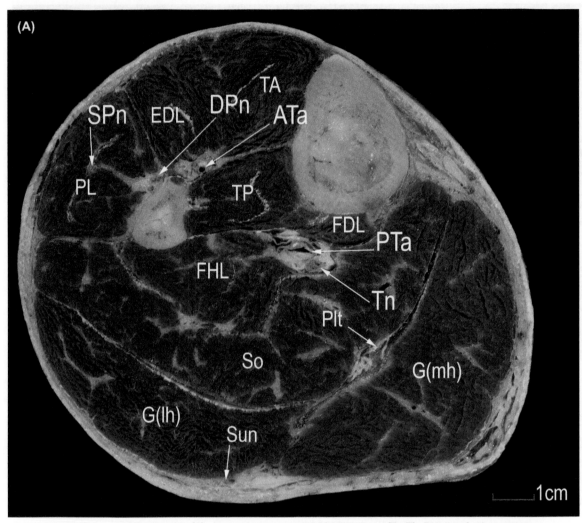

FIG. 18.14 Axial section 56. **(A)**: Anatomical structures of lower limb. **(B–D)**: Details of microanatomy. Studied area within the axial section in Fig. 18.25. *ATa*, anterior tibial artery; *DPn*, deep peroneal nerve; *EDL*, extensor digitorum longus; *FDL*, flexor digitorum longus; *FHL*, flexor hallucis longus; *G(lh)*, gastrocnemius lateral head; *G(mh)*, gastrocnemius medial head; *PB*, peroneus brevis; *PL*, peroneus longus; *Plt*, plantaris tendon; *PTa*, posterior tibial artery; *So*, soleus; *SPn*, superficial peroneal nerve; *Sun*, sural nerve; *TA*, tibialis anterior; *Tn*, tibial nerve; *TP*, tibialis posterior.

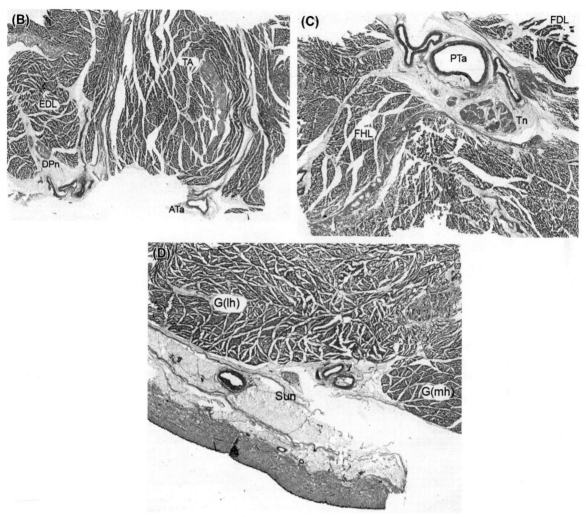

FIG. 18.14 cont'd.

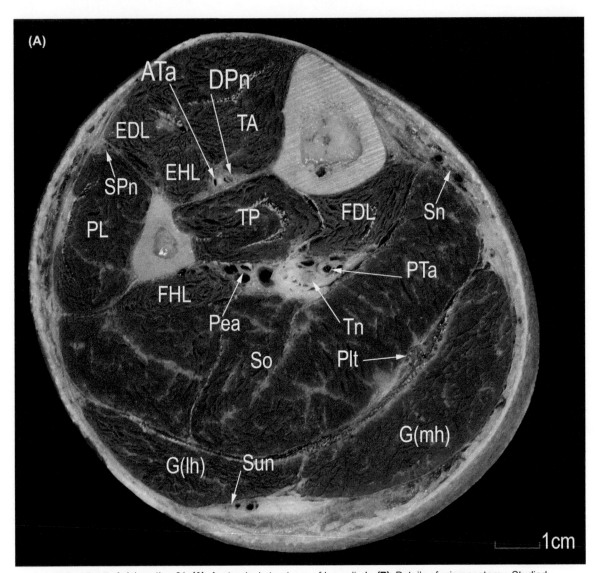

FIG. 18.15 Axial section 61. **(A)**: Anatomical structures of lower limb. **(B)**: Details of microanatomy. Studied area within the axial section in Fig. 18.25. *ATa*, anterior tibial artery; *DPn*, deep peroneal nerve; *EDL*, extensor digitorum longus; *FDL*, flexor digitorum longus; *FHL*, flexor hallucis longus; *G(lh)*, gastrocnemius lateral head; *G(mh)*, gastrocnemius medial head; *PB*, peroneus brevis; *Pea*, peroneal artery; *PL*, peroneus longus; *Plt*, plantaris tendon; *PTa*, posterior tibial artery; *So*, soleus; *Sn*, saphenous nerve; *SPn*, superficial peroneal nerve; *Sun*, sural nerve; *TA*, tibialis anterior; *Tn*, tibial nerve; *TP*, tibialis posterior.

(B)

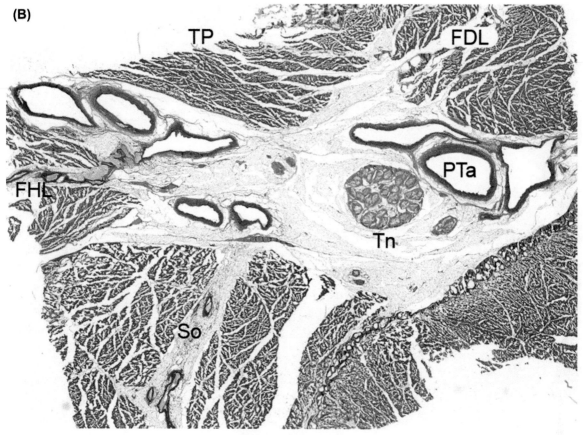

FIG. 18.15 cont'd.

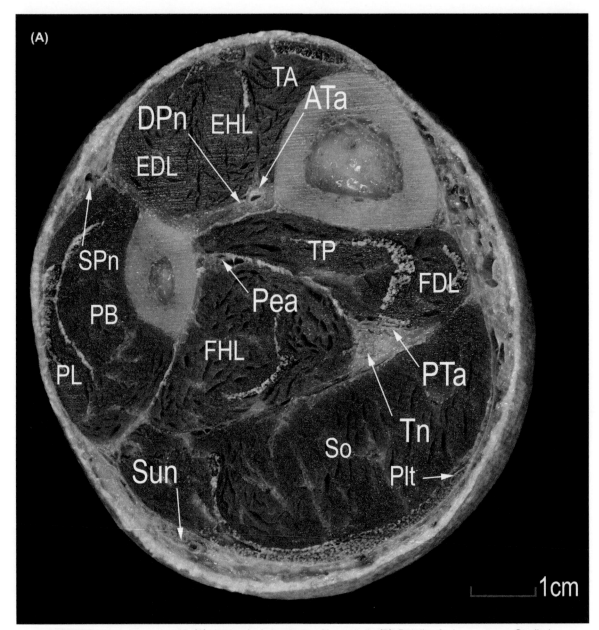

FIG. 18.16 Axial section 69. **(A)**: Anatomical structures of lower limb. **(B)**: Details of microanatomy. Studied area within the axial section in Fig. 18.25. *ATa*, anterior tibial artery; *DPn*, deep peroneal nerve; *EDL*, extensor digitorum longus; *EHL*, extensor hallucis longus; *FDL*, flexor digitorum longus; *FHL*, flexor hallucis longus; *PB*, peroneus brevis; *Pea*, peroneal artery; *PL*, peroneus longus; *Plt*, plantaris tendon; *PTa*, posterior tibial artery; *Sn*, saphenous nerve; *So*, soleus; *SPn*, superficial peroneal nerve; *Sun*, sural nerve; *TA*, tibialis anterior; *Tn*, tibial nerve; *TP*, tibialis posterior.

(B)

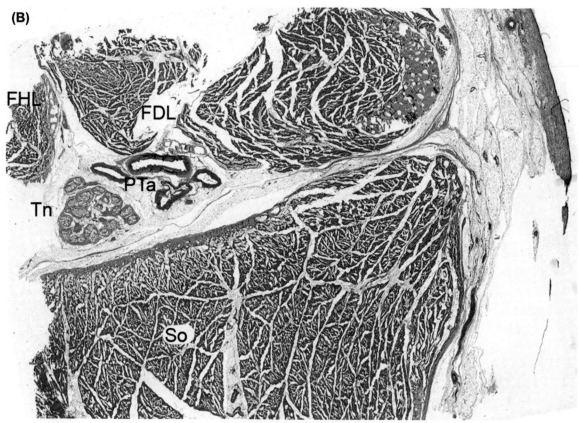

FIG. 18.16 cont'd.

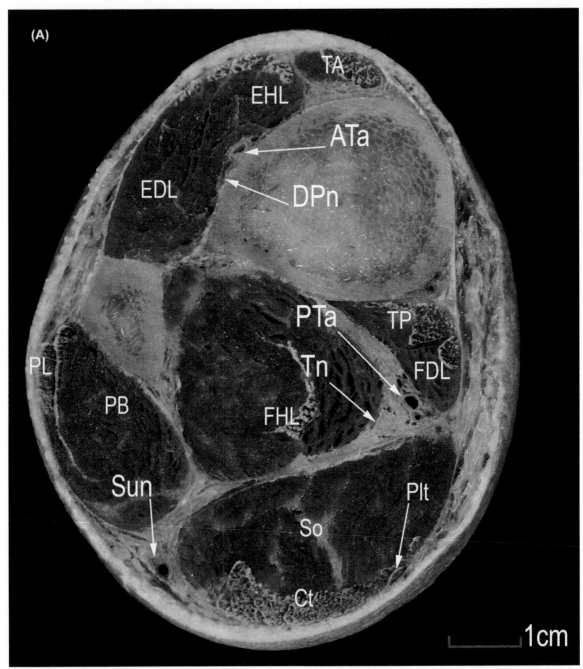

FIG. 18.17 Axial section 73. **(A)**: Anatomical structures of lower limb. **(B and C)**: Details of microanatomy. Studied area within the axial section in Fig. 18.25. *ATa*, anterior tibial artery; *Ct*, calcaneal tendon; *DPn*, deep peroneal nerve; *EDL*, extensor digitorum longus; *EHL*, extensor hallucis longus; *FDL*, flexor digitorum longus; *FHL*, flexor hallucis longus; *PB*, peroneus brevis; *Pea*, peroneal artery; *PL*, peroneus longus; *Plt*, plantaris tendon; *PTa*, posterior tibial artery; *So*, soleus; *Sn*, saphenous nerve; *SPn*, superficial peroneal nerve; *Sun*, sural nerve; *TA*, tibialis anterior; *Tn*, tibial nerve; *TP*, tibialis posterior.

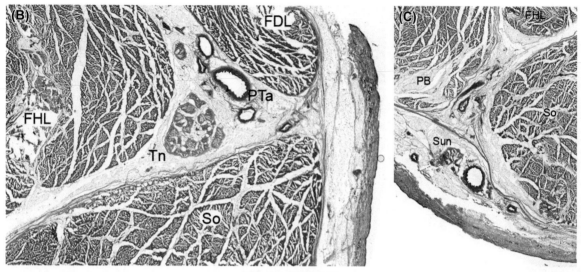

FIG. 18.17 cont'd.

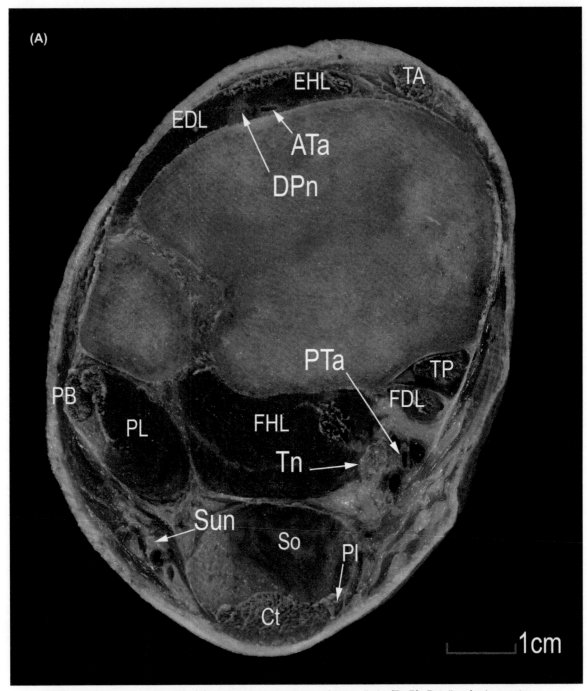

FIG. 18.18 Axial section 76. **(A)**: Anatomical structures of lower limb. **(B–D)**: Details of microanatomy. Studied area within the axial section in Fig. 18.25. *ATa*, anterior tibial artery; *Ct*, calcaneal tendon; *DPn*, deep peroneal nerve; *EDL*, extensor digitorum longus; *EHL*, extensor hallucis longus; *FDL*, flexor digitorum longus; *FHL*, flexor hallucis longus; *PB*, peroneus brevis; *Pea*, peroneal artery; *PL*, peroneus longus; *Plt*, plantaris tendon; *PTa*, posterior tibial artery; *So*, soleus; *Sun*, sural nerve; *TA*, tibialis anterior; *Tn*, tibial nerve; *TP*, tibialis posterior.

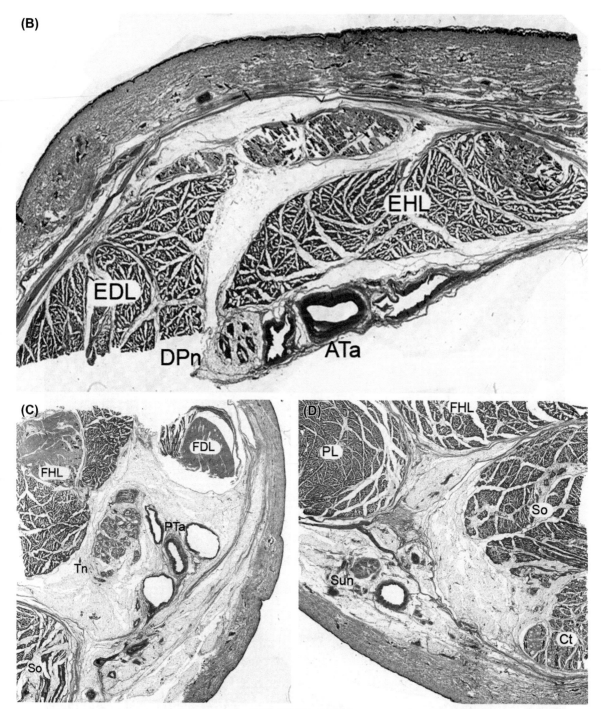

FIG. 18.18 cont'd.

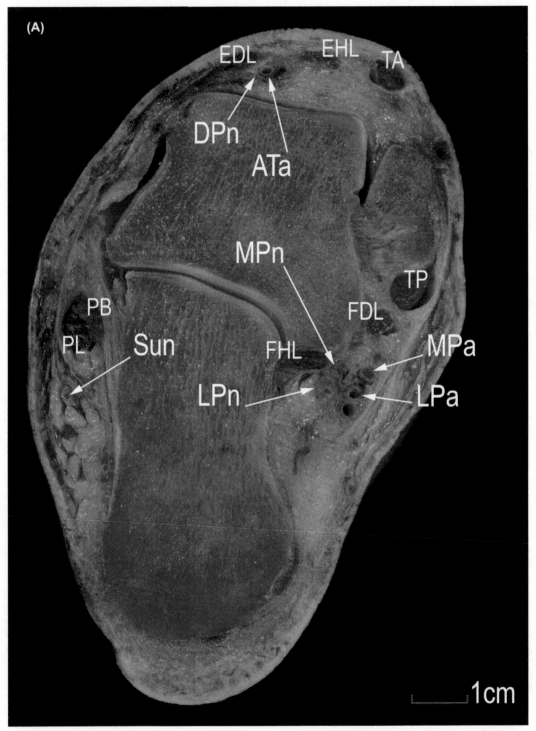

FIG. 18.19 Axial section 79. **(A)**: Anatomical structures of lower limb. **(B–D)**: Details of microanatomy. Studied area within the axial section in Fig. 18.25. *ATa*, anterior tibial artery; *DPn*, deep peroneal nerve; *EDL*, extensor digitorum longus; *EHL*, extensor hallucis longus; *FDL*, flexor digitorum longus; *FHL*, flexor hallucis longus; *LPa*, lateral plantar artery; *LPn*, lateral plantar nerve; *MPa*, medial plantar artery; *MPn*, medial plantar nerve; *PB*, peroneus brevis; *PL*, peroneus longus; *Sun*, sural nerve; *TA*, tibialis anterior; *TP*, tibialis posterior.

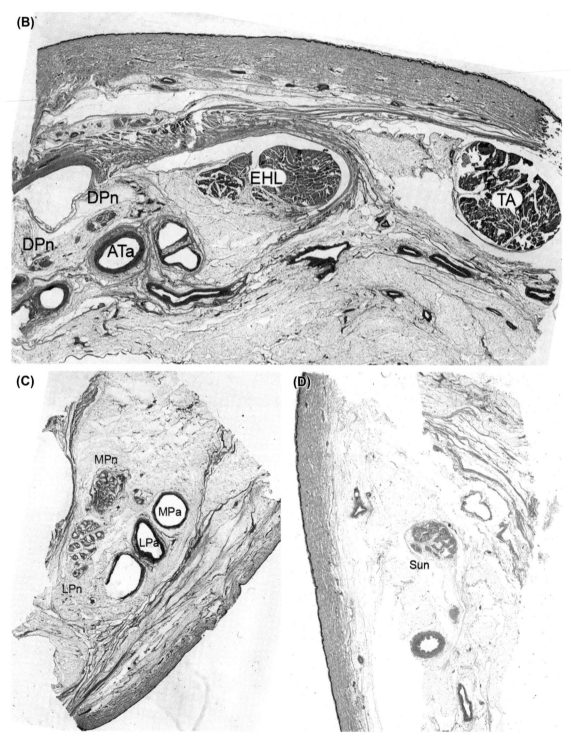

FIG. 18.19 cont'd.

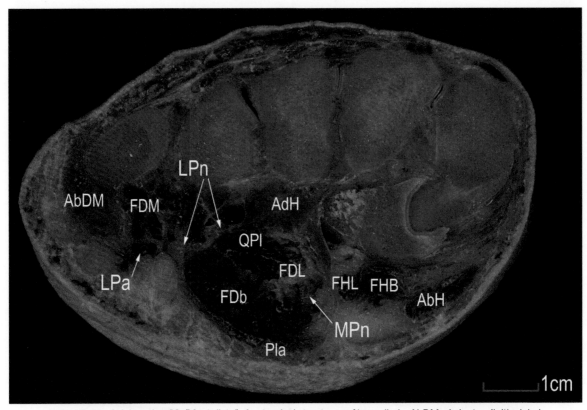

FIG. 18.20 Axial section 86. (Most distal). Anatomical structures of lower limb. *AbDM*, abductor digiti minimi; *AbH*, abductor hallucis; *AdH*, adductor hallucis; *FDB*, flexor digitorum brevis; *FDL*, flexor digitorum longus; *FDM*, flexor digiti minimi; *FHB*, flexor hallucis longus; *FHL*, flexor hallucis longus; *LPa*, lateral plantar artery; *LPn*, lateral plantar nerve; *MPn*, medial plantar nerve; *Pla*, plantaris aponeurosis ; *QPI*, quadratus plantae.

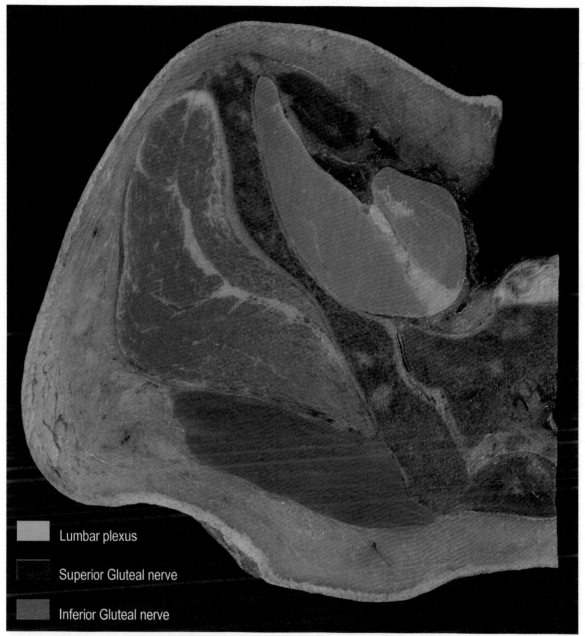

FIG. 18.21 Axial section 5. Muscular innervation of the lower limb.

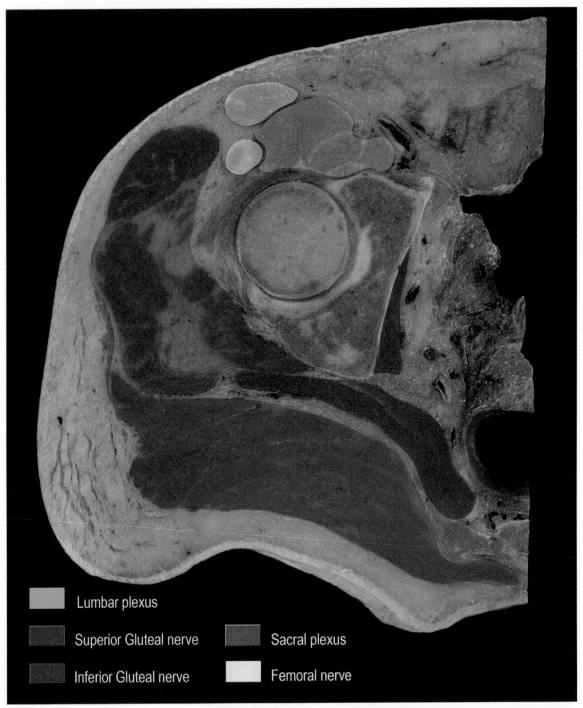

Lumbar plexus

Superior Gluteal nerve   Sacral plexus

Inferior Gluteal nerve   Femoral nerve

FIG. 18.22 Axial section 10. Muscular innervation of the lower limb.

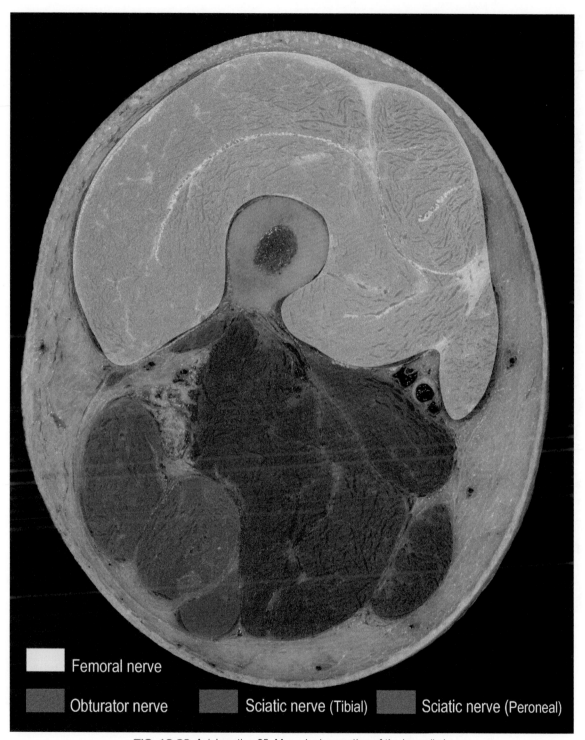

Femoral nerve

Obturator nerve   Sciatic nerve (Tibial)   Sciatic nerve (Peroneal)

FIG. 18.23 Axial section 25. Muscular innervation of the lower limb.

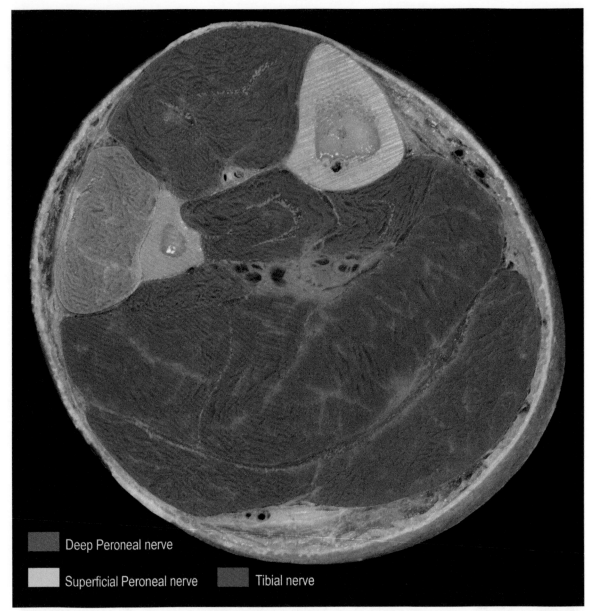

FIG. 18.24 Axial section 61. Muscular innervation of the lower limb.

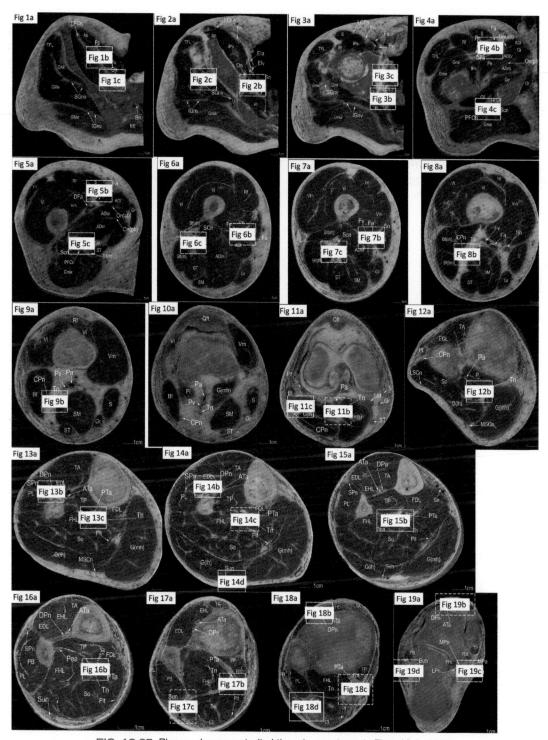

FIG. 18.25 Places where we studied the microanatomy in Figs. 18.1–18.19.

In the popliteal region, the tibial and common peroneal nerves provide branches that form the **sural nerve**. The tibial nerve gives off the **medial sural cutaneous nerve**. This nerve runs with the small saphenous vein, superficially between the two muscular bellies of the gastrocnemius muscle (Figs. 18.12 and 18.13, *axial* sections 50 and 53). The common peroneal nerve gives off the **lateral sural cutaneous nerve** that innervates the posterolateral aspect of the leg (Fig. 18.12, *axial* section 50). The **peroneal communicating branch** originates from the lateral sural cutaneous nerve, and it unites with the medial sural cutaneous nerve to form the sural nerve. This union takes place at variable points along the posterior aspect of the leg. Once formed, the sural nerve courses distally and laterally. It passes dorsally (posterior) to the lateral malleolus and supplies the skin of the lateral part of the foot (Fig. 18.19, *axial* section 79). Muscular innervation was shown in Figs. 18.21–18.24 (*axial* sections 5, 10, 25, and 61).

REFERENCE

Sarrafian, S.K., 1993. Anatomy of the Foot and Ankle, second ed. J.B. Lippincott Company, Philadelphia, pp. 385–386.

CHAPTER 19

Comparative Anatomy of the Lumbosacral Plexus

MALCON ANDREI MARTINEZ-PEREIRA

The peripheral nerves comprise cranial and spinal nerves that link the central nervous system to the peripheral tissues. Spinal nerves emerge from all regions of the spinal cord and can be organized by networks and anastomoses of various branches, which constitute neural plexuses (Getty, 1975; Dyce et al., 2009). In particular, there are more cells and nerve fibers in the cervical and lumbar regions of the spinal cord, called enlargements. Considering only the caudal end of the spinal cord (lumbar enlargement and conus medullaris: Getty, 1975; Dyce et al., 2009), which innervates the pelvic cavity and hindlimbs, the topography varies widely among mammals and other vertebrates. This is of considerable interest for clinical and surgical medicine and for experimental models (Orosz et al., 2007; Rigaud et al., 2008), which is why morphological and morphometric descriptions of this structure in many species have been published.

Peripheral nerve lesions and plexopathies are very common in emergency hospital care. Injuries to the lumbar region of spinal cord can compromise quality of life and incapacitate the patient. This part of the spinal cord is also very important for epidural anesthesia or analgesia procedures (Hall and Clarke, 1991; Jones, 2001), collection of cerebrospinal fluid (Elias and Brown, 2008), and injection of opaque substances for imaging (Paithanpagare et al., 2001; Lu et al., 2011). In fact, epidural anesthesia has become an alternative anesthetic procedure for surgeries caudal to the diaphragm (Najman, 2011). Knowledge of the relevant anatomy (spinal cord location and origin, route and destination of plexus components) is therefore important for developing new techniques or procedures to treat pathologies. It is also necessary to reduce the risk of iatrogenic injury during treatment and for rehabilitation from various diseases.

The comparative approach to the neuroanatomy of the peripheral nerves taken in this chapter helps us to understand the functional aspects of neural structure. The anatomical descriptions include mammals used in experimental procedures for studies of plexopathies and nerve injuries, such as the rat (*Rattus norvegicus*), guinea pig (*Cavia porcellus*), chinchilla (*Chinchilla lanigera*), rabbit (*Oryctolagus cuniculus*), dogs, cats, pigs, and nonhuman primates. A comparative perspective on mammalian plexus design includes an analysis of lower tetrapods, although fewer reports are available on amphibians and reptiles or even birds than on mammals. These descriptive accounts illustrate the remarkable variation in limb shapes and modes of locomotion among tetrapods.

LUMBOSACRAL SPINAL CORD AND NERVES

Although the neuroanatomy and cytoarchitecture of the mammalian cerebral cortex (pallial domains) differ considerably from that of lower tetrapods, the spinal cord and peripheral nervous system are very similar in cytoarchitectural features and anatomical arrangement.

The number of lumbar and sacral spinal segments varies among species according to the number of vertebrae. Among mammals, for example, humans have five lumbar segments and nerves (Standring, 2009); nonhuman primates range between four and seven (Hepburn, 1892a,b; Hill, 1953, 1957, 1960, 1966, 1972); dogs have seven (Getty, 1975; Dyce et al., 2009). From Th1, all spinal nerves emerge below their corresponding vertebrae. The diameter of the lumbar spinal cord is not uniform owing to the lumbar enlargement characterized by the increased number of cells and nerve fibers. However, the end of the spinal cord is tapered to form the conus medullaris, which continues with a thin meningeal filament, the filum terminale. The numbers of vertebrae, lumbar and sacral spinal segments, and nerves that correspond to spinal segments for some species are shown in Table 19.1.

Surgical Anatomy of the Sacral Plexus and Its Branches. https://doi.org/10.1016/B978-0-323-77602-8.00019-2

189

TABLE 19.1
Number of Vertebrae, Medullary Segments, and Lumbar Spinal Nerve Ventral Rami in the Lumbar and Sacral Regions of Some Vertebrates.

Species	LUMBAR REGION			SACRAL REGION		
	Vertebrae	Spine Segment	Lumbar Nerves	Vertebrae	Spine Segment	Sacral Nerves
Human	5	5	6	5	5	5
NONHUMAN PRIMATES						
Ateles	4	4	6	3	3	3
Cebus	5–6	5–6	5	3	5	5
Chimpanzee	4	4	6	6	6	6
Cynomolgus	6–7	6–7	5	3–4	3–4	3–4
Gibbon	5	5	6	5	5	5
Gorilla	4	4	6	5	5	5
Lagothrix	4	4	6	3	3	3
Orangutan	4	4	5	5	5	5
Rhesus	6–7	6–7	6–7	3–4	3–4	3–4
OTHER MAMMALS						
Cat	6	7	7	3	3	3
Chinchilla	6	6	7	4	4	4
Dog	7	7	7	3	3	3
Guinea pig	6	6	6	4	4	4
Swine	6–7	6	6	4	4	4
Rabbit	7	7	7	4	4	4
Rat	6	6	6	4	4	4
OTHER TETRAPODS						
Alligator	22-24 PSV	22-24 PSS	3	2	2	2
Iguana	23-25 PSV	23-25 PSS	3	2	2	2
Varanus	27-29 PSV	27-29 PSS	3	2	2	2
Turtles	16-18 PSV	16-18 PSS	3	2	2	2
Red-footed tortoise	13 PSV	13 PSS	1	4–5	4–5	4–5
Anurans	4 PSV	4 PSS	5 PSSN	1	1	1

PSV, presacral vertebrae; *PSS*, presacral medullary segments; *PSSN*, presacral spinal nerves.

The spinal cord in birds extends throughout the entire vertebral canal including the coccygeal region; however, the diameter decreases caudally (Baumel, 1975; Nickel et al., 1977; Dubbeldam, 1993). In contrast to the spinal cord in mammals, the cervical, sacral, and coccygeal regions are longer and more variable among avians, while the thoracic portion is very short. Although its segmentation is the same as in mammals, the *Nomina Anatomica Avium* (Dubbeldam, 1993) suggests that the best method to determine the number of spinal segments is to count the number of vertebrae, starting at the base of the skull and proceeding caudally. Because the number of vertebral segments differs widely among taxa and distinct regional boundaries are lacking, this same method is used for other tetrapods such as amphibians and reptiles (Table 19.1). The spinal cord has two enlargements in birds, cervical and lumbar, as in mammals, but only birds have a glycogen body in the lumbosacral sinus (Baumel, 1975; Nickel et al., 1977; Dubbeldam, 1993). Glycogen body cells are of glial origin, possibly from astrocytes, and have undergone extreme differentiation; but neither the origin of these cells nor the functions of the glycogen body are wholly clear.

The reptilian spinal cord has a segmented organization, as in other vertebrates; however, it lacks some of the functional regionalization seen in mammals. It tends to be larger near the brainstem, and the cervical and sacral regions are larger in cross section, corresponding to the brachial and lumbosacral plexuses. In alligators, it fills 50% of the lumen, and 29%–34% in several lizard species (Wyneken, 2003, 2007). Although it extends throughout the vertebral canal, there is no lumbar region in turtles (Ashley, 1962; Kadota et al., 2009), lizards, or crocodiles (Rowe, 1986; Wyneken, 2003, 2007), and snakes and limbless lizards lack cervical and sacral enlargements (Wyneken, 2003, 2007). In reptiles, no lateral horn can be distinguished, but the large area of gray matter between the horns is composed of interneurons (Wyneken, 2003, 2007). However, in testudines, the ventral horn is reduced in the midtrunk because there are fewer motor neurons, since trunk musculature is lacking (Ashley, 1962; Kadota et al., 2009).

The spinal cord of amphibians is more differentiated in anurans than urodeles. Anurans have a relatively short spinal cord with 11 segments and exhibit cervical and lumbar enlargements (Underhill, 1969). The spine cord terminates in a relatively long and slender cone, which represents the remnant of the premetamorphosis caudal portion (Akita, 1992a; Underhill, 1969).

The topography of the caudal end of the spinal cord (lumbar enlargement and conus medullaris) differs widely among mammals and other taxa, as mentioned above. The topographies of these regions are described between the last lumbar (basis) and first sacral (apex) vertebrae, varying with species and age. For example, in dogs the conus medullaris lies between L3 and L7, although Santiago (1974), Fletcher (1970), and Evans and De Lahunta (2010) reported that in large dogs the conus ends at the rostral margin of L4, while in small dogs is more elongated, ending at L6. The topographies of these structures in different species are compared in Table 19.2. However, owing to the differential growth rates of vertebral column and spinal cord, the increase in caudal lumbar nerves forms the cauda equina. This consists of nerve roots located inside the spinal canal of the lumbar and sacral spine, together laterocaudally with the conus medullaris and filum terminale, with variation of this position among species.

Therefore, injuries to the cauda equina can involve several nerves because there are numerous nerve roots in the small area between L3 and S3, including the main nerves of the lumbosacral plexus. However, birds, reptiles, and amphibians have no cauda equina (Ashley, 1962; Underhill, 1969; Baumel, 1975; Nickel et al., 1977; Rowe, 1986; Akita, 1992 a,b; Dubbeldam, 1993; Wyneken, 2003, 2007).

TABLE 19.2
Levels of Lumbar Enlargement and Conus Medullaris in Spinal Cords of Some Vertebrates.

Species	Lumbar Enlargement	Conus Medullaris
Human	Th11-L1	L1-3
NONHUMAN PRIMATES		
Ateles	L1-4	L5-S2
Cebus	L1-4	L5-S3
Chimpanzee	Th11-L1	L1-3
Cynomolgus	L1-4	L5-S3
Gibbon	L1-4	L3-S3
Gorilla	Th11-L1	L1-3
Lagothrix	L1-4	L1-S2
Orangutan	Th11-L1	L1-3
Rhesus macaque	L1-4	L1-S3
OTHER MAMMALS		
Cat	L3-5	L5-S3
Chinchilla	L2-L5	L6-S2
Dog	L4-6	L3-7
Guinea pig	Th12-L2	L5-S2
Swine	L6-7	L5-S3
Rabbit	Th12-L2	L5-S4
Rat	Th11-L1	L1-3
OTHER TETRAPODS		
Birds	Synsacrum	Synsacrum
Iguana	PS25-28	PS28-S2
Varanus	PS28-30	PS30-S2
Tortoise	Th6-S1-5-Co1	No present
Turtles	PS16-18	No present
Anurans	SN7-10	S1-Urostyle

PS, presacral segments; *SN*, spinal nerve.

LUMBOSACRAL PLEXUSES

Although Getty (1975) considers the lumbar and sacral plexuses to be distinct in large animals, other authors consider the denomination "lumbosacral plexus" more pertinent. According to Nomina Anatomica Veterinaria (2017), the lumbosacral plexus is a somatic nerve plexus formed by intercommunications among the ventral rami of the lumbar segments (lumbar plexus) and the first sacral segments (sacral plexus). Differences in plexus formation are due to the different segmental participations of certain nerves, and to their participation in tissue innervation, as with the brachial plexus on the periphery. Lumbar nerves spread similarly to nerves from the medial and lateral fascicles of the brachial plexus, and sacral nerves spread similarly to nerves from the posterior fascicle of the brachial plexus, providing sensory and motor innervations to the gluteal region, pelvis and pelvic limb.

Anatomy textbooks mention three possible configurations of the lumbosacral plexus: (1) separate lumbar plexus (iliohypogastric, ilioinguinal, genitofemoral, lateral femoral cutaneous, femoral, and obturator nerves) and sacral plexus (cranial gluteal, caudal gluteal, sciatic, pudendal, and inferior rectal nerves), their formations not being considered together; (2) only the lumbar nerves and the sciatic nerve are constituents of the lumbosacral trunk; (3) the cranial (superior) and caudal (inferior) gluteal nerves grouped with the tibial and common fibular nerves are components of the plexus (Getty, 1975; Frandson, 1979; Lacerda et al., 2006; Dyce et al., 2009). However, some axons that innervate the pelvic limb via lumbar and/or sacral nerves could originate from various spinal segments, with greater or less participation by each segment in forming three consecutive trunks: cranial or superior (middle lumbar segments), medium (last lumbar and first sacral segments), and caudal or inferior (only sacral segments).

On the other hand, several studies describe variations in the formation and distribution of the lumbosacral nerves. Since the terms "prefixed" (proximal or superior or cranial), "ordinary" (normal or median-fixed), and "postfixed" (distal or inferior or caudal) were introduced by Sherrington (1892), variations in the lumbar and sacral plexuses and nerve origins in humans have been extensively reviewed. When a communicating branch from L4-5 joins the first lumbar trunk (L6), it constitutes a prefixed plexus (Bardeen and Elting, 1901; Severeano, 1904; Webber, 1961). Post-fixed plexuses include S3-4 in forming the more caudal lumbosacral nerves, the sciatic, pudendal, and rectal caudal (Bardeen and Elting, 1901; Severeano, 1904;

Webber, 1961). Nevertheless, Gomez-Amaya and colleagues (2015) proposed a classification of a mixed pre-post-fixed lumbosacral plexus (L3-S2) in dogs because these animals possess a high degree of variability, irrespective of breed.

However, experimental approaches to the lumbosacral plexus should consider details of plexus formation because both injuries and variations in formation are frequent (Rigaud et al., 2008). Indications for reconstructive operations on the plexus are exceedingly rare because the structures that form it are located further from each other than the brachial plexus. Therefore, less significant neurological failures result from injuries to the lumbar and sacral plexuses. Also, owing to the variable locations of the conus medullaris and cauda equina (Table 19.2), occasional lesions cranial to L4-5 produce signs of lumbosacral disease (Di Dio, 2002; Standring, 2009). Disease in the lumbosacral articulations or the sacrum produces sensory and motor deficits of the caudal hindlimb (sciatic and cranial and caudal gluteal), the perineal region (pudendal), and the pelvic viscera (autonomic). For example, a lesion affecting the L4-6 roots produces partial effects on the gluteal nerves, even though the major signals are observed in the femoral and obturator nerve territories.

The pelvic visceral autonomic innervation, which is responsible for controlling tone and contractility, is frequently affected by lesions of the lumbosacral plexus (Di Dio, 2002; Standring, 2009). Severe caudal lumbar lesions block central inhibition of micturition and result in urinary incontinence, while the parasympathetic reflex of bladder emptying is usually intact. On the other hand, parasympathetic loss associated with maintenance of sympathetic innervation results in detrusor sphincter dysynergy, loss of detrusor muscle activity, and abnormally strong contractions of the sphincter urethrae muscle. Another important factor is the effect of epidural anesthesia on the sympathetic and parasympathetic nervous systems.

Human and Nonhuman Primates

Human anatomy textbooks describe the caudal branches of the spinal cord as divided into three main trunks: (1) first trunk or lumbar plexus (Th12 and L1-4); (2) second trunk or sacral or lumbosacral plexus (L4-5 and S1-3); and (3) third trunk or pudendal plexus (S2-5 and Co1, Di Dio, 2002; Standring, 2009). The first trunk was well detailed in the textbook *Surgical Anatomy of the Lumbar Plexus* (Tubbs et al., 2018), while the anatomy of the remaining trunks is described in other chapters of the present volume. However, a descriptive summary is necessary to contextualize the comparative anatomy. Thus, the second trunk formed from L4-5 and S1-3 can be called sciatic plexus or trunk because all roots constitute this nerve, which branches into the other nerves to the inferior limb (Di Dio, 2002; Standring, 2009). The sciatic nerve trunk emits proximal branches (superior and inferior gluteal nerves, and two branches to the obturator internus and piriformis muscles) and terminal branches (tibial and common fibular nerves). The inferior trunk, also called the pudendal plexus, is usually formed by branches from S2-5 and Co1 and gives off the following nerves: perforating cutaneous (S2-3), pudendal (S2-4), inferior rectal (S3-4), nerve to levator ani, nerve to coccygeus and external anal sphincter (S4), and the anococcygeal nerve (S4-5 and Co1, Di Dio, 2002; Standring, 2009).

The innervation in nonhuman primates is very similar to that in humans, being described a lumbar plexus, which originates from L1-4 (Champneys, 1871; Hepburn, 1892a,b; Raven and Hill, 1950; Zaluska and Urbanowicz, 1972), and a sacral plexus, constituted by L5-6 (or L7 when present) and S1-2 (Fig. 19.1: Hill, 1953, 1957, 1960, 1972). The lumbar and sacral plexuses are anastomosed by a bifurcated nerve, which delimits the end and beginning of each (Piasecka-Kacperska and Gladykowska-Rzeckzycka, 1972). This nerve is described in apes (L5: ; Hepburn, 1892a,b; Raven and Hill, 1950) and *Cebus* (L4: Hill, 1960; Barros et al., 2003), but is absent in the rhesus macaque (Hartmann and Straus, 1932; Krechowiecki et al., 1972; Pietrzk et al., 1964), *Cynomolgus* (Urbanowicz and Zaluska, 1969; Zaluska and Urbanowicz, 1972), and *Ateles* (Chang and Ruch, 1947, 1949; Hill, 1957; El Assy, 1966). In some species, the sacral plexus is divided into sacral and pudendal plexuses. The lumbar and sacral plexuses are almost always connected in prosimians and primates (Pietrzk et al., 1964; El Assy, 1966). There is a functional correspondence between the lumbosacral plexus in humans and some monkeys, although in many cases the medullary segments do not correspond numerically; for example, L4 in humans corresponds to L5 in macaques (Pietrzk et al., 1964; El Assy, 1966). In humans, the first root engaged in the plexus is L4, while in apes it is L3, L4, or L5, as observed in chimpanzees and gorillas (Eisler, 1890; El Assy, 1966).

In nonhuman primates there are various degrees of pre- and postfixation of the lumbosacral plexus reflecting the number of presacral vertebrae and probable shortening of the thoracic region (Pietrzk et al., 1964; Piasecka-Kacperska and Gladykowska-Rzeckzycka, 1972). Reduction of the presacral vertebral column is more pronounced in orangutans and other primates,

resulting in a prefixation process, whereas the postfixed condition is caused by stretching of this portion (Schultz and Straus, 1945). Primates with 13 thoracic vertebrae are considered evolutionarily primitive, a condition observed in arboreal shrews, the common ancestor of all primates (Schultz and Straus, 1945). Likewise, six is the original number of lumbar vertebrae in primates, being observed the *Plathyrrhinos*, *Alouattinae*, *Atelinae*, and higher primates (Hill, 1957, 1960;

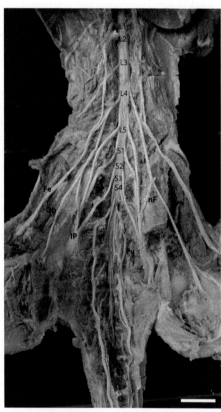

FIG. 19.1 Ventral view of the vertebral column showing the spinal roots of the lumbosacral plexus in Platyrrhini, Atelidae, Alouattinae, *Alouatta guariba*. The nerves shown are the femoral (Fe) and obturator (Ob), originating from the union of the (L2) L3, and L4 spinal nerves; the furcal (nF) emerging from the L4 spinal nerve; the sciatic plexus (IP) arising from (L4) L5 and S1-2; and the pudendal (Pu), which is constituted by the combination of S2-4. The sacrococcygeal (SC) innervation is formed by the combination of S3-4 and the six coccygeal nerves. The filum terminale (ft) of the spinal cord is also shown. Scale bar: 2 cm. (Personal collection. Dissected by Matheus Cândano de Brito and photographed by Victoria Cristina dos Santos, Applied Animal Anatomy Laboratory, Federal University of Santa Catarina, Brazil.)

1972; Schultz and Straus, 1945). On the other hand, three sacral vertebrae are characteristic of primate ancestors, predominating in most current primates, although the average number can range from three to six (Schultz and Straus, 1945). These observations show a tendency toward inferior displacement of the lumbosacral plexus (postfixed condition) in all primate genera, with exception of Hominoidea (Zaluska and Urbanowicz, 1972). In the prefixed plexus, the third lumbar nerve (L3) participates in forming the lumbar plexus, while it is always present in the postfixed plexus. Long-tailed monkeys (*Haplorrhini*) have interconnected coccygeal nerves forming a plexus on each side of the length of tail, as in *Ateles*, which has eight coccygeal spinal segments involved in innervating this region (Hill, 1957).

Some authors have distinguished two groups of lumbosacral nerves in these animals because of their muscular territories and functions. Thus, a flexor group (branches of the tibial and common fibular, pubioisquiofemoral, and pudendal nerves) and an extensor group (piriform, superior and inferior gluteal, sciatic and posterior femoral cutaneous nerves: Urbanowick and Zaluska, 1969; El Assy, 1966, Zaluska and Urbanowicz, 1972; Pietrzk, Piasecka-Kacperska and Gladykowska-Rzeckzycka, 1972) can be identified. Although pertinent, this functional classification does not correspond to real territories of innervation in primates; these animals have lower limbs of both lifting and carrier types. It is more relevant to humans, which have only carrier-type limbs.

In fact, an anatomical lumbosacral plexus has been described only in *Cynomolgus*, rhesus macaques, and *Ateles*; the lumbar and sacral plexuses are distinct in other primates. The plexus in *Cynomolgus* and the rhesus macaque is formed from L1-7-S1-2 (Hartmann and Straus, 1932; Pietrzk et al., 1964; Urbanowicz and Zaluska, 1969), while in *Ateles* is formed from L3-5 and S1-2 (Hill, 1957; Chang and Ruch, 1947; 1949; El Assy, 1966). In chimpanzees, orangutans, and gorillas, the sacral plexus emerges from L5-6 and S1-2 and is joined to the lumbar plexus by the furcal nerve (L4: Champneys, 1871; Eisler, 1890; Hepburn, 1892a,b; Raven and Hill, 1950). However, in the gibbon, the plexus arises from L5-S1-2 (Hepburn, 1892 a; b), as in humans, while in *Cebus* it emerges from L5-S1 with the furcal nerve in L4 (Hill, 1960; Barros et al., 2003). *Cebus* also has a coccygeal plexus originating from S2-5-Co1-2 (Hill, 1960; Barros et al., 2003).

The lumbosacral trunk formed in humans and nonhuman primates shows a slight asymmetry between the right and left antimers (Zaluska and Urbanowicz, 1972). All apes except the chimpanzee have a prefixed lumbosacral trunk, originating from L4-5-S1-2 (Champneys, 1871; Eisler, 1890; Hepburn, 1892a; b). However, the degree of pre- and postfixation of the plexus in other species varies according to the first or last root involved in their formation. In the chimpanzee and *Ateles* the trunk is formed by L3-5-S1-2 (Champneys, 1871; Hepburn, 1892a,b; Hill, 1957; Chang and Ruch, 1947, 1947; El Assy, 1966, respectively), while in the rhesus it is formed from L4-6-S1-2 (Urbanowicz and Zaluska, 1969; Zaluska and Urbanowicz, 1972; Krechowiecki et al., 1972), and in *Cynomolgus* from L5-7-S1-2 (Hartmann and Straus, 1932). In *Cebus*, a lumbosacrococcygeal trunk is constituted from L2-5-S1-5-Co1-3, prefixed in L1 and postfixed in L5 (Hill, 1960; Barros et al., 2003).

The nerves that arise from the lumbosacral plexus can be distinguished as short and long branches. Short branches (piriform, obturator internus, iliopsoas, pubioisquiofemoral, gluteal, and tensor fasciae latae) emerge directly of the lumbosacral trunk or indirectly from the long nerves, e.g., the sciatic, caudal cutaneous femoral, tibial, and common fibular. Among the short nerves, the piriformis emerges from L4-S1 in anthropoids (Champneys, 1871; Eisler, 1890; Hepburn, 1892a; b; El Assy, 1966), L7-S1-2 in the rhesus (Hartmann and Straus, 1932; Urbanowicz and Zaluska, 1969; Zaluska and Urbanowicz, 1972; Krechowiecki et al., 1972), L6-7 in *Cynomolgus* (Urbanowicz and Zaluska, 1969), L5-S1-2 in *Ateles* (Chang and Ruch, 1947; Hill, 1957), and as plexus branches in *Cebus* (El Assy, 1966; Hill, 1960; Barros et al., 2003). Three gluteal nerves (superior, medium, and inferior) arise from the union of L4-5 in *Cebus* (El Assy, 1966; Hill, 1960; Barros et al., 2003), L4-S1-2 in *Ateles* (Chang and Ruch, 1947; El Assy, 1966), and L3-4 in apes (Champneys, 1871; Eisler, 1890; El Assy, 1966), but are branches of the sciatic nerve in the rhesus and *Cynomolgus* (Hartmann and Straus, 1932; Pietrzk et al., 1964; El Assy, 1966; Urbanowicz and Zaluska, 1969). The origin of the pubioischiofemoral nerve varies among Hominoidea primates. In the chimpanzee it arises from L3-4-S1 (Champneys, 1871; El Assy, 1966), but in *Ateles* it is from L4-S1 (Chang and Ruch, 1947; Hill, 1957; El Assy, 1966), while in the rhesus and *Cynomolgus* it is from L5-7 (Urbanowicz and Zaluska, 1969; Zaluska and Urbanowicz, 1972; Krechowiecki et al., 1972). This nerve runs near to the nerve of the flexor muscles, innervating the pubioisquiofemoralis, gemelli, obturator internus, and quadratus femoris.

The typical sciatic nerve is not observed in most nonhuman primates; the common fibular and tibial nerves originate directly from the lumbosacral trunk.

However, there is disagreement among authors about the origin and existence of the sciatic nerve. In the rhesus and *Cynomolgus*, three possible configurations for this nerve are mentioned: from L5-S1-7 in prefixed plexuses, from L6-7-S1-2 in postfixed plexuses, and from L5-S1-6 in animals with six lumbar vertebrae, the common fibular nerve originating from L5-7 and the tibial from L5-7-S1-2 (El Assy, 1966; Hill, 1966). The chimpanzee and orangutan have a sciatic nerve formed from L3-4, receiving fibers from S1 to form the common fibular nerve or S1-2 for the tibial nerve (Champneys, 1871; El Assy, 1966; Hill, 1966). In the gorilla (Eisler, 1890; El Assy, 1966; Hill, 1966) and gibbon (Hepburn, 1892 a; b), the trunk divides into the common fibular nerve formed from L4-5-S1 and the tibial nerve (L4-5-S1-2), whereas in *Ateles* the trunk is formed from L3-4-S1-3, constituting the common fibular nerve, and from L3-4-S1-2 constituting the tibial nerve (Chang and Ruch, 1947; Hill, 1957; El Assy, 1966). Only in *Cebus* is there a sciatic nerve, originating from L4-5-S1-2, which divides into the common fibular and tibial nerves (Hill, 1960; Barros et al., 2003).

Nonhuman primates have no pudendal plexus as in humans. In those animals, the plexus of the lumbosacral trunk emerges from S1-3 in *Cebus* (Hill, 1960; Barros et al., 2003), L4-S1-3 in *Ateles* (Chang and Ruch, 1947; El Assy, 1966), L7-S1-2 in the rhesus monkey and *Cynomolgus* (El Assy, 1966; Pietrzk et al., 1964; Urbanowicz and Zaluska, 1969; Piasecka-Kacperska and Gladykowska-Rzeczzycka, 1972), and S2-3 in anthropoids (El Assy, 1966). In *Cebus*, *Ateles*, rhesus, and *Cynomolgus*, the final portion of the sacrococcygeal plexus gives rise to the nerves to the tail, innervating a developed coccygeal musculature. These nerves and muscles are important in these species because they are used in locomotion and prehension of objects.

Other Mammals

Several experimental models can be used for studying injury to the lumbosacral plexus, mimicking the different lesions observed in humans (Rigaud et al., 2008). Among the methods widely studied are those that produce mechanical trauma, with special reference to the sciatic nerve.

In general, the lumbosacral plexus is described as being formed by the union of L3-7 and S1-3 in dogs (Miller et al., 1964; Dyce et al., 2009; Evans and De Lahunta, 2010, Fig. 19.2), T13 and L1-6 and S1-S2 in rats (Hunt, 1924; Greene, 1968; Chiasson, 1980; Vejsada and Hnik, 1980; Asato et al., 2000), L4-7 and S1-3 in cats (Ghoshal, 1972; Getty, 1975; Crouch, 1985) and rabbits (Bensley and Craigie, 1938; Barone et al.,

1973; Mclaughlin, 1987), L3-6 and S1-3 in guinea pigs (Cooper and Schiller, 1975), L4-6 and S1-3 in the chinchilla (Martinez-Pereira and Rickes, 2011), and L4-6(7) to S1-2 in pigs (Bosa and Getty, 1969; Ghoshal, 1975; Massone, 1988; Miheliae et al., 2004; Chagas et al., 2006, Fig. 19.3). However, as previously mentioned, zoological anatomy textbooks describe various formations of the lumbosacral plexus for each species. If some species have undergone selective pressures to generate experimental lineages (Ernst, 2016),

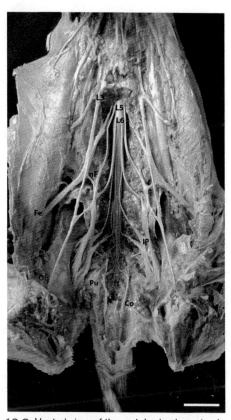

FIG. 19.2 Ventral view of the vertebral column to show the spinal roots of the lumbosacral plexus in mongrel dogs. The nerves shown are the femoral (Fe) and obturator (Ob) originating from the union of L3 and L4 spinal nerves; the furcal (nF) emerging from the L4 spinal nerve; the sciatic plexus (IP) arising from (L4) L5-7 and S1; the pudendal (Pu) constituted by the union of S1-3; and the coccygeal (Co), formed by the union of S3-4 and the four to seven coccygeal nerves. The filum terminale (ft) of the spinal cord is also shown. Scale bar: 2 cm. (Personal collection. Dissected and photographed by Victoria Cristina dos Santos, Applied Animal Anatomy Laboratory, Federal University of Santa Catarina, Brazil.)

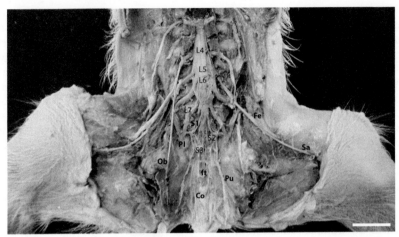

FIG. 19.3 Ventral view of the vertebral column to show the spinal roots of the lumbosacral plexus of the pig. The nerves shown are the femoral (Fe) and obturator (Ob) originating from the union of L4-6 spinal nerves; the furcal (nF) emerging from L5 spinal nerve; the sciatic plexus (IP) arising from L4-6(7) and S1-2; the pudendal (Pu) constituted by the union of S1-3; and the coccygeal (Co), formed by the union of S3-4 and the four to seven coccygeal nerves. The filum terminale (ft) of the spinal cord is also shown. Scale bar: 2 cm. (Personal collection. Dissected by Matheus Cândano de Brito and photographed by Victoria Cristina dos Santos, Applied Animal Anatomy Laboratory, Federal University of Santa Catarina, Brazil.)

the anatomical plexus model can be more variable. On the other hand, everyone agrees that the lumbosacral plexus invariably consists of the most caudal lumbar nerve roots (lumbar plexus) associated with the more cranial sacral nerve roots (sacral plexus: Getty, 1975; Frandson, 1979). Moreover, some consider that in all these species the lumbosacral plexus generates two trunks: cranial (responsible for the formation of the femoral and obturator nerves) and caudal (from which cranial and caudal gluteal, caudal cutaneous femoral, and sciatic nerves emerge). Thus, in many mammals, in contrast to primates, the caudal lumbar nerves (femoral and obturator) are described as originating from the cranial trunk of the lumbosacral plexus (Getty, 1975; Frandson, 1979; Lacerda et al., 2006; Dyce et al., 2009), but this is very debatable.

The constitution of the cranial trunk varies among the species described because more caudal lumbar and/or sacral segments are involved in the formation of the obturator nerve in the guinea pig (L5-6: Cooper and Schiller, 1975) and rabbit (L5-S3: Bensley and Craigie, 1938; Barone et al., 1973; Mclaughlin, 1987). However, Nascimento and colleagues (2019) recently showed that the obturator nerve is formed from the ventral spinal branches of L6 and L7 in New Zealand rabbits, with a variation between L5 and S1. In rats, the cranial trunk is formed by L2-4 or L5 while the

femoral nerve originates from L2-4 (Hunt, 1924; Greene, 1968; Chiasson, 1980) and the obturator from (L2) L3-5 (Chiasson, 1980; Greene, 1968). In the dog (Miller et al., 1964; Dyce et al., 2009; Evans and De Lahunta, 2010), pig (Bosa and Getty, 1969; Ghoshal, 1975; Massone, 1988; Miheliae et al., 2004; Chagas et al., 2006), and chinchilla (Martinez-Pereira and Rickes, 2011), both nerves emerge from a common trunk formed by L3-6 and L3-4, respectively. The femoral nerve arises from L4-5 in the guinea pig (Cooper and Schiller, 1975), mostly from L6 with contributions from L5 and L7 in rabbits (Bensley and Craigie, 1938; Barone et al., 1973; Mclaughlin, 1987; Malik, 2011) and from L5-6 in the cat; and the obturator emerges from L6-7 in the cat (Ghoshal, 1972). The innervation territories of the femoral nerve include the psoas major and minor and the deep lumbar muscles, and upon reaching the femoral space the nerve emits branches to the quadriceps muscle (Getty, 1975; Dyce et al., 2009). The saphenous nerve arises more caudally and innervates the gracilis, pectineus, and sartorius muscles, branching to supply the skin and fascia in the medial femoral region. The obturator nerve, after leaving the pelvic cavity through the obturator foramen, supplies the branches of the adductor, pectineus, gracilis, and obturator internus and externus muscles (Getty, 1975; Dyce et al., 2009).

The pelvic limb is innervated by the caudal trunk, formed by the union of L5-7 and S1(2) in dogs (Miller et al., 1964; Dyce et al., 2009; Evans and De Lahunta, 2010), L4-7 and S1-2 in cats (Ghoshal, 1972; Getty, 1975), L6 and S1-2 in guinea pigs (Cooper and Schiller, 1975), L5-7 and S1-3 in rabbits (Bensley and Craigie, 1938; Barone et al., 1973; Mclaughlin, 1987; Malik, 2011), and L5-6 and S1-2 in the pig and chinchilla (Bosa and Getty, 1969; Ghoshal, 1975; Martinez-Pereira and Rickes, 2011, respectively). Nevertheless, Miheliae (2004) and colleagues, like Chagas and contributors (2006), observed that some pig lineages have a seventh lumbar segment and nerve that participates in the plexus (Fig. 19.3). However, L4 and L5 always, and L6 rarely, contribute to the formation of the common root in the rat, and L4-6 and S1-2 contribute to this trunk (Hunt, 1924; Greene, 1968; Chiasson, 1980; Vejsada and Hnik, 1980). In more recent studies, the common caudal trunk has been referred to as the sciatic plexus (Martinez-Pereira and Rickes, 2011; Martinez-Pereira and Zancan, 2015; Lorenzão et al., 2016) because it constitutes a common root, originating from different spinal nerves and branching into the cranial gluteal, caudal gluteal, caudal cutaneous femoral and sciatic nerves. The sciatic plexus was indirectly described in dogs (Miller et al., 1964) and cats (Ghoshal, 1972) as the origin of the cranial (L6-7 and S1) and caudal (L7) gluteal nerves with the sciatic nerve. This plexus covers the iliac region dorsocaudally, reaching the femoral region caudally and ramifying into their four branches. However, some peculiarities of each nerve in each species should be considered. (1) The cranial gluteal nerves arise from different nerves in the guinea pig (L6 and S1: Cooper and Schiller, 1975), rat (L4-6 and S1: Hunt, 1924; Greene, 1968; Chiasson, 1980; Vejsada and Hnik, 1980), and cat (L6-7: Ghoshal, 1972), or from a common root with the caudal gluteal in the rabbit (L6-7: Bensley and Craigie, 1938; Barone et al., 1973; Mclaughlin, 1987; Malik, 2011) and pig (L5-6 and S1: Bosa and Getty, 1969; Ghoshal, 1975). On the other hand, in dogs, the cranial gluteal nerve arises only from L6-7-S1 or both nerves arise from L6-7-S1 (Miller et al., 1964), while in the chinchilla both nerves originate from the sciatic plexus (Martinez-Pereira and Rickes, 2011). This nerve, after leaving the pelvic cavity through the greater sciatic foramen, supplies the branches of the deep gluteal, piriformis, and tensor fasciae latae muscles. (2) When the caudal gluteal nerve originates alone it is reported to arise from L7 in dogs (Miller et al., 1964), from S1 in the guinea pig (Cooper and Schiller, 1975), and from the peroneal nerve in rats (L6-S1-4-Co1-2: Mckenna and

Nadelhaft, 1986). It arises from the caudal portion of the sciatic plexus and innervates the superficial gluteal, the cranial part of the biceps femoris, the abductor muscle of the thigh, and the vertebral head of semitendinosus and semimembranosus muscles. However, the medial gluteal muscle is innervated by the two gluteal nerves. (3) In the guinea pig, the sciatic nerve gives rise to the caudal nerve (Cooper and Schiller, 1975), but in dogs it arises mostly from L4, with contributions from L3 and L5 (Miller et al., 1964), while in cat it arises from S2-3 (Ghoshal, 1972; Crouch, 1985). It innervates the biceps femoris and semitendinosus muscles, and then between those muscles it supplies the skin over the tuber sciaticum, the caudal portion of the femur and, through a union with the pudendal nerve, the perineum.

The roots that constitute the sciatic nerve differ among species owing to variations in the numbers of lumbar and sacral vertebrae. Nevertheless, these nerve roots can be considered the last spinal nerves that form the plexus, except in cats (L6-7 and S1-2: Ghoshal, 1972; Crouch, 1985) and rats (L4-6: Hunt, 1924; Greene, 1968; Chiasson, 1980; Vejsada and Hnik, 1980). The sciatic is the largest nerve in the body, often suffering injuries that result in insensitivity and motor dysfunction in all regions of the affected limb. It ramifies into several muscular branches and forms the tibial, common fibular, and lateral and caudal cutaneous sural nerves. The proximal muscular branch supplies the obturator internus, gemelli, and quadratus femoris muscles, and, after innervating the caudal portion of the biceps femoris, semitendinosus, and semimembranosus muscles, it extends to the skin. The lateral sural cutaneous nerve innervates the hypodermis and skin in the cranial sural region, while the caudal sural cutaneous nerve crosses the caudal sural region and innervates the skin of this region and the common calcaneal tendon. The tibial is a muscular and cutaneous nerve that crosses to the tarsal joint level, emitting slender branches to the skin in this region and dividing into the dorsal digital and common digital plantar V nerves. After this branching, the tibial nerve supplies a distal muscular branch that extends to the flexor muscles, between the two heads of the gastrocnemius and the popliteus, and continues as branches to the muscles of the plantar surface of the metatarsus and dividing into the common digital plantar II, III, and IV nerves. The common fibular nerve innervates the muscles and skin of the cranial surface of the tibia, tarsus, metatarsus, and digits. It passes over the lateral head of the gastrocnemius muscle and enters the sulcus between the fibularis longus and extensor digitorum lateralis, then divides into the superficial and deep fibular nerves. The superficial fibular nerve innervates the skin of the dorsum of the tarsus and metatarsus and the extensor digitorum lateralis, while the deep fibular nerve innervates the cranial tibial, long and short fibular, and extensor digitorum longus muscles and forms the common dorsal digital III and IV nerves.

The pudendal plexus is described only in rats, being formed by the union of L6, S1-4, and Co1-2 with the cranial gluteal nerve (Mckenna and Nadelhaft, 1986). However, the pudendal and caudal rectal nerves originate together in guinea pigs (S2-4), rabbits (S1-4), dogs (S1-3: Miller et al., 1964; Dyce et al., 2009; Evans and De Lahunta, 2010), and cats (S2-3: Ghoshal, 1972; Crouch, 1985), while in the chinchilla (Martinez-Pereira and Rickes, 2011) both nerves emerge separately from S1-2 (pudendal) and S2-3 (rectal caudal), and in the pig from S2-3 (pudendal) and S4 (rectal caudal). The pudendal nerve crosses toward the caudal pelvic aperture and divides into the dorsal nerve of the penis or clitoris and the superficial and deep perineal nerves. The former of these innervates the ischiocavernosus, bulbospongiosus, and retractor penis muscles, and the preputium in males and the constrictor vulvae, clitoris, and vulva in females. The superficial and deep perineal nerves innervate the skin and muscles of the anal and perianal regions. The rectal caudal nerve innervates up to the end of the rectum, the sphincter muscles of the anus, and the skin of the anal region.

BIRDS
Lumbar, Sacral, and Pudendal Plexuses

Before we describe the innervation of the pelvic region, hindlimb and tail, it is important to note that the caudal region of the vertebral column is differentiated in birds. It comprises 14−15 vertebrae, depending on the species, which are fused to form the synsacrum. The connection between the synsacrum and the ilium bone, which reaches far into the thoracic region, is crucial for the shape of the trunk in birds. The bony connection is accomplished cranially by spines and transverse processes and caudally by the transverse processes of the synsacrum, which are fused into a continuous bony plate that permits the passage of nerves and blood vessels. The following vertebrae are differentiated in the synsacrum, from cranial to caudal: synsacrothoracic, synsacrolumbar, primary sacral, and synsacrocaudal (Getty, 1975; Nickel et al., 1977). If we consider that the lumbar to coccygeal segments of the spinal cord are located in the canal of the synsacrum, the spinal nerves arising from it can be called synsacral nerves (Sy).

Among the anatomical characteristics of birds that differ from mammals, the pelvic region, hindlimb, and tail are innervated by mixed nerves from the lumbar, sacral, and pudendal plexuses (Baumel, 1975; Nickel et al., 1977; Dubbeldam, 1993). The division of this innervation into plexuses is more didactic than anatomical. Thus, these regions are innervated by (1) a lumbar plexus formed by the last two lumbar ventral (L6-7 or SN23-24) and one sacral (S1 or SN25) strand, also called the furcal nerve, that connects this plexus to the next; (2) a sacral plexus constituted by the ventral strands of S1-S5(6) or SN26-30 (31), with 5-7 roots, which emit the bigeminal nerve to communicate from the last plexus. Because this plexus has so many roots, three trunks can be recognized: (1) cranial (formed by the first three roots); (2) medium (fourth root alone) and caudal (fifth and sixth roots united); and (3) a pudendal plexus originating from S9-12 (SN31-34). Nevertheless, the furcal and bigeminal nerves are sometimes not visible. However, these descriptions refer mainly to domestic birds (chicken, duck, and goose: Baumel, 1975; Nickel et al., 1977; Dubbeldam, 1993, Fig. 19.4). For example, in the ostrich (*Struthio camelus*: El-Mahdy et al., 2010), the lumbar plexus is formed by the union of four roots (Sy2-5) and the sacral plexus by the union of seven (Sy5-11). Sy5-9 form the cranial trunk of the plexus, whereas Sy10-11 constitute its caudal trunk and Sy5 constitutes the furcal nerve. In contrast, in Kyrgyz pheasant (*Phasianus colchicus mongolicus*: İstanbullugil et al., 2013), the sacral plexus is formed by the ventral branches of S1-5 and is located between the lumbar and pudendal plexuses. In this species, the sacral plexus gives rise to three trunks: a cranial trunk formed by the union of S1-3, a medium trunk formed by S4 and a caudal trunk comprising S5 only. The cranial and medium trunks connect in a single root. In a study of the merlin (*Falco columbarius*), Akalan and colleagues (2019) observed that the lumbrosacral plexus was formed by six ventral rami of the Sy2-7 nerves, divided into lumbar (Sy2-4) and sacral (Sy4-7) plexuses joined by the furcal nerve (Sy4).

For better understanding, the description of the nerves is based only on the didactic division of the plexus. Thus, the nerves of the lumbar plexus comprise the iliohypogastric and ilioinguinal (both to the ventral muscles of the trunk), obturator (obturator externus and adductor muscles), cutaneous femoral (sartorius muscles and cutaneous branch in the lateral surface of the thigh), femoral (larger lumbar branch that innervates the iliacus, quadriceps femoris or femorotibial, gracilis, and tensor fasciae latae muscles), cranial gluteal (gluteus medius and deep muscles), and saphenous

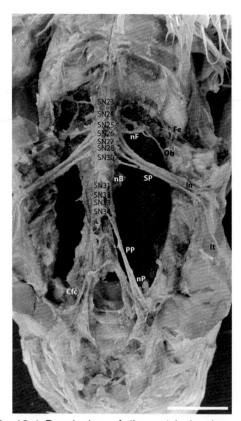

FIG. 19.4 Dorsal view of the vertebral column and synsacrum showing the spinal roots of the lumbosacral plexus in *Gallus gallus domesticus*. The lumbar plexus (LP) is formed by spinal nerves 23–24, with the furcal nerve (nF) represented by SN25, while the sacral plexus (SP) is constituted by spinal nerves 26–30, with the bigeminal nerve (nB) represented by SN30. SN31-34 constitute the pudendal plexus (PP). From the LP the femoral (Fe) and obturator (Ob) nerves arise, the sciatic (In) and iliotibial (It) originate from the SP, and the pudendal (nP) and caudal cutaneous femoral (Cfc) come from the PP. Scale bar: 2 cm. (Personal collection. Dissected and photographed by Guilherme José Parizzi, Applied Animal Anatomy Laboratory, Federal University of Santa Catarina, Brazil.)

(innervates the knee joint and the inner surface of the leg: Baumel, 1975; Nickel et al., 1977; Dubbeldam, 1993). However, in the ostrich the cranial femoral nerve originates from the union of Sy2-3, supplies the cranial iliotibial muscle, and divides into the lateral and cranial femoral cutaneous nerves, which supply the skin of the lateral and cranial surfaces of the thigh (El-Mahdy et al., 2010). The obturator nerve is the smallest branch of the lumbar plexus formed by Sy3-5 in the ostrich (El-Mahdy et al., 2010), while in the chicken it is formed

by two lumbar roots (Baumel, 1975; Nickel et al., 1977). The sacral nerves include the caudal gluteal (superficial gluteal and biceps femoris); nerve branches to the biceps femoris, semitendinosus, semimembranosus, quadratus femoris and gemelli, caudal femoral cutaneous (skin of the caudal surface of thigh), and sciatic muscles, while the pudendal plexus innervates the ventral muscles of the tail, the muscles of the cloaca, and the skin in both regions (Baumel, 1975; Nickel et al., 1977). In the merlin, the lateral cutaneous femoral (Sy2-3), femoral (Sy2-4, which emits the saphenous, cranial cutaneus femoris cranialis and *coxalis cranialis*) and obturator (Sy3-4) nerves emerge from the lumbar plexus, while the sacral plexus emits each Sy5 and Sy6 nerve separately, after which they unite with Sy7 to form the sciatic nerve. The sciatic nerve ramifies into the *coxalis caudalis*, caudal cutaneous femoral, sural cutaneous, tibial, and fibular nerves (the last-named branches into the third, superficial and deep fibular: Akalan et al., 2019).

Among the nerves present in these regions, the sciatic is important for diagnosing Marek's disease. This widespread avian infection causes swelling of peripheral nerves, loss of striated mass, and lethargy. The sciatic, the largest nerve of the sacral plexus, arises from S1-4 in domestic birds and the Kyrgyz pheasant (İstanbullugil et al., 2013), and from Sy5-9 in the ostrich (El-Mahdy et al., 2010). It gives rise to the lateral cutaneous crural (skin of the lateral surface of the tibiotarsus, but this is present only in the ostrich, not in domestic birds), tibial (larger terminal branch of this nerve, which bifurcates to form the medial and lateral sural to supply the flexor muscles of the leg and toes), medial tibial (which innervates the gastrocnemius and popliteus muscles, then continues as the parafibular and medial plantar), and fibular nerve, which is divided into superficial fibular (supplies the extensor brevis digiti II, fibularis longus, fibularis brevis, and extensor digitorum brevis III and IV muscles), and deep fibular (continues as the medial dorsal metatarsal nerve and innervates the extensor hallucis longus and abductor digiti II: Rowe, 1986).

REPTILES

The lumbosacral plexus is formed by up to six branches of the ventral spinal nerves, which supply the inguinal, pelvis, and pelvic limb muscles. In general, a cranial root (the crural, tibial, and femoral nerves, which provide major innervation to the inguinal, thigh adductors and limb extensors) and a caudal root (providing the obturator and sciatic nerves before dividing into the fibular nerve and sciatic nerve branches) are described. Mivart and Clarke (1877), in contrast, observed that the lumbar plexus in lizards can be formed by 2-3 presacral roots, while the sacral nerves are constituted by a root of the sciatic plexus (Fig. 19.5). Owing to the wide variation in lumbosacral plexus formation among reptiles, the description in this chapter is based on studies of the iguana (*Iguana iguana*: Akita, 1992a,b; Arantes, 2016), varanus (*Varanus dumerilii*: Akita, 1992a,b),

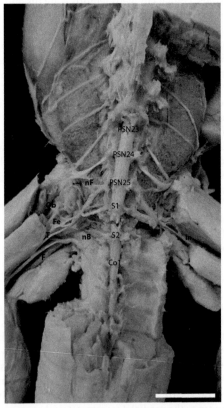

FIG. 19.5 Dorsal view of the vertebral column showing the spinal roots of the lumbosacral plexus in Sauria, Squamata, and Teiidae. The plexus is formed by spinal nerves 23-24 and includes the PSN23-25 and S1-2 nerves and the first coccygeal nerve (Co1). The plexus is divided into a cranial trunk (PSN23-24), joined to the medium trunk (PSN25-S1) by the furcal nerve (nF) from PSN24, and a caudal trunk (S2-Co1), united to the second by the bigeminal nerve (nB). The cranial trunk emits the femoral (Fe) and obturator (Ob) nerves, while the medium trunk originates the fibular (F), tibial (T), and sciatic (In) nerves. Scale bar: 2 cm. (Personal collection. Dissected and photographed by Guilherme José Parizzi, Applied Animal Anatomy Laboratory, Federal University of Santa Catarina, Brazil.)

alligator (Wyneken, 2007), turtle (*Trachemys scripta elegans* and sea turtles: Kusuma et al., 1979; Ashley, 1962; Wyneken, 2003, respectively), and red-footed tortoise (*Geochelone carbonaria*) Carvalho et al., 2011.

There are about 4800 species of lizard ranging in size from 3-cm-long lizards to the Komodo dragon, which at maturity is 3 meters long and weighs 75 kg. Some aspects of vertebral column should be considered: (1) there is a disagreement about the presence of lumbar vertebrae because ribs are associated with all vertebrae in the trunk; (2) the absence of space between vertebral arches makes anesthesia and puncture for cerebrospinal fluid difficult; (3) the number and morphology of sacral vertebrae, pelvic limb conformation, body framework, and environmental adaptation all vary among species; (4) there is a bone distinct from the caudal vertebrae (hemal arch) that both protects nerves and regional blood vessels and stabilizes the tail (Wyneken, 2007; Arantes, 2016). In view of these differences, this chapter considers the number of presacral vertebrae to determine the spinal nerves that contribute to formation of the lumbosacral plexus.

The iguana has 24 presacral and two sacral vertebrae, and the plexus is constituted by SN23-29, beginning with the 23 presacral nerves including two sacral and the first and second coccygeal nerves. However, prefixation in SN22 and the second coccygeal nerve is more frequent in males than females (Akita, 1992b; Arantes, 2016). In varanus, the first author found 29 presacral vertebrae and two sacral vertebrae, with the plexus constituted by SN27-31. Wyneken (2007) found that SN22-26 generates the plexus in the alligator. However, all these animals have a plexus organized into three trunks: the cranial trunk formed by SN23-24 in the iguana (Akita, 1992b; Arantes, 2016), SN27-28 in varanus (Akita, 1992a), and SN23-26 in the alligator (Wyneken, 2007); a medium trunk or sacral plexus (from SN25-27 in the iguana, SN28-30 in the varanus, and SN24-25 in the alligator); and a caudal trunk (from 27 to 28 in the iguana, SN30-31 in the varanus and by SN25-26 in the alligator). The cranial trunk gives rise to the femoral and obturator nerves and two nerve branches to the abdominal wall. Four nerves arise from the medium trunk: dorsal (fibular or peroneal), ventral (tibial), ventralmost (pubioischiotibilal), and the thin caudoiliofemoral (Akita, 1992b). The pubioischiofemoral and caudoiliofemoral nerves are analogous to the sciatic nerve, described in the alligator (Wyneken, 2007) as in other vertebrates, mainly considering their innervation territories (laterocaudal surface and muscles of the thigh, including the flexor muscles of the tibia and the pelvic muscles, with the exception of the obturator nerve's territory). On the other hand, in *Uromastyx hardwickii*, SN20-21 forms the origin of the sciatic nerve (Malik, 2011), being more cranial than in the other animals mentioned above. The fibular nerve innervates the calf and foot extensor muscles, whereas the tibial nerve supplies the flexor muscles of the same region. The caudal trunk of the lumbosacral plexus forms the caudofemoral, pudendal, and caudosciatic nerves and innervates the musculature of the caudal body wall (Rowe, 1986). The pudendal nerve has a wide innervation territory, including the cranial pudendal (muscles of the tail) and caudal pudendal (muscles of the penis and cloaca) divisions. Although the iguana, varanus, and *Uromastyx* are of the same class and order, they have different numbers of vertebrae, altering the location of the lumbosacral plexus.

Like other reptiles, testudines present a variable number of presacral and sacral vertebrae. Turtles (*Trachemys scripta elegans*, previously called *Pseudemys*) have 18 presacral, two sacral, and about 16 caudal vertebrae (Kusuma et al., 1979; Ashley, 1962; Wyneken, 2003), the lumbosacral plexus arising from SN16-18 (presacral), S1-2 (sacral), and the first coccygeal nerve (Ruigrok and Crowe, 1984; Mortin and Stein, 1985, 1989; Wyneken, 2003). However, Ashley (1962) described only SN16-18 (presacral) and S1-2 (sacral) as constituting the lumbosacral plexus. In contrast, Carvalho and colleagues (2011) observed 13 presacral, four sacral, and about 23-25 coccygeal vertebrae in females or 27−29 in male of red-footed tortoise (*Geochelone carbonaria*). Three origins of the lumbosacral plexus are described in the red-footed tortoise, from SN13-S5, SN13-Ca1 or S1-5. However, up to eight or nine spinal nerves are scattered in the skin and musculature of the thigh. The plexus can be divided into three trunks: (1) cranial, constituted by the femoral (triceps femoris, pars iliotibialis, ambiens and femorotibial, a knee extensor, hip protractor, and hip abductor muscles) and obturator (nerves to the hip protractor, which include the puboischiofemoralis internus, pars anteroventralis, a hip protractor, and femoral rotator muscles); (2) sciatic, innervating the flexor cruris, pars flexor tibialis internus, and several other muscles that retract the hip and flex the knee, and one muscle that adducts the hip); and (3) caudal, involving no nerve roots from the caudal and/or pudendal plexuses. The pelvic girdle and respiratory muscles are innervated by a distal ramus of SN11 (Mortin and Stein, 1985, 1989). The sciatic nerve of each species arises from the last presacral nerve and S1-2 and divides into three sciatic nerves in the turtle. This finding suggests that the functional significance of a caudal and/or pudendal plexus in this species is questionable and this is important for anesthesia practice in testudines.

AMPHIBIANS

In amphibians, adaptation to terrestrial life involved the development of limbs and CNS modifications subserving tetrapod locomotion. Nevertheless, some species are limbless (the cecilians of Order Gymnophonia) or possess rudimentary extremities (e.g., *Amphiuma*, a genus of aquatic salamander). The vertebral column and spinal cord differ among amphibians. While urodeles have a coccygeal region, anurans or tailless amphibians have a relatively short spinal cord with 10 segments and a conspicuous lumbar enlargement (Underhill, 1969). The spine cord terminates in a relatively long and slender cone in anurans, which represents the remnant of the caudal portion premetamorphosis. The lumbosacral plexus in frogs arises from SN7-10 and forms two trunks (Underhill, 1969; Malik, 2011): one from SN7-8 that gives rise to the iliohypogastric, femoral, and crural nerves; the other after the union of SN8 with the junction between SN9 and S10 (Fig. 19.6). This major trunk forms the sciatic nerve, divided into the tibial and fibular nerves. The coccygeal nerve emerges from SN10 (Underhill, 1969; Malik, 2011). Gaupp (1896) noted the same in bullfrogs (*Rana catesbeiana*), where SN8-10 constitute the lumbosacral plexus. The nerves arising were crural (which emits three branches to the adductor longus and pectineus, iliacus internus and externus, and tensor fasciae latae muscles, respectively; this nerve is analogous to the cranial gluteus in other vertebrates); deep anterior (also with three muscular branches to the cruralis, gluteus magnus and iliofibularis, respectively; these are analogous to the femoral and caudal gluteal); deep posterior (divided into four branches supplying the semimembranosus, adductor magnus and sartorius, semitendinosus and dorsal head of semitendinosus, gracilis maior and minor, and adductor magnus, quadratus femoris and obturator externus muscles; these territories correspond to innervation by the caudal cutaneous femoral caudalis, obturator, and sciatic nerves.); tibial (to the gastrocnemius and other muscles of foot); and peroneal or fibular (innervation of muscles in the toes).

On the other hand, Akita (1992a) described the lumbosacral plexus as comprising SN19-22, SN20 being called the furcal nerve in the Japanese giant

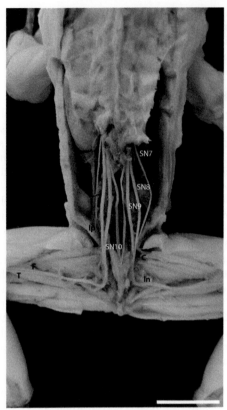

FIG. 19.6 Dorsal view of the vertebral column showing the spinal roots of the lumbosacral plexus in Amphibia, Anura, *Leptodactylus latrans*. The lumbosacral plexus originates from SN7-10. The first trunk is formed by SN7-8 and emits the iliohypogastric (Ip) and crural (C) nerves; the second is constituted after the union of SN8 with the junction between SN9-10 and forms the sciatic (In) nerve, which divides into the tibial (T) and fibular (F) nerves, while the coccygeal nerve emerges from SN10. Scale bar: 2 cm. (Personal collection. Dissected and photographed by Guilherme José Parizzi, Applied Animal Anatomy Laboratory, Federal University of Santa Catarina, Brazil.)

salamander (*Megalobatracus japonicus*). The nerves are divided into four groups: (1) those that innervate the caudofemoral muscle (SN19-21, common fibular and tibial nerves); (2) those passing between the caudofemoral and caudoisquiadic muscles (SN20-22, pubioischiotibial and pudendal nerves); (3) those that follow ventrally to the caudosciatic muscle (SN21-22 and nerve to the caudosciatic muscle); and (4) terminal nerves of the limb (sciatic from SN20, femoral from SN19-20, and obturator from SN19-20).

REFERENCES

Akalan, M.A., Çevik Demirkan, A., Türkmenoğlu, İ., Demirkan, İ., 2019. Macroanatomic structure of spinal nerves forming the plexus lumbosacralis in the merlin (*Falco columbarius*). Atatürk Üniversitesi Veteriner Bilimleri Dergisi 14 (1), 15–22.

Akita, K., 1992a. An anatomical investigation of the muscles of the pelvic outlet in Japanese giant salamander (Cryptobranchidae *Megalobatrachus japonicus*) with special reference to their nerve supply. Ann. Anat. 174, 235–243.

Akita, K., 1992b. An anatomical investigation of the muscles of the pelvic outlet in Iguanas (Iguanidae *Iguana iguana*) and Varanus (Varanidae Varanus (dumerillii)) with special reference to their nerve supply. Ann. Anat. 174, 119–129.

Arantes, R.C., 2016. Ossos da coluna vertebral e origens dos plexos braquial e lombossacral da iguana *Iguana iguana*. Tese (doutorado). Universidade Federal de Uberlândia, Programa, de Pós-Graduação em Ciências Veterinárias, 47 pp.

Asato, F., Butler, M., Blomberg, H., Gordh, T., 2000. Variation in rat sciatic nerve anatomy: implications for a rat model of neuropathic pain. J. Peripher. Nerv. Syst. 5, 19–21.

Ashley, L.M., 1962. Laboratory Anatomy of the Turtle. WM C. Brown Company Publishers, Iowa.

Bardeen, C.R., Elting, A.W., 1901. A statistical study of the variations in the formation and position the lumbo-sacral plexus in man. Anat Anz 19, 209–239.

Barone, R., Pavaux, C., Blin, P.C., Cuq, P., 1973. Atlas of Rabbit Anatomy. Masson & Cie, Paris.

Barros, R.A.C., Prada, I.L.S., Silva, Z., Ribeiro, A.R., Silva, D.C.O., 2003. Lumbar plexus formation of the *Cebus apella* monkey. Braz. J. Vet. Res. Anim. Sci. 40, 373–381.

Baumel, J.J., 1975. Aves nervous system. In: Getty, R. (Ed.), Sisson and Grossman's. The Anatomy of the Domestic Animals, fifth ed., vol. 2. W.B. Saunders Company, Philadelphia, PA, USA, pp. 2044–2052.

Bensley, B.A., Craigie, E.H., 1938. Practical Anatomy of the Rabbit an Elementary Text-Book in Mammalian Anatomy, sixth ed. The University of Toronto Press, Toronto.

Bosa, Y.M., Getty, R., 1969. Somatic and autonomic nerves of the lumbar, sacral and coccygeal regions of the domestic pig (*Sus scrofa domesticus*). Iowa State J. Sci. 44, 45–77.

Carvalho, R.C., Sousa, A.L., Oliveira, S.C.R., Pinto, A.C.B.F., Fontenelle, J.H., Cortopassi, S.R.G., 2011. Morphology and topographic anatomy of the spinal cord of the red-footed tortoise (*Geochelone carbonaria* Spix, 1824). Pesqui. Vet. Bras. 31, 47–52.

Chagas, R.G., Drummond, S.S., Silva, F.O.C., Eurides, D., Alves, E.C.M., Miranda, R.L., 2006. Origem e distribuição do nervo obturatório em suínos (*Sus scrofa domesticus* – Linnaeus, 1758) da linhagem AG-1050. Arquivos de Ciências Veterinárias e Zoologia 9, 15–20.

Champneys, F., 1871. The muscles and nerves of a chimpanzee (*Troglodytes niger*) and a *Cynocephalus anubis*. J. Anat. Physiol. 6, 176–211.

Chang, H.-T., Ruch, T.C., 1947. Morphology of the spinal cord, spinal nerves, caudal plexus, tail segmentation, and caudal musculature of the spider monkey. Yale J. Biol. Med. 19 (3), 345–377.

Chang, H.-T., Ruch, T.C., 1949. The projection of the caudal segments of the spinal cord to the lingula in the spider monkey. J. Anat. 83 (Pt 4), 303–307.

Chiasson, R.B., 1980. Laboratory Anatomy of the White Rat. Brown Company Publisher, Iowa.

Cooper, G., Schiller, A.L., 1975. Anatomy of the guinea Pig. Harvard, University Press, Cambridge, Massachusetts.

Crouch, J.E., 1985. Text-atlas of Cat Anatomy. Lea & Febiger, Philadelphia.

Di Dio, L.J.A., 2002. Tratado de anatomia aplicada, second ed. Póluss Editorial, São Paulo.

Dubbeldam, J.L., 1993. Systema nervosum periphericum. In: Baumel, J.J. (Ed.), Handbook of Avian Anatomy: Nomina Anatomica Avium, second ed. Nuttall Ornithological Club, Cambridge, pp. 555–584.

Dyce, K.M., Sack, W.O., Wensing, C.J.G., 2009. Textbook of Veterinary Anatomy, fourth ed. Elsevier.

Eisler, P., 1890. Das Gefass- und Periphere Nervensystem des Gorilla. Tausch & Grosse, Halle.

El Assy, Y.S., 1966. Beitrage zur morphologie des peripheren nervensystems der primaten. Gegenbaurs Morphol. Jahrb. 27, 476–567. Frankfurt.

El-Mahdy, T., El-Nahla, S.M., Abbott, L.C., Hassan, S.A.M., 2010. Innervation of the pelvic limb of the adult ostrich (*Struthio camelus*). Anat. Histol. Embryol. 39, 411–425.

Elias, A., Brown, C., 2008. Cerebellomedullary cerebrospinal fluid collection in the dog. Lab. Anim. 37 (10), 457–458. https://doi.org/10.1038/laban1008-457.

Ernst, W., 2016. Humanized mice in infectious diseases. Comp. Immunol. Microbiol. Infect. Dis. 49, 29–38.

Evans, H.E., DeLahunta, A., 2010. The nervous system. In: Evans, H.E., DeLahunta, A. (Eds.), Guide to the Dissection of the Dog, seventh ed. Saunders Elsevier, Missouri, pp. 263–288.

Fletcher, T.F., 1970. Lumbosacral plexus and pelvic limb myotomes of the dog. Am. J. Vet. Res. 31, 35–41.

Frandson, R.D., 1979. Anatomia e fisiologia dos animais domésticos, second ed. Guanabara Koogan, Rio de Janeiro. 61 pp.

Gaupp, E., 1896. A. Ecker's und R. Wiedersheim's Anatomie des Frosches. Vieweg, Braunschweig.

Getty, R., 1975. Sisson and Grossman's the Anatomy of the Domestic Animals, fifth ed. W. B. Saunders Company, Philadelphia.

Ghoshal, N.G., 1972. The lumbosacral plexus (Plexus lumbosacrales) of the cat (*Felis domestica*). Anat. Anzeiger 131, 272–279.

Ghoshal, N.G., 1975. Spinal nerves of the swine. In: Getty, R. (Ed.), Sisson and Grossman's the Anatomy of the Domestic Animals, fifth ed. WB. Saunders Company, Philadelphia.

Gomez-Amaya, S.M., Ruggieri, M.R.S., Arias Serrato, S.A., Massicotte, V.S., Barbe, M.F., 2015. Gross anatomical study of the nerve supply of genitourinary structures in female mongrel Hound dogs. Anat. Histol. Embryol. 44, 118–127.

Greene, E.C., 1968. Anatomy of the Rat. Hafner Publishing Company, New York and London.

Hall, L.W., Clarke, K.W., 1991. Veterinary Anaesthesia, ninth ed. Bailliere Tindall, London, pp. 183–187 (Chapter 10).

Hartmann, C.G., Straus Junior, W.L., 1932. Anatomy of the Rhesus Monkey. Editora, New York.

Hepburn, D., 1892a. The comparative anatomy of the muscles and nerves of the superior and inferior extremities of the anthropoid apes. Part I. J. Anat. Physiol. 26, 149–186.

Hepburn, D., 1892b. The comparative anatomy of the muscles and nerves of the superior and inferior extremities of the anthropoid apes Part II. J. Anat. Physiol. 26, 324–356.

Hill, W.C.O., 1953. Primates Comparative Anatomy and Taxonomy I Strepsirhini. Edinburgh.

Hill, W.C.O., 1957. Primates: Comparative Anatomy and Taxonomy III Pithecoidea – Platyrrhini – Hapalidae. Edinburgh University Press, Edinburgh.

Hill, W.C.O., 1960. Primates: Comparative Anatomy and Taxonomy IV Cebidae: Part A. Edinburgh University Press, Edinburgh.

Hill, W.C.O., 1966. Primates: comparative anatomy and taxonomy VI Catarrhini-Cercopithecoidea - Cercopithecinae. Edinburgh University Press, Edinburgh.

Hill, W.C.O., 1972. Primates: Comparative Anatomy and Taxonomy V Cebidae: Part B. Edinburgh University Press, Edinburgh.

Hunt, H.R.A., 1924. Laboratory Manual of the Anatomy of the Rat. Macmillan Company, New York.

İstanbullugil, F.R., Karadağ, H., Sefergil, S., İnce, N.G., Alpak, H., 2013. Formation of the plexus sacralis in pheasants (*Phasianus colchicus mongolicus*) and macroanatomic investigation of the nerves originating from the plexus sacralis. Turk. J. Vet. Anim. Sci. 37, 160–163.

Jones, R.S., 2001. Epidural analgesia in the dog and cat. Vet. J. 161 (2), 123–131.

Kadota, T., Nakano, M., Atobe, Y., Goris, R.,C., Funakoshi, K., 2009. The chelonian spinal nerve ganglia are a conglomerate of the spinal nerve ganglia proper and the sympathetic ganglia. Brain Behav. Evol. 73, 165–173.

Krechowiecki, A., Goscicka, D., Samulak, S., 1972. The lumbosacral plexus and lumbar enlargement in *Macaca mulatta*. Folia Morphol. 31, 11–19.

Kusuma, A., ten Donkelaar, H.J., Nieuwenhuvs, R., 1979. Intrinsic orgazation of the spinal corh. In: Gans, C., Northcutt, R.G., Ulinski, P. (Eds.), Biology of the Reptila, vol. 10. Academic, New York, pp. 59–109.

Lacerda, P.M.O., Moura, C.E.B., Miglino, M.A., Oliveira, M.F., Albuquerque, J.F.G., 2006. Origin of lumbar sacral plexus of rock cavy (*Kerodon rupestris*). Braz. J. Vet. Res. Anim. Sci. 43, 620–628.

Lorenzão, C.J., Zimpel, A.V., Novakoski, E., Silva, A.A., Martinez-Pereira, M.A., 2016. Comparison of the lumbosacral plexus nerves formation in pampas fox (*Pseudalopex gymnocercus*) and crab-eating fox (*Cerdocyon thous*) in relationship to plexus model in dogs. Anat. Rec. 299, 361–369.

Lu, S., Chang, S., Zhang, Y.-Z., Ding, Z.-H., Xu, X.M., Xu, Y.-G., 2011. Clinical anatomy and 3D virtual reconstruction of the lumbar plexus with respect to lumbar surgery. BMC Muscoskel. Disord. 12, 76–84.

Malik, S., Ahmed, S., Azeem, M.A., Noushad, S., Sherwani, S.K., 2011. Comparison of sciatic nerve course in amphibians, reptiles and mammals. FUUAST J. Biol. 1 (2), 7–14.

Martinez-Pereira, M.A., Rickes, E.M., 2011. The spinal nerves that constitute the lumbosacral plexus and their distribution in the chinchilla. J. S. Afr. Vet. Assoc. 82, 150–154.

Martinez-Pereira, M.A., Zancan, D.M., 2015. Comparative anatomy of the peripheral nerves. In: Tubbs, R.S., Rizk, E., Shoja, M., Loukas, M., Spinner, R.J. (Eds.), Nerves and Nerves Injuries. Academic Press Elsevier, London, pp. 55–77.

Massone, F., 1988. Técnica anestésica em suínos. In: Anestesiologia veterinária. Editora Guanabara, Rio de Janeiro, pp. 132–141.

Mckenna, K.E., Nadelhaft, I., 1986. The organization of the pudendal nerve in the male and female rat. J. Comp. Neurol. 248, 532–549.

Mclaughlin, C.A., Chiasson, R.B., 1987. Laboratory Anatomy of the Rabbit. W. C. Brown Company, Iowa.

Miheliae, D., Gjurèeiae-Kantural, V., Markovinoviae, S., Damjanoviae, A., Trbojeviae-Vukièeviae, T., 2004. Variations of formation of n. femoralis, n. obturatorius and n.sciatic in pigs. Vet. Arh. 74, 261–270.

Miller, M., Christensen, G., Evans, H., 1964. Anatomy of the Dog. W. B. Saunders Company, Philadelphia.

Mivart, G., Clarke, R., 1877. On the sacral plexus and sacral vertebrae of lizards. Zool. J. Linn. Soc. 13 (70), 370–373. https://doi.org/10.1111/j.1096-3642.1877.tb00185.x.

Mortin, L.I., Stein, P.S.G., 1985. Segmental properties of three forms of scratch reff ex in the spinal turtle: localization of input dermatomes and central pattern generating elements. Soc. Neurosci. Abstr. 11, 1021.

Mortin, L.I., Stein, P.S.G., 1989. Spinal cord segments containing key elements of the central pattern generators for three forms of scratch reflex in the turtle. J. Neurosci. 9 (7), 2285–2298.

Najman, I.E., Frederico, T.N., Segurado, A.V.R., Kimachi, P.P., 2011. Caudal epidural anesthesia: an anesthetic technique exclusive for pediatric use? Is it possible to use it in adults? What is the role of the ultrasound in this context? Rev. Bras. Anestesiol. 61 (1), 95–109.

Nascimento, R.M., Estruc, T.M., Pereira, J.L.A., Souza, E.C., Souza Júnior, P., Abidu-Figueiredo, M., 2019. Origin and antimeric distribution of the obturator nerves in the New Zealand rabbits. Ciência animal brasileira, Goiânia 20, 1–11. https://doi.org/10.1590/1089-6891v20e-55428.

Nickel, R., Schummer, A., Seiferle, E., 1977. Peripheral nervous system. In: Nickel, R., Schummer, A., Seiferle, E. (Eds.), Anatomy of the Domestic Birds. Parey, Berlin, pp. 131–139.

Nomina Anatomica Veterinaria, 2017. Copyright by the World Association of Veterinary Anatomists. Editorial Committee, sixth ed. (revised version). Hanover, Germany.

Orosz, S.E., Bradshaw, G.A., 2007. Avian neuroanatomy revisited: from clinical principles to avian cognition. Vet. Clin. Exot. Anim. Pract. 10, 775–802.

Paithanpagare, Y.M., Tank, P.H., Mankad, M.Y., Shirodkar, K., Derashri, H.J., 2001. Myelography in dogs. Vet. World 1 (5), 152–154.

Piasecka-Kacperska, K., Gladykowska-Rzeckzycka, J., 1972. The sacral plexus in primates. Folia Morphol. 31, 21–33.

Pietrzk, K., Urbanowick, Z., Zaluska, S., 1964. Nerwy pachowy i promieniowy. U macacus Rhesus. Folia Morphol. 15, 425–436.

Raven, H.C., Hill, J.E., 1950. Regional anatomy of the Gorilla. In: Gregory, W.K. (Ed.), The Anatomy of the Gorilla. Columbia University Press, New York.

Rigaud, M., Gemes, G., Barabas, M.-E., Chernoff, D.I., Abram, S.E., Stucky, C.L., Hogan, Q.H., 2008. Species and strain differences in rodent sciatic nerve anatomy: implications for studies of neuropathic pain. Pain 136, 188–201.

Rowe, T., 1986. Homology and evolution of the deep dorsal thigh musculature. in birds and other reptilia. J. Morphol. 189, 327–346.

Ruigrok, T.J.H., Crowe, A., 1984. The organization of motoneurons in the turtle lumbar spinal cord. J. Comp. Neurol. 228, 24–37.

Santiago, W., 1974. Esqueletopia do cone medular em *Canis familiaris*, vol. 4. Arquivo da Universidade Federal Rural Rio de Janeiro, Seropédica, pp. 67–69.

Schultz, A.H., Straus Jr., W.L., 1945. The numbers of vertebrae in primates. Proc. Am. Phil. Soc. 89, 601–626.

Severeano, G., 1904. Du plexus lombaire. Biblio Anatomique 12, 299–313.

Sherrington, C.S., 1892. Notes on the arrangement of some motor fibres in the lumbo-sacral plexus. J. Physiol. 13, 621–772.

Standring, S., 2009. Gray's Anatomy: The Anatomical Basis of Clinical Practice, Expert Consult, fortieth ed. Elsevier.

Tubbs, R.S., Loukas, M., Hanna, A.S., Oskouian, R.J., 2018. Surgical Anatomy of the Lumbar Plexus. Thieme Publishers, New York.

Underhill, R.A., 1969. Laboratory Anatomy of the Frog. WM C. Brown Company Publishers, Iowa.

Urbanowicz, Z., Zaluska, S., 1969. Arrangement of lumbar plexus in man and macaca. Folia Morphol. (Wars.) 28, 285–299.

Vejsada, R., Hnik, P., 1980. Radicular innervation of hind-limb muscles of the rat. Physiol. Bohemoslov. 29, 385–392.

Webber, R.H., 1961. Some variations in the lumbar plexus of nerves in man. Acta Anat. 44, 336–345.

Wyneken, J., 2003. The external morphology, musculoskeletal system, and neuroanatomy of sea turtles. In: Lutz, P.L., et al. (Eds.), The Biology of Sea Turtles, Volume 2. CRC Marine Biology Series, vol. 4, pp. 39–77.

Wyneken, J., 2007. Reptilian neurology: anatomy and function. Vet. Clin. Exot. Anim. Pract. 10, 837–853.

Zaluska, S., Urbanowicz, Z., 1972. Origin of the sacral plexus in man and in *Macacus*. Acta Biol. Med. 17, 93–107.

CHAPTER 20

High-Resolution MR Neurography Anatomy of the Sacral Plexus

CLAUDIA CEJAS • MERCEDES SERRA

INTRODUCTION

Magnetic resonance neurography (MRN), a noninvasive technique using high-resolution magnetic resonance imaging to diagnose peripheral nerve disorders, has been added to the diagnostic armamentarium of the neuromuscular specialist relatively recently (Chhabra et al., 2011a, 2011b). Supplementing the history and the clinical and electrophysiological examination, MRN aids in the diagnosis and management of peripheral nerve disease by enabling peripheral nerve lesions to be located precisely and characterized in detail, often in areas inaccessible to standard electrophysiology (Evans and Manji, 2013).

MRN requires deep knowledge and dedicated analysis of the imaging anatomy of the sacral plexus and adjacent structures (Cejas et al., 2015). To date, few papers have been published on standard lumbar sacral root size measurement using MRN in patients (Tazawa et al., 2008; Gürkanlar et al., 2005; Chaves et al., 2018). However, normal peripheral nerves are similar in size to the adjacent arteries, and the size and signal are nearly symmetrical bilaterally (Zoccali et al., 2015).

MRN uses high-resolution imaging combined with 2- and three-dimensional (2D and 3D) fast suppression turbo spin echo (TSE) sequences for multiplanar depiction of peripheral nerves. At present, 3.0 T (3T) scanners provide better signal-noise ratio and spatial resolution than 1.5T scanners. This converts into superior anatomical characterization of the sacral plexus and its tributaries (Chhabra, 2016; Cejas and Pineda, 2017).

TECHNICAL ASPECTS

MRN adjusts conventional imaging techniques to enhance visualization of peripheral nerves. It includes isometric high-resolution T1- and T2-WI with fat-suppressed sequences (Chhabra et al., 2011a; Du et al., 2010).

New technologies such as 3T scanners, phase-array surface coils, and robust accelerated acquisition methods allow 3D sequences with isotropic voxel size and thinner slices (less than 1 mm) to be incorporated routinely in short imaging times. These isometric high-resolution techniques involve a variety of TSE sequences such as VISTA (Phillips, Best, the Netherlands), SPACE (Siemens, Erlangen, Germany), and CUBE (GE, Waukeesha, WI). These sequences allow maximum intensity projection (MIP), multiplanar (MPR), and curved-planar reconstructions that increase the signal-to-noise ratio and improve delineation of the complex sacral anatomy (Delaney et al., 2014; Eppenberger et al., 2014). Other sequences available for studying peripheral nerves are 3D diffusion-weighted (DW) fast imaging, which takes advantage of the anisotropic diffusion of water within nerve fibers, preferentially paralleling the course of axonal bundles (Zhang et al., 2008).

Normal peripheral nerves have isointense T1-WI and hyperintense T2-WI signals in contrast to the adjacent muscles. Nowadays, it is possible to determine the fascicular pattern, epineural fat plane, and the structures surrounding the nerve (Soldatos et al., 2013). Administration of intravenous contrast agents enhances conventional structural imaging techniques, particularly T2-WI sequences, with fat suppression due to the shortening effect of adjacent venous vessels.

LUMBOSACRAL TRUNK

The lumbosacral trunk connects the lumbar and sacral plexuses. It is formed by a minor branch of L4 and the ventral ramus of L5 and runs on the medial side of the psoas major muscle (Neufeld et al., 2015). It descends over the sacral ala and joins the S1, S2, and S3 roots to form the sciatic nerve (SN) (Delaney et al., 2014). Developmental differences underlie the variable contributions of L4 and L5 to the lumbosacral trunk; sometimes, the contribution of L4 is absent (Schmidt et al., 2017).

Because of its width, the lumbosacral trunk is easily identified on MRN medial to the psoas major and over the sacral ala. On T1- and T2-weighted sequences, the perineural fat helps delimit the lumbosacral trunk and distinguish it from adjacent structures (Figs. 20.1–20.3).

S1 TO S4 NERVE ROOTS

Along with the lumbosacral trunk (L4 and L5), the sacral plexus is formed by the S1 to S4 anterior rami. The sacral nerve roots exit the spinal canal through the sacral foramina in an inferolateral direction. Each successive nerve is progressively smaller in diameter

and locates itself more medially than the preceding nerve (Gierada et al., 1992).

Most sacral nerve roots lie close to the anterior surface of the sacroiliac joint and the ala of the sacrum (Waikakul et al., 2010). Their relationship to the pyramidal muscle (PM) is variable. The S1 nerve root usually courses above the PM; the S2 and S3 nerve roots can travel above or through that muscle as common anatomical variations; and the S4 nerve root usually courses below the PM (Russell et al., 2008).

Because of their width and location, the first and second sacral nerve roots are usually identified exiting through the sacral foramina on MRN (Figs. 20.1–20.3); the most caudal roots can be less evident after exiting the spinal

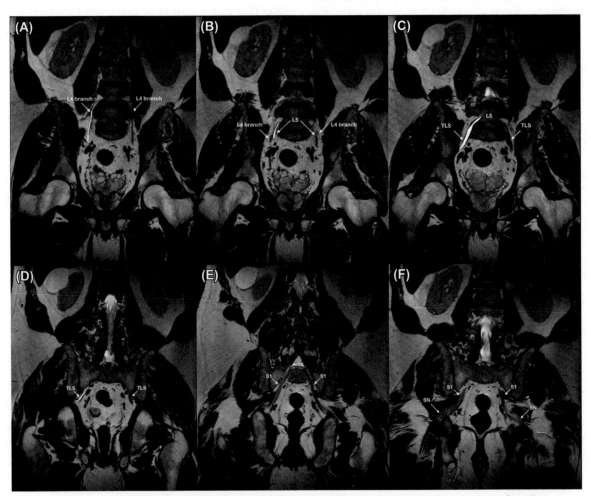

FIG. 20.1 T2-WI Hyper-Cube, coronal reconstruction. **(A and B)** L4 and L5 contributions joining to form the lumbosacral trunk (LST). **C** and **D:** LST is identified over the sacral ala and easily distinguished from adjacent structures by perineural fat. **E** and **F:** On a posterior plane, we see the S1 nerve root joining the LST to form the sciatic nerve (SN).

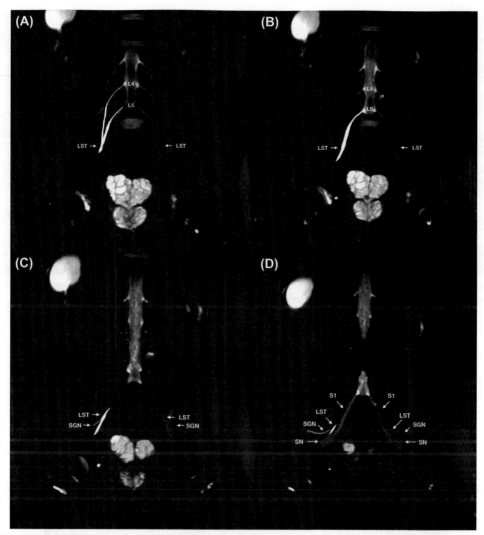

FIG. 20.2 T2-WI Hyper-Cube DIR with intravenous gadolinium, coronal reconstruction. Note the hyperintense signal of the nerves in contrast to the suppressed signal of the vessels given by the intravenous contrast agent. **(A)**: L4 and L5 contributions joining to form the lumbosacral trunk (LST). **(B and C)** The LST is identified over the sacral ala. **(D)** On a posterior plane, we can see the S1 nerve root joining the LST to form the SN. The superior gluteal nerve (SGN) origin is easily identified on **(C and D)**.

canal (Fig. 20.4). On T1-WI with intravenous gadolinium injection, healthy nerves do not enhance owing to the blood-nerve barrier, but it is important to remember that nerve ganglia normally enhance owing to their rich peripheral microvasculature (Demondion et al., 2002).

SUPERIOR GLUTEAL NERVE

The superior gluteal nerve (SGN) is a motor nerve that arises from the dorsal rami of L4, L5, and S1 nerve roots of the sacral plexus (Lung and Lui, 2019). The SGN,

accompanied by the vessel's superior gluteal artery and vein, exits the pelvis through the greater sciatic foramen superior to the PM (Lung and Lui, 2019).

Collinge et al. (Collinge et al., 2015) studied the positional anatomy of the SG vessels and nerve at the greater sciatic notch by cadaveric dissection of 23 hemipelves. They noted more than one SGN branch in the sciatic notch in all specimens, including an inferior branch that exited caudal or caudal-superficial to the SG vessels. The most caudal portion of the SGN was adjacent to the bony notch's periosteum in 65% of specimens.

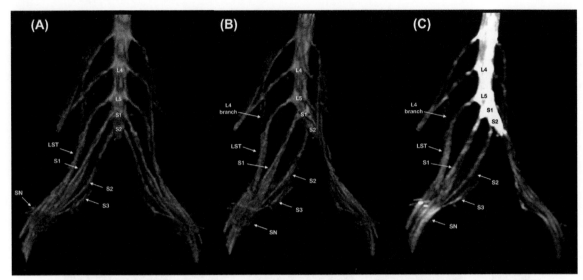

FIG. 20.3 T2-WI Hyper-Cube DIR with intravenous gadolinium. **(A** and **B)** Volume rendering (VR) reconstruction. **(C)** Maximum intensity projection (MIP) reconstruction. The L4 and L5 contributions are easily identified joining to form the lumbosacral trunk (LST). The S1, S2, and S3 nerve roots join the LST to form the SN.

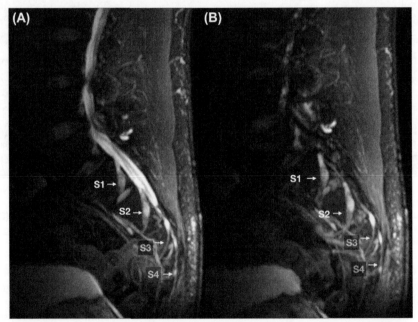

FIG. 20.4 T2-WI Hyper-Cube DIR, sagittal maximum intensity projection (MIP) reconstruction. The sacral nerve roots are shown exiting the spinal canal through the sacral foramina, with an inferior direction. Successive nerves are progressively smaller in diameter.

The SGN innervates the gluteus medius, gluteus minimus, and tensor fasciae latae muscles (Lung and Lui, 2019). However, Iwanaga et al. (Iwanaga et al., 2019) studied 20 sacral plexus from 10 fresh frozen cadavers via anterior dissection and demonstrated that in 70% cases the PM was also innervated by the SGN (Fig. 20.5).

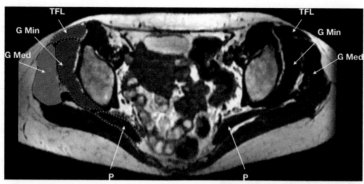

FIG. 20.5 Superior gluteal nerve (SGN): Axial Hyper-Cube sequence on T2 WI shows the muscles innervated by the SGN in orange: the gluteus medius (G Med), gluteus minimus (G Min), and tensor fasciae latae (TFL). The Pyramidal (P) muscle is included by some anatomists (dotted line).

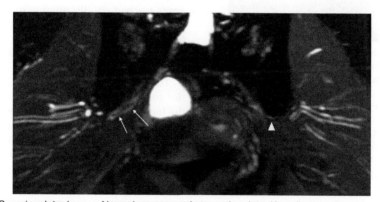

FIG. 20.6 Superior gluteal nerve: Normal neurovascular superior gluteal bundles are shown in a coronal Cube DIR sequence (arrows); the artery is easily distinguished from the nerve and vein by their lack of flow voids (arrowhead).

On MRN, the SGN forms part of the neurovascular bundle, and the nerve and the adjacent artery usually have similar caliber (Mirilas and Skandalakis, 2010). It is important to differentiate normal neurovascular bundles from isolated nerves. Current high-resolution MRN enables the SGN to be easily distinguished from the surrounding artery because of the lack of flow voids (Fig. 20.6). However, it is more difficult to distinguish the adjacent vein because both nerve and vein show hyperintense signals in T2-WI. Sequences that use double inversion recovery acquisitions before intravenous contrast injection allow the vein signal to be suppressed, enhancing the appearance of the normal nerve. The nerve caliber gradually decreases along its distal course and the size and signal are nearly symmetrical bilaterally (Figs. 20.2C and D, 20.7).

INFERIOR GLUTEAL NERVE

The inferior gluteal nerve (IGN) exits the pelvis between the PM and the coccygeus muscle-sacrospinous ligament (C-SSL) complex and supplies the gluteus maximus and the overlying skin (Roshanravan et al., 2007). An anatomical study by Florian Rodriguez et al. (Florian-Rodriguez et al., 2016) showed the IGN lying approximately 3 cm superior to the midpoint of the SSL and ischial spine.

On MRN, the IGN runs medial to the SN and exits the pelvis through the lower part of the greater sciatic foramen, under the PM (Fig. 20.8). Distal to the PM, it divides into a variable number of branches that enter the undersurface of the gluteus maximus. The deep surface of the gluteus maximus is the reference for identifying the IGN (Roshanravan et al., 2007) (Fig. 20.9).

The IGN has traditionally been described as a solely motor branch innervating the gluteus maximus

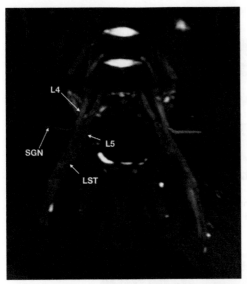

FIG. 20.7 Superior gluteal nerve (SGN): Coronal Hyper-Cube DIR sequences that use double inversion recovery times before intravenous contrast injection (gadolinium) allow the signal vein to be suppressed and show the appearance of the normal SGN (orange line). *LST*, lumbosacral trunk.

(Fig. 20.10). However, during routine dissection of 12 gluteal regions in six fresh-frozen adult cadaveric specimens, Iwanaga et al. (Iwanaga et al., 2018) identified a cutaneous branch of the IGN in all 12.

SCIATIC NERVE

The SN, the largest nerve in the human body, is formed in the pelvis by contributions from the ventral rami of L4 to the S3 spinal roots (Adibatti and Sangeetha, 2014). It exits the pelvis through the greater sciatic foramen as the most lateral structure within it. It courses below the PM, along with the pudendal nerve and vessels, the IGN and vessels, the nerve to the obturator internus, and the posterior cutaneous nerve (Giuffre and Jeanmonod, 2019). It then runs through the subgluteal space, which is limited posteriorly by the gluteus maximus muscle; laterally by the linea aspera and the lateral fusion of the middle and deep gluteal aponeurosis layers, extending up to the tensor fasciae latae muscle via the iliotibial tract; and anteriorly by the posterior border of the femoral neck and the greater and lesser trochanters. Its inferior margin continues into the posterior thigh. This space contains, from superior to inferior, the piriformis, superior gemellus, obturator internus, inferior gemellus, and quadratus femoris muscles (Carro et al., 2016).

The SN then progresses downward within the posterior compartment of the thigh, where it travels deep to the long head of the biceps femoris muscle, superficial to the adductor magnus and the short head of the biceps femoris, and lateral to the semitendinosus and semimembranosus muscles (Ribeiro et al., 2018). Its anatomy varies with respect to the PM (Smoll, 2010).

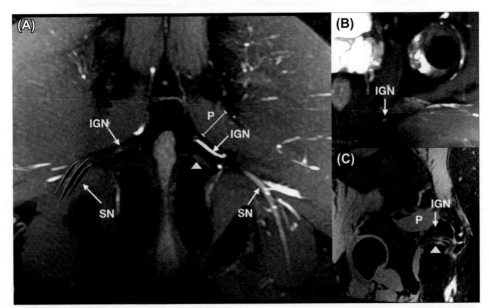

FIG. 20.8 Inferior gluteal nerve (IGN): Hyper-Cube DIR sequence in coronal plane **(A)**, in axial plane **(B)**, and 3D SPGR T1-WI in sagittal-oblique reconstruction **(C)** show the IGN (arrow and yellow line) between the pyramidal muscle (P) and the coccygeous muscle-sacrospinous ligament (C-SSL) complex (arrowhead). The SN is shown in blue.

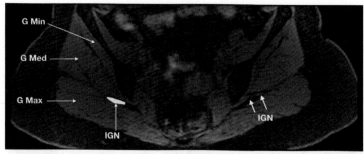

FIG. 20.9 Inferior gluteal nerve (IGN): Axial 3D SPGR T1-WI sequence shows the distal IGN (arrows and yellow line) between the fasciae of the maximus (G Max) and middle (G Med) gluteus muscles. *SPGR*, fat-suppressed spoiled gradient recalled echo imaging.

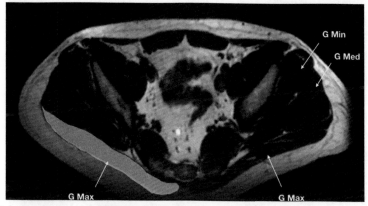

FIG. 20.10 Inferior gluteal nerve (IGN): 3D SPGR T1-WI in axial plane shows the muscle innervated by the IGN: Gluteus maximus (in yellow). *SPGR*, fat-suppressed spoiled gradient recalled echo imaging.

Tomaszewski et al. (Tomaszewski et al., 2016) analyzed the prevalence of PM and SN variants in humans in a systematic review and meta-analysis. Patterns of SN exit and relationships to the PM were classified with a modified Beaton and Anson classification (Beaton and Anson, 1937) as follows:

Type A: The SN exits the pelvis undivided below the PM.

Type B: The SN divides in the pelvis, the common peroneal nerve (CPN) pierces the PM, and the tibial nerve (TN) lies below the PM.

Type C: The SN divides in the pelvis, the CPN courses over the PM, and the TN lies below the PM.

Type D: The SN exits the pelvis undivided, piercing the PM.

Type E: The SN divides in the pelvis, the CPN courses over the PM, and the TN pierces the PM.

Type F: The SN exits the pelvis undivided, coursing over the PM.

Type G: The SN divides in the pelvis, both the CPN and TN coursing separately below the PM.

The normal Type A variation, where the SN exits the pelvis as a single entity below the PM, was most common with a pooled prevalence of 85.2% (95%CI: 78.4−87.0). This was followed by Type B, with a pooled prevalence of 9.8% (95%CI: 6.5−13.2), where the SN bifurcated in the pelvis with the exiting CPN piercing, and the TN coursing below, the PM.

On MRN, the SN is the most evident nerve of the pelvis owing to its diameter (Figs. 20.1F, 20.2D, 20.3 and 20.11).

Eastlack et al. (Eastlac et al., 2017) examined the frequency of the relationship of sciatic neuromuscular variants and the PM on MRN. They simplified the Beaton and Anson classification:

Type 1: The common peroneal division exits through the muscle, and the tibial division exits below the muscle.

Type 2: The common peroneal division exits above the muscle, and the tibial division exits below the muscle.

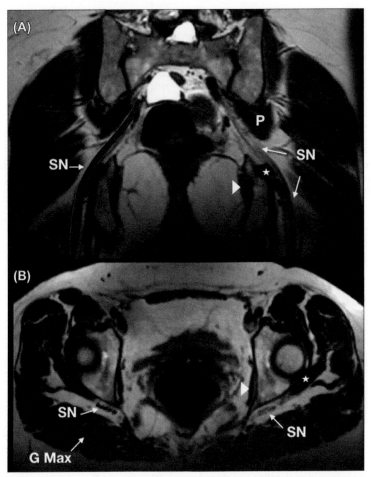

FIG. 20.11 Sciatic nerve (SN) in the subgluteal space: Hyper-Cube T2-WI sequence in coronal **(A)** and axial **(B)** plane shows the SN (blue line in **(A)** and dotted in **(B)**); its posterior limit is the gluteus maximus muscle (G Max) and its anterior limit is formed by the posterior border of the acetabulum and femoral bone. Within the space, superior to inferior, the piriformis (P), the obturator internus (arrowhead), and the quadratus femoris (asterisk) muscles are included.

Type 3: An undivided SN exits through the muscle.
Type 4: The common peroneal and tibial divisions exit below the muscle but are divided by a fibrous slip.

In the pelvis, the SN innervates the PM and the quadriceps femoris (Fig. 20.12). In the thigh, the tibial division of the SN innervates the long head of the biceps femoris and the semitendinosus, semimembranosus, and the adductor magnus muscles. The fibular division innervates the short head of the biceps femoris (Cejas et al., 2012) (Fig. 20.13).

Apparently, SN fascicles maintain a clearly arranged spatial position within the nerve cross section depending on their origin from the spinal nerve roots, not only within the proximal nerve trunk but even up to the bifurcation of the SN into the CPN and TN (Bäumer et al., 2015) (Fig. 20.14A).

COMMON FIBULAR NERVE

The fibular (peroneal) and tibial divisions of the SN are divided at or above the popliteal fossa to give origin to the CPN and TN. The CPN is the lateral division of the SN. Its courses from the posterolateral side of the knee around the biceps femoris tendon and the fibular head to the anterolateral side of the lower leg (La Rocca Vieira et al., 2007).

The first segment of CPN descends obliquely along the lateral side of the popliteal fossa; it is easily

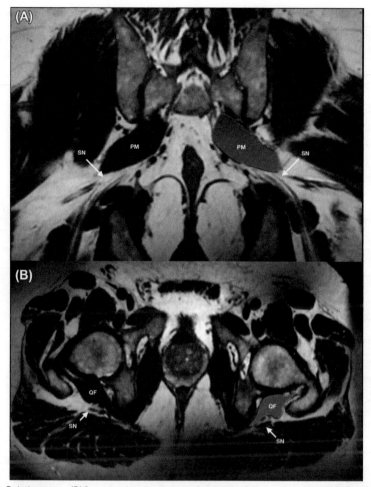

FIG. 20.12 Sciatic nerve (SN) motor innervation at the level of the pelvis. T2-WI Hyper-Cube coronal reconstruction **(A)**, where the pyramidal muscle (PM) is observed above the SN. Axial reconstruction **(B)**, where the quadratus femoris (QF) can be observed anterior to the sciatic nerve.

visualized in T2-WI and T1-WI owing to the rich peri-neural fat at this level. The distal segment of the CPN has a lateral and superficial course around the fibular neck, in the fibular tunnel, between the muscular-aponeurotic arch of the peroneus longus and soleus tendon and the bony floor of the proximal fibula. Within this narrow tunnel, this segment of the nerve is better depicted with 3D sequences and MPR or MIP reconstructions (Van den Bergh et al., 2010; Pineda et al., 2014) (Fig. 20.14).

The CPN typically trifurcates into the deep peroneal nerve (DPN) and superficial peroneal nerve (SPN) and a smaller articular or recurrent branch when it exits the fibular tunnel (Donovan et al., 2010). This division

commonly occurs at or distal to the fibular neck but can also occur above or up to 3 cm below the knee joint (Trappeniers et al., 2003) (Fig. 20.15). The CPN and its branches innervate the anterior and lateral compart-ments of the lower leg. The DPN provides motor inner-vation to the muscles of anterior compartment: the tibialis anterior, extensor hallucis longus, extensor digi-torum longus, and peroneus tertius. The SPN provides motor innervation to the muscles of the lateral compartment of the leg, the peroneus longus and bre-vis; and sensory innervation to the anterolateral side of the lower leg, where it pierces the crural fascia, and to the dorsum of the foot (Deutsch et al., 1999) (Fig. 20.16).

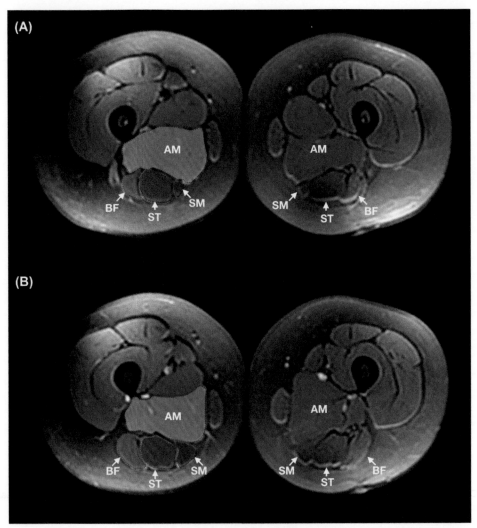

FIG. 20.13 Sciatic nerve (SN) motor innervation at the level of the thigh. Axial PD Fat-Sat **(A** and **B)**, where the adductor magnus (AM), long head of the biceps femoris (BF), semitendinosus (ST), and semimembranosus muscles are easily identified.

TIBIAL NERVE

The TN originates from the anterior division of the L4-S3 nerve roots via the medial trunk of the SN. The SN bifurcates into the TN and CPN at or above the popliteal fossa, the TN being the larger of the two terminal branches (Fig. 20.14A and C). In the popliteal fossa, the TN is located deep to the soleus, plantaris, and gastrocnemius muscles. It supplies branches to the gastrocnemius, popliteus, soleus, and plantaris muscles and an articular branch to the knee joint (Fig. 20.16). Additionally, it gives a medial cutaneous nerve of the calf, a cutaneous branch that joins fibers from the lateral

cutaneous nerve of the calf (from the CPN) to constitute the sural nerve (Spinner et al., 2012).

The soleus muscle has a bipennate origin from the posterior aspects of the tibia and fibula. Its fascial sling between the two heads lies directly on top of the tibial neurovascular bundle as it divides the posterior superficial and deep compartments. An anatomical study by Williams et al. (Williams et al., 2009) found that three (8%) of 36 cadaver limbs had focal narrowing of the TN diameter at the level of the soleus fascial sling.

When the TN leaves the popliteal fossa, it continues distally toward the calf to supply the lateral aspect of the

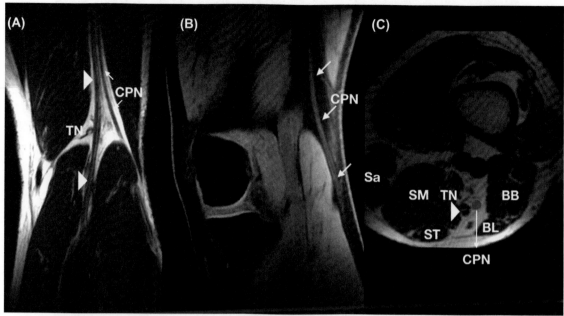

FIG. 20.14 The first segment of common peroneal nerve (CPN) (arrows) descends obliquely along the lateral side of the popliteal fossa, easily visualized in Hyper-CUBE T2-WI in coronal **(A)** and axial **(C)** plane and 3D SPGR T1-WI **(B)**, owing to the large amount of surrounding fatty tissue. Tibial nerve (*arrowhead*); *BB*, biceps femoris muscle short head; *BL*, biceps femoris muscle long head; *Sa*, sartorius muscle ; *SM*, semimembranosus muscle; *ST*, semitendinosus muscle.

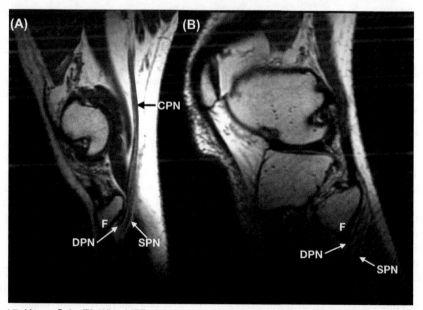

FIG. 20.15 Hyper-Cube T2-WI in MPR oblique reconstruction **(A** and **B)** shows the distal common peroneal nerve (CPN) (*green line*) trifurcating into the deep peroneal nerve (DPN), superficial peroneal nerve (SPN), and a smaller articular or recurrent branch (not shown) when exiting the fibular tunnel. In this case the division occurs up to the fibular neck (F).

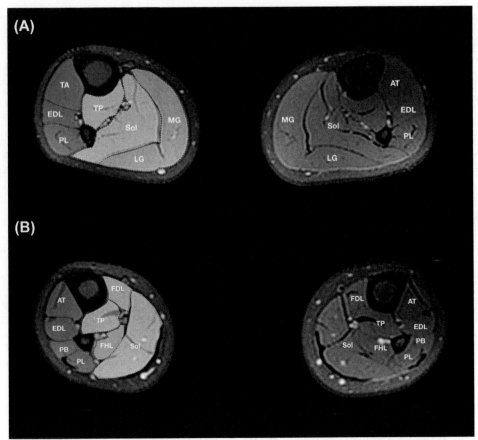

FIG. 20.16 FSE T2-WI in axial plane **(A, B)** shows innervation by the peroneal nerve and its branches, and the tibial nerve. The peroneal deep nerve innervates the muscles of the anterior compartment of the leg: the tibialis anterior (TA), extensor hallucis longus (EHL), extensor digitorum longus (EDL), and peroneus tertius muscles. The superficial peroneal nerve innervates the muscles of the lateral compartment of the leg: the peroneus longus (PL) and brevis (PB) muscles. The tibial nerve supplies branches to the posterior compartment of the leg: the gastrocnemius (G), popliteus, soleus (Sol), plantaris, tibialis posterior (TP), flexor digitorum longus (FDL), and flexor hallucis longus (FHL) muscles.

foot. In the calf, it runs down beside the posterior tibial vessels and supplies motor innervation to all of the above muscles (Fig. 20.16). Approximately 15 cm above the ankle it acquires a superficial course, crosses medial to the Achilles tendon, and then enters the tarsal tunnel (Chhabra et al., 2011c).

The tarsal tunnel, a fibro-osseous anatomical space, is divided into upper (tibiocalcaneal) and lower (talocalcaneal) compartments on the basis of a bony landmark, the sustentaculum talus. It contains the TN and its branches. In the lower tarsal tunnel, the medial and lateral plantar nerves and the calcaneal nerves course in their own tunnels separated by fibrous septations. The posterior TN provides motor function to the plantar muscles of the foot and sensation to the plantar aspect of the foot and toe (Beltran et al., 2010).

Owing to its caliber, the TN is easily seen in the popliteal fossa, close to the popliteal vessels, on MRN (Fig. 20.17). In the calf, its caliber decreases as it descends to the ankle, where its straight path makes it easier to recognize (Fig. 20.18). On the ankle, when the division into medial and lateral plantar nerves occurs, it is essential to obtain 3D sequences with MIP, MPR, or reconstruction (Fig. 20.19).

POSTERIOR FEMORAL CUTANEOUS NERVE

The posterior femoral cutaneous nerve (PFCN), or posterior cutaneous nerve of the thigh, is a sensory nerve that arises from the ventral rami of the S1 to S3 roots (Fritz et al., 2013). It exits the pelvic cavity via the greater sciatic notch, below the PM, and descends under

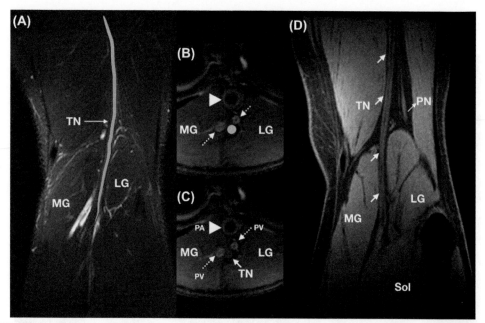

FIG. 20.17 Tibial nerve (TN): Dixon Water Ideal T2-WI sequence in coronal plane (A), FSE DP FS in axial plane (B and C), SPGR Water T1-WI (D) show the TN (*light green line* in (A and B); *arrows* in (C and D)) in the popliteal fossa, its location deep to the soleus and gastrocnemius muscles, close to the popliteal vessels (veins: *dotted arrow*; artery: *arrowhead*. MG, medial gatrocnemius; LG, lateral gastrocnemius; Sol, soleus. Common peroneal nerve in dark green (D).

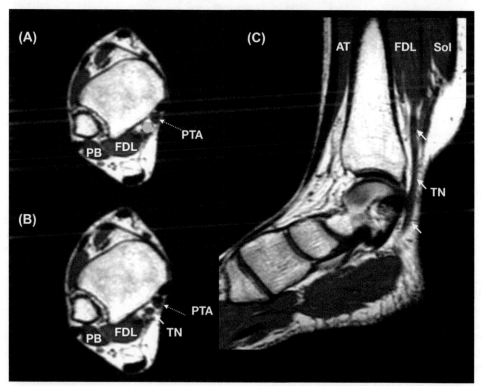

FIG. 20.18 Tibial nerve: Hyper-Cube T2 WI on the ankle in axial plane (A and B), and multiplanar sagittal-oblique (C) show the TN (*light green* in (A), *arrow* in (B and C)) is located behind the tibial posterior artery (PTA, *dotted arrow* in (A and B)). AT, tibialis anterior muscle; FDL, flexor digitorum longus muscle; PB, peroneus brevis muscle; Sol, soleus muscle.

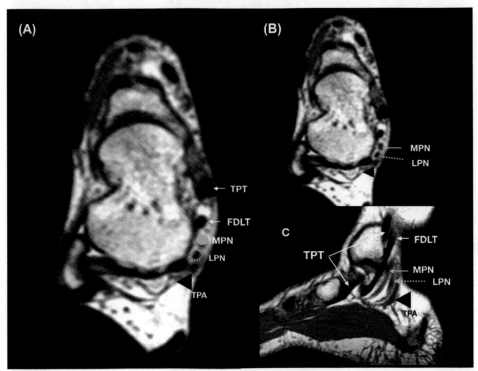

FIG. 20.19 Hyper-Cube T2-WI on the ankle in axial plane **(A and B)** and sagittal-oblique multiplanar reconstruction show the division of the TN into the medial plantar (MPN, *light green circle* in **(A)** and *green arrow* in **(B and C)**) and lateral plantar (LPN, *dotted green circle* in **(A)** and *dotted green arrow* in **(B and C)**) nerves. Tibial posterior artery (*black arrowhead* in **(A–C)**); *TPT*, tibialis posterior tendon; *FDLT*, flexor digitorum longus tendon.

the gluteus maximus medial or posterior to the SN (Ploteau et al., 2017a). After reaching the subgluteal region, the PFCN gives rise to the inferior cluneal/gluteal branches, which provide cutaneous sensory innervation to the inferior buttock, and perineal branches that provide sensory innervation to the proximal medial thigh, lateral perineum, and posterolateral surface of the external genitalia (Tubbs et al., 2009). It then continues descending superficial to the long head of the biceps femoris, deep to the fascia lata, providing sensory innervation to the back and medial surfaces of the thigh. At the level of the popliteal fossa, the PFCN pierces the fascia and gives rise to terminal branches that communicate with the sural nerve and innervate the popliteal fossa (Meng et al., 2015).

Anatomical variations include variable contributions from as high as the L4 and as low as the S4 roots, and variable extensions into the calf, occasionally all the way into the calcaneal region (Murinova et al., 2016).

On MRN, the normal PFCN is difficult to identify owing to its caliber. It can be seen intermittently on axial and coronal reconstructions, exiting the pelvic region medial or posterior to the SN (Figs. 20.20 and 20.21) and sometimes along the posterior thigh. Because of their caliber, the cluneal and perineal branches are not easily seen.

PUDENDAL NERVE

The pudendal nerve is a mixed sensory, motor, and autonomic nerve derived from contributions of the S2, S3, and S4 roots (Wadhwa et al., 2017). It provides motor innervation to the external anal and striated urethral sphincters, and the urogenital triangle muscles (transverse perineal, ischiocavernosus, and bulbospongiosus) (Fig. 20.22) and sensory cutaneous innervation to the perineum and external genitalia of both men and women (Soldatos et al., 2013). The main pudendal nerve exits the pelvic cavity through the greater sciatic notch, between the PM and coccygeus muscle, entering the gluteal region between the SN and PFCN (Elkins et al., 2017). At this point, the pudendal nerve lies between the sacrotuberous and sacrospinous ligaments, adjacent and posterior to the ischial spine (Ploteau

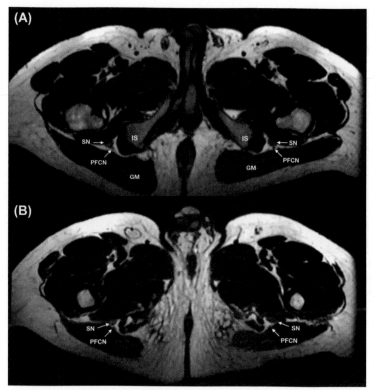

FIG. 20.20 T2-WI Hyper-Cube, axial reconstruction. The posterior femoral cutaneous nerve (PFCN) is identified descending under the gluteus maximus (GM), medial and posterior to the sciatic nerve (SN).

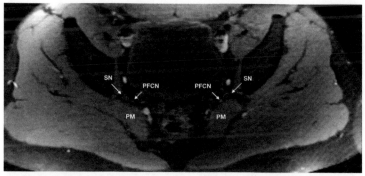

FIG. 20.21 Axial PD Fat-sat. The posterior femoral cutaneous nerve (PFCN) is identified on the axial plane, anterior to the pyramidal muscle (PM) and medial to the sciatic nerve (SN).

et al., 2017b). It passes through the lesser sciatic notch, entering the perineal region, and continues in a ventral direction through the pudendal (Alcock's) canal along the medial ischial tuberosity, under the fascia of the obturator internus muscle. The inferior rectal branch can arise before the pudendal nerve enters Alcock's canal or, more commonly, in its proximal portion (Weissman et al., 2017). Then it gives the superficial perineal branches and concludes with the dorsal nerve of the penis or clitoris, and the posterior scrotal or labial nerves (Chhabra et al., 2016). Along its full course, the nerve is accompanied by the internal pudendal artery and veins (Muniz Neto et al., 2018).

Anatomical variations include pudendal branches originating directly from the sacral plexus, separate pudendal trunks along Alcock's canal, and branching

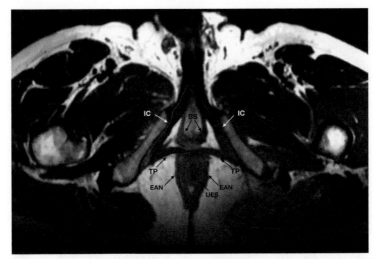

FIG. 20.22 Pudendal nerve motor innervation. T2-WI Hyper-Cube, axial reconstruction. **(A)** External anal sphincter (EAN) and urogenital triangle muscles; **(C)** transverse perineal (TP), ischiocavernosus (IC) and bulbospongiosus (BS); **(B)** urethral striated sphincter (UES).

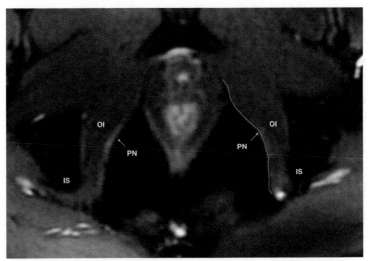

FIG. 20.23 T2-WI Cube DIR, Axial minimum intensity projection reconstruction. The pudendal nerve (PN) is identified medial to the obturator interns (OI) muscle, at the level of Alcock's canal.

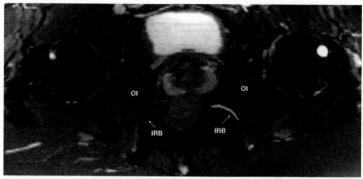

FIG. 20.24 Pudendal nerve branches. T2-WI Cube DIR, Axial minimum intensity projection (MIP) reconstruction. **(A)** The inferior rectal (IRB) branch is identified coursing through the ischiorectal fossa in a curvilinear fashion toward the external anal sphincter. **(B)** Perineal branches are identified along the urogenital triangle. Note the higher signal of the satellite vein adjacent to the left perineal branch in this Cube DIR sequence without intravenous contrast.

variations including a rectal-perineal trunk, dorsal-perineal nerve trunk, and rectal-dorsal trunk (Wadhwa et al., 2017).

On MRN, the normal pudendal nerve can best be depicted on both axial and coronal planes posterior to the ischial spine and through the Alcock's canal (Fig. 20.23) (Chhabra, 2016). The sacrotuberous and sacrospinous ligaments can serve as references to locate it on MRN (Muniz Neto et al., 2018). The inferior rectal branch can be seen coursing through the ischiorectal fossa in a curvilinear fashion toward the external anal sphincter, and the dorsal nerve of the clitoris or penis can be identified immediately under the pubic symphysis (Wadhwa et al., 2017). Because of their caliber, the perineal branches are not easily seen (Fig. 20.24).

REFERENCES

Adibatti, M., Sangeetha, V., 2014. Study on variant anatomy of sciatic nerve. J. Clin. Diagn. Res. 8. https://doi.org/10.7860/JCDR/2014/9116.4725.

Bäumer, P., Weiler, M., Bendszus, M., Pham, M., 2015. Somatotopic fascicular organization of the human sciatic nerve demonstrated by MR neurography. Neurology 84, 1782–1787. https://doi.org/10.1212/WNL.0000000000001526.

Beaton, L.E., Anson, B.J., 1937. The relation of the sciatic nerve and of its subdivisions to the piriformis muscle. Anat. Rec. 70, 1–5. https://doi.org/10.1002/ar.1090700102.

Beltran, L.S., Bencardino, J., Ghazikhanian, V., Beltran, J., 2010. Entrapment neuropathies III: lower limb. Semin. Muscoskel. Radiol. 14, 501–511. https://doi.org/10.1055/s-0030-1268070.

Carro, L.P., Hernando, M.F., Cerezal, L., et al., 2016. Deep gluteal space problems: piriformis syndrome, ischiofemoral impingement and sciatic nerve release. Muscles Ligaments Tendons J. 6, 384–396. https://doi.org/10.11138/mltj/2016.6.3.384.

Cejas, C., Pineda, D., 2017. Imaging of pain in the peripheral nerves. In: Neuroimaging of Pain. Springer International Publishing, Cham, pp. 215–265.

Cejas, C., Aguilar, M., Falcon, L., et al., 2012. High resolution (3T) magnetic resonance neurography of the sciatic nerve. Radiologia. https://doi.org/10.1016/j.rx.2012.04.004.

Cejas, C., Escobar, I., Serra, M., Barroso, F., 2015. Neurografía de alta resolución del plexo lumbosacro en resonancia magnética 3 T magneteic resonance imaging. Radiología 57, 22–34. https://doi.org/10.1016/j.rx.2014.07.006.

Chaves, H., Bendersky, M., Goñi, R., et al., 2018. Lumbosacral plexus root thickening: establishing normal root dimensions using magnetic resonance neurography. Clin. Anat. 31, 782–787. https://doi.org/10.1002/ca.23073.

Chhabra, A., 2016. Incremental value of magnetic resonance neurography of Lumbosacral plexus over non-contributory lumbar spine magnetic resonance imaging in radiculopathy: a prospective study. World J. Radiol. 8, 109. https://doi.org/10.4329/wjr.v8.i1.109.

Chhabra, A., Andreisek, G., Soldatos, T., et al., 2011a. MR neurography: past, present, and future. Am. J. Roentgenol. 197, 583–591. https://doi.org/10.2214/AJR.10.6012.

Chhabra, A., Lee, P.P., Bizzell, C., Soldatos, T., 2011b. 3 Tesla MR neurography – technique, interpretation, and pitfalls. Skeletal Radiol. 40, 1249–1260.

Chhabra, A., Williams, E.H., Subhawong, T.K., et al., 2011c. MR neurography findings of soleal sling entrapment. Am. J. Roentgenol. 196, 290–297. https://doi.org/10.2214/AJR.10.4925.

Chhabra, A., McKenna, C.A., Wadhwa, V., et al., 2016. 3T magnetic resonance neurography of pudendal nerve with cadaveric dissection correlation. World J. Radiol. 8, 700. https://doi.org/10.4329/wjr.v8.i7.700.

Collinge, C.A., Ziran, N.M., Coons, D.A., 2015. Relationship between the superior gluteal vessels and nerve at the greater sciatic notch. Orthopedics 38, e929—e933.

Delaney, H., Bencardino, J., Rosenberg, Z.S., 2014. Magnetic resonance neurography of the pelvis and lumbosacral plexus. Neuroimaging Clin. N. Am. 24, 127—150.

Demondion, X., Leroy, X., Lapègue, F., et al., 2002. Lumbar spinal ganglia enhancement after Gadolinium chelate administration: a radio-histological correlation. Surg. Radiol. Anat. 23, 415—419. https://doi.org/10.1007/s00276-001-0415-1.

Deutsch, A., Wyzykowski, R.J., Victoroff, B.N., 1999. Evaluation of the anatomy of the common peroneal nerve: defining nerve- at-risk in arthroscopically assisted lateral meniscus repair. Am. J. Sports Med. 27, 10—15. https://doi.org/10.1177/03635465990270010201.

Donovan, A., Rosenberg, Z.S., Cavalcanti, C.F., 2010. MR imaging of entrapment neuropathies of the lower extremity: Part 2. the knee, leg, ankle, and foot. Radiographics 30, 1001—1014. https://doi.org/10.1148/rg.304095188.

Du, R., Auguste, K.I., Chin, C.T., et al., 2010. Magnetic resonance neurography for the evaluation of peripheral nerve, brachial plexus, and nerve root disorders: clinical article. J. Neurosurg. 112, 362—371. https://doi.org/10.3171/2009.7.JNS09414.

Eastlac, J.K., Tenorio, L., Wadhwa, V., et al., 2017. Sciatic neuromuscular variants on MR neurography: frequency study and interobserver performance. Br. J. Radiol. 90 https://doi.org/10.1259/bjr.20170116.

Elkins, N., Hunt, J., Scott, K.M., 2017. Neurogenic pelvic pain. Phys. Med. Rehabil. Clin 28, 551—569. https://doi.org/10.1016/j.pmr.2017.03.007.

Eppenberger, P., Andreisek, G., Chhabra, A., 2014. Magnetic resonance neurography. Diffusion tensor imaging and future directions. Neuroimaging Clin. N. Am. 24, 245—256. https://doi.org/10.1016/j.nic.2013.03.031.

Evans, M., Manji, H., 2013. Progress in peripheral nerve disease research in the last two years. J. Neurol. 260, 3188—3192. https://doi.org/10.1007/s00415-013-7121-x.

Florian-Rodriguez, M.E., Hare, A., Chin, K., et al., 2016. Inferior gluteal and other nerves associated with sacrospinous ligament: a cadaver study. Am. J. Obstet. Gynecol. 215 https://doi.org/10.1016/j.ajog.2016.06.025, 646.e1—646.e6.

Fritz, J., Bizzell, C., Kathuria, S., et al., 2013. High-resolution magnetic resonance-guided posterior femoral cutaneous nerve blocks. Skeletal Radiol. 42, 579—586. https://doi.org/10.1007/s00256-012-1553-8.

Gierada, D.S., Erickson, J., Estkowski, D., Nowicki, H., 1992. Pictorial Essay MR Imaging of the Sacral Plexus: Normal and Lloydia, pp. 655—659 (Cincinnati).

Giuffre, B.A., Jeanmonod, R., 2019. Anatomy, Sciatic Nerve.

Gürkanlar, D., Ozan, H., Gönül, E., Çal)flma, A., 2005. Yusuf (ZC(The Morphological Aspects of Lumbar Plexus and Roots an Anatomical Study Lomber Pleksus ve Köklerin Morfolojik Özellikleri.

Iwanaga, J., Simonds, E., Vetter, M., et al., 2018. The inferior gluteal nerve often has a cutaneous branch: a discovery with application to hip surgery and targeting gluteal pain syndromes. Clin. Anat. 31, 937—941. https://doi.org/10.1002/ca.23232.

Iwanaga, J., Eid, S., Simonds, E., et al., 2019. The majority of piriformis muscles are innervated by the superior gluteal nerve. Clin. Anat. 32, 282—286. https://doi.org/10.1002/ca.23311.

La Rocca Vieira, R., Rosenberg, Z.S., Kiprovski, K., 2007. MRI of the distal biceps femoris muscle: normal anatomy, variants, and association with common peroneal entrapment neuropathy. Am. J. Roentgenol. 189, 549—555. https://doi.org/10.2214/AJR.07.2308.

Lung, K., Lui, F., 2019. Anatomy, Abdomen and Pelvis, Superior Gluteal Nerve. StatPearls.

Meng, S., Lieba-Samal, D., Reissig, L.F., et al., 2015. High-resolution ultrasound of the posterior femoral cutaneous nerve: visualization and initial experience with patients. Skeletal Radiol. 44, 1421—1426. https://doi.org/10.1007/s00256-015-2177-6.

Mirilas, P., Skandalakis, J.E., 2010. Surgical anatomy of the retroperitoneal spaces, part IV: retroperitoneal nerves. Am. Surg.

Muniz Neto, F.J., Kihara Filho, E.N., Miranda, F.C., et al., 2018. Demystifying MR neurography of the lumbosacral plexus: from protocols to pathologies. BioMed Res. Int. 2018 https://doi.org/10.1155/2018/9608947.

Murinova, N., Krashin, D., Trescot, A.M., 2016. Posterior femoral cutaneous nerve entrapment: low back. In: Trescot, A.M. (Ed.), Peripheral Nerve Entrapments. Springer, Cham.

Neufeld, E.A., Shen, P.Y., Nidecker, A.E., et al., 2015. MR imaging of the lumbosacral plexus: a review of techniques and pathologies. J. Neuroimaging 25, 691—703. https://doi.org/10.1111/jon.12253.

Pineda, D., Barroso, F., Cháves, H., Cejas, C., 2014. High resolution 3T magnetic resonance neurography of the peroneal nerve. Radiologia 56, 107—117. https://doi.org/10.1016/j.rxeng.2014.04.005.

Ploteau, S., Salaud, C., Hamel, A., Robert, R., 2017a. Entrapment of the posterior femoral cutaneous nerve and its inferior cluneal branches: anatomical basis of surgery for inferior cluneal neuralgia. Surg. Radiol. Anat. 39, 859—863. https://doi.org/10.1007/s00276-017-1825-z.

Ploteau, S., Perrouin-Verbe, M.A., Labat, J.J., et al., 2017b. Anatomical variants of the pudendal nerve observed during a transgluteal surgical approach in a population of patients with pudendal neuralgia. Pain Physician 20, E137—E143.

Ribeiro, F.S., Bettencourt Pires, M.A., da Silva, E.X., et al., 2018. Rethinking sciatica in view of a bilateral anatomical variation of the sciatic nerve, with low origin and high division: historical, anatomical and clinical approach. Acta Med. Port. 31, 568—575. https://doi.org/10.20344/amp.10567.

Roshanravan, S.M., Wieslander, C.K., Schaffer, J.I., Corton, M.M., 2007. Neurovascular anatomy of the sacrospinous ligament region in female cadavers: implications in sacrospinous ligament fixation. Am. J. Obstet. Gynecol. 197. https://doi.org/10.1016/j.ajog.2007.08.061, 660.e1—660.e6.

Russell, J.M., Kransdorf, M.J., Bancroft, L.W., et al., 2008. Magnetic resonance imaging of the sacral plexus and piriformis muscles. Skeletal Radiol. 37, 709–713. https://doi.org/10.1007/s00256-008-0486-8.

Schmidt, C.K., Iwanaga, J., Yilmaz, E., et al., 2017. Absence of the lumbosacral trunk. Cureus 9, 10–13. https://doi.org/10.7759/cureus.1809.

Smoll, N.R., 2010. Variations of the piriformis and sciatic nerve with clinical consequence: a review. Clin. Anat. 23, 8–17. https://doi.org/10.1002/ca.20893.

Soldatos, T., Andreisek, G., Thawait, G.K., et al., 2013. High-resolution 3-T MR neurography of the lumbosacral plexus. Radiographics 33. https://doi.org/10.1148/rg.334115761.

Spinner, R.J., Binaghi, D., Socolovsky, M., et al., 2012. Entrapment neuropathies of the lower extremity. Med. Clin. N. Am. 41, 371–382. https://doi.org/10.1007/s00256-011-1146-y.

Tazawa, K.-I., Matsuda, M., Yoshida, T., et al., 2008. Spinal Nerve root hypertrophy on MRI: clinical significance in the diagnosis of chronic inflammatory demyelinating polyradiculoneuropathy. Intern. Med 47. https://doi.org/10.2169/internalmedicine.47.1272.

Tomaszewski, K.A., Graves, M.J., Henry, B.M., et al., 2016. Surgical anatomy of the sciatic nerve: a meta-analysis. J. Orthop. Res. 34, 1820–1827. https://doi.org/10.1002/jor.23186.

Trappeniers, L., De Maeseneer, M., Van Roy, P., et al., 2003. Peroneal nerve injury in three patients with knee trauma: MR imaging and correlation with anatomic findings in volunteers and anatomic specimens. Eur. Radiol. 13, 1722–1727. https://doi.org/10.1007/s00330-003-1833-8.

Tubbs, R.S., Miller, J., Loukas, M., et al., 2009. Surgical and anatomical landmarks for the perineal branch of the posterior femoral cutaneous nerve: implications in perineal pain syndromes — laboratory investigation. J. Neurosurg. 111, 332–335. https://doi.org/10.3171/2008.11.JNS081248.

Van den Bergh, P.Y.K., Hadden, R.D.M., Bouche, P., et al., 2010. European Federation of Neurological Societies/Peripheral Nerve Society guideline on management of chronic inflammatory demyelinating polyradiculoneuropathy: report of a joint task force of the European Federation of Neurological Societies and the Peripher. Eur. J. Neurol. 17, 356–363. https://doi.org/10.1111/j.1085-9489.2005.10302.x.

Wadhwa, V., Hamid, A.S., Kumar, Y., et al., 2017. Pudendal nerve and branch neuropathy: magnetic resonance neurography evaluation. Acta Radiol. 58, 726–733. https://doi.org/10.1177/0284185116668213.

Waikakul, S., Chandraphak, S., Sangthongsil, P., 2010. Anatomy of L4 to S3 nerve roots. J. Orthop. Surg. 18, 352–355. https://doi.org/10.1177/230949901001800319.

Weissman, E., Boothe, E., Wadhwa, V., et al., 2017. Magnetic resonance neurography of the pelvic nerves. Semin. Ultrasound CT MRI 38, 269–278. https://doi.org/10.1053/j.sult.2016.11.006.

Williams, E.H., Williams, C.G., Rosson, G.D., Dellon, L.A., 2009. Anatomic site for proximal tibial nerve compression: a cadaver study. Ann. Plast. Surg. 62, 322–325. https://doi.org/10.1097/SAP.0b013e31817e9d81.

Zhang, Z.W., Song, L.J., Meng, Q.F., et al., 2008. High-resolution diffusion-weighted MR imaging of the human lumbosacral plexus and its branches based on a steady-state free precession imaging technique at 3T. Am. J. Neuroradiol. 29, 1092–1094. https://doi.org/10.3174/ajnr.A0994.

Zoccali, C., Skoch, J., Patel, A., et al., 2015. The surgical neurovascular anatomy relating to partial and complete sacral and sacroiliac resections: a cadaveric, anatomic study. Eur. Spine J. 24, 1109–1113. https://doi.org/10.1007/s00586-015-3815-3.

CHAPTER 21

Pathologies Affecting the Sacral Plexus

DIA R. HALALMEH • MARC MOISI

INTRODUCTION

Sacral plexus pathologies are relatively rare but potentially debilitating phenomena and can cause significant morbidity. Usually, the sacral plexus is considered together with the lumbar plexus as the lumbosacral plexus. However, this chapter highlights largely the various lesions that tend to affect the sacral plexus. The chapter begins with a brief review of some of the sacral plexus and its branches' basic anatomy, which provides a foundation for the subsequent discussion of the diseases related to this plexus.

ANATOMY

The sacral plexus is one of the five spinal plexuses (cervical, brachial, lumbar, sacral, and coccygeal), and is a major contributor to the motor and sensory functions of the lower limbs and parts of the pelvis. It is situated on the posterolateral pelvic wall anterior to the piriformis muscle (Cramer and Ro, 2017). It is composed of the merging of the ventral rami of L4-S4, with a minor contribution from L4 and L5 through the lumbosacral trunk (Petchprapa et al., 2010). The sacral and lumbar plexuses form the larger lumbosacral plexus. The sacral plexus' ventral rami emerge from the anterior sacral foramina and are joined by the fourth and fifth lumbar roots, the lumbosacral trunk. Most of the sacral plexus' nerves enter the lower limbs via the greater sciatic foramen and pass either above or below the piriformis muscles. Other nerves remain within the pelvis to innervate the pelvic muscles, organs, and perineum. The remainder of the branches leave the pelvis via the greater sciatic foramen and reenter the lesser sciatic foramen by looping around the sacrospinous ligament to supply lateral pelvic and perineal structures (Drake et al., 2010).

BRANCHES

The sacral plexus' five major branches are the superior and inferior gluteal nerves, sciatic nerve, posterior femoral cutaneous nerve, and pudendal nerve, which is the perineum's nerve. In addition, there are numerous smaller branches that innervate the pelvic wall, floor, and individual muscles of the gluteal region.

Sciatic Nerve (L4-S3)

The sciatic nerve forms from two major components' convergence: the tibial and common fibular. The sacral plexus' upper nerve roots (ventral divisions of L4 to S3) unite near the greater sciatic foramen and contribute to the sciatic nerve's tibial component. The common fibular component is formed from the dorsal divisions of L4 to S2. Initially, a band of connective tissue encloses the tibial and common fibular components together and forms the sciatic nerve, which then separates at another variable point. After forming on the piriformis muscle's anterior aspect, the sciatic nerve exits the pelvis inferior to the piriformis via the greater sciatic foramen (Petchprapa et al., 2010). At this level, the superior gluteal artery, the internal iliac artery's (IIA) largest branch, runs just medial to the nerve.

With respect to motor function, the sciatic nerve's tibial portion innervates all of the muscles in the thigh's posterior compartment, except for the short head of the biceps femoris. It also innervates the adductor magnus muscle's hamstring portion. In addition, the tibial component innervates all muscles in the leg's posterior compartment and in the sole of the foot. The common fibular portion innervates the short head of the biceps femoris, all muscles of the leg's anterior and lateral compartments, and the extensor digitorum brevis muscle. With respect to sensory function, the tibial portion carries sensory fibers from the skin of the posterolateral leg as well as the sole of the foot. The common fibular portion innervates the skin on the leg's anterolateral and dorsal aspects.

Superior Gluteal Nerve (L4-S1)

This nerve originates from dorsal divisions of L4, L5, and S1. It leaves the pelvis by passing through the greater sciatic foramen and enters the gluteal region

Surgical Anatomy of the Sacral Plexus and Its Branches. https://doi.org/10.1016/B978-0-323-77602-8.00021-0

superior to the piriformis muscle. It is accompanied by the superior gluteal artery and vein throughout most of its course, and supplies the gluteal medius and minimus, and the tensor fasciae latae muscles.

Inferior Gluteal Nerve (L5-S2)

The inferior gluteal nerve originates from dorsal divisions of L5, S1, and S2. It exits the pelvis through the greater sciatic foramen inferior to the piriformis muscle and innervates the gluteus maximus muscle. The inferior gluteal artery and vein accompany it along its course.

Posterior Femoral Cutaneous Nerve (S1-S3)

The posterior femoral cutaneous nerve, which branches from the ventral rami of S1, S2, and S3, leaves the pelvic cavity through the greater sciatic foramen and enters the gluteal region inferior to the piriformis muscle. It innervates the skin on the thigh and leg's posterior surfaces, and on the perineum through perineal branches distributed over the upper and medial side of the thigh.

Pudendal Nerve (S2-S4)

The pudendal nerve derives from the ventral divisions of S2, S3, and S4. Both the pudendal nerve and the nerve to the obturator internus leave the pelvic cavity via the greater sciatic foramen inferior to the piriformis muscle and reenter the lesser sciatic foramen by looping around the sacrospinous ligament and taking the nerve into the perineum. The pudendal nerve innervates the skeletal muscles in the perineum, the external urethral and external anal sphincters, and the levator ani muscle. With respect to sensory function, it innervates the skin on the penis and clitoris and most of the perineal region's skin.

Other Branches

In addition to the sacral plexus' primsary branches, there are a number of smaller branches. These tend to be nerves that supply the muscles directly, with the exception of the perforating cutaneous nerve, which supplies the skin over the inferior gluteal region, and the pelvic splanchnic nerves, which innervate the abdominal viscera. The perforating cutaneous nerve originates from the S2 and S3 nerve roots. After leaving the pelvis through the greater sciatic foramen inferior to the piriformis muscle, it perforates the sacrotuberous ligament to supply the skin covering the gluteal folds. The nerve to the piriformis is formed from S2 and occasionally S1, and innervates the piriformis muscle directly. The nerve to the obturator internus originates from L5 through S2. Like the pudendal nerve, this nerve leaves the pelvis by passing through the greater sciatic foramen, wraps around the sacrospinous ligament,

and reenters the lesser sciatic foramen to innervate the obturator internus and superior gemellus muscles directly. The nerve to the quadratus femoris formed from L4 through S1 leaves the pelvis via the greater sciatic foramen inferior to the piriformis muscle to innervate the quadratus femoris as well as the inferior gemellus muscles.

CLINICAL PRESENTATION

Clinical manifestations usually help clinicians confine the lesion to a specific location within the lumbosacral plexus. Lesions that involve the sacral plexus and the lumbosacral trunk tend to cause foot drop and weak knee flexion. Depending upon the lesion's extent, sensory disturbances may vary; typically, however, they involve the dorsum of the foot, posterior aspect of the leg and thigh, and perineum.

DIAGNOSTIC EVALUATION

A thorough history and physical exam with focused neurological examination are necessary to limit the differential diagnosis. Nevertheless, clinical presentation usually is insufficient to differentiate between plexopathies and radiculopathies. Therefore, electrophysiology is essential to distinguish lumbosacral plexopathies from the more prevalent radiculopathies. In summary, accurate diagnosis and the lesion's specific localization depend on laboratory studies, including electromyography (EMG) and appropriate imaging, such as MRI and CT.

SACRAL PLEXOPATHY ETIOLOGIES

Lumbosacral plexopathy is relatively rare. However, if untreated, vulnerable patients can experience debilitating pain and potentially, paralysis. Given these lesions' wide array of etiologies, physicians should maintain an organized approach to localize and manage these conditions accurately and effectively. Therefore, it is important to stratify etiologies into major broad categories when evaluating patients with signs and symptoms suspicious for sacral plexopathies.

Injuries

Unlike the brachial plexus, which is susceptible to injury, the pelvic bones and vertebral column protect the sacral plexus, and thus, direct injury is an unusual cause of sacral plexopathy. In fact, only high-impact pelvic injuries usually affect the sacral plexus. The mechanisms of injuries may include posterior hip dislocation, hyperextension of the thigh, and flexion-abduction of the hip (Lang et al., 2004; Tonetti et al., 2004; Kutsy et al., 2000; Schmal et al., 2010). In a prospective review of 44 patients treated surgically for pelvic injuries, the estimated incidence of lumbosacral plexopathy was 52%; however, only 21% suffered permanent deficits (Tonetti et al., 2004). As a result of the multiple injuries and involvement of multiple organs in these patients, lumbosacral injuries usually go unnoticed (Kutsy et al., 2000). Many risk factors influence the development of neurological deficits after pelvic injuries, including complex, unstable fractures that involve the sacrum (Schmal et al., 2010), longitudinal displacement of the pelvis, and suicidal jumps (Sugimoto et al., 2010). Consequently, the sacral plexus typically is involved in pelvic injuries that result in neurologic manifestations.

Lumbosacral plexopathy attributable to obstetric complications has been reported. Nevertheless, other causes of intrapartum/postpartum neurological complications, such as nerve block procedure-associated injuries (De Tommaso et al., 2002) and fibular nerve compression (Qublan and Al-Sayegh, 2000; Colachis III et al., 1994), should be excluded first. In cases in which obstetrical lumbosacral plexopathy is suspected, it is challenging to confirm the location of the nerve roots affected without electrophysiologic testing, particularly during the intrapartum/postpartum period. However, based upon patients who had electrodiagnostic studies, numerous of these have shown that the lumbosacral trunk (L4 and L5) and S1 nerve root are most likely to be affected in intrapartum lumbosacral plexopathy (Feasby et al., 1992). This appears to be attributable to the fact that psoas muscle does not cover the lumbosacral trunk's terminal portion near the pelvic brim. As a result, this trunk is more susceptible to injury by fetal presentation at this level, where it is adjacent to the pelvic inlet's bony edge (Katirji et al., 2002). Recovery and prognosis depend upon the severity of axonal injury and continuity of the nerve fibers after the trauma. The symptoms of nearly all patients with neuropraxia (nerve contusion with temporary conduction block or diminished signal transmission) resolve completely.

Vascular Etiologies

Familiarity with the anatomy of the sacral plexus' blood supply is essential to evaluate vascular causes of lumbosacral plexopathies.

The vascular supply to the sacral plexus comes predominantly through branches of the IIA and the deep iliac circumflex artery (Day, 1964). The internal iliac vessels are anterior to the sacral plexus. As a result, these vessels' enlargement attributable to aneurysms/pseudoaneurysms may affect the plexus. The entities described here include ischemic plexopathy, compression by aneurysm/pseudoaneurysms, and retroperitoneal hematoma.

Ischemic pathology of the sacral plexus secondary to vascular occlusion is an uncommon phenomenon because of the rich blood supply and the presence of good collaterals. However, occlusion of the terminal arteries that lack sufficient collateral blood supply may lead to ischemic injury (Kim et al., 2014). Patterns of neurologic deficits are unpredictable, but symptoms range from intermittent claudication and sensory disturbances to progressive paraplegia, and bowel and bladder dysfunction late in the course (Wohlgemuth et al., 1999). It is worth mentioning that such ischemic plexopathies are more likely to occur after major surgeries that involve vascular reconstruction, such as kidney transplantation, particularly in those with a history of atherosclerotic disease (Dhillon and Sarac, 2000; Hefty et al., 1990). Moreover, aortic dissection (Lefebvre et al., 1995) and inadvertent intra-arterial gluteal injection of vasoactive drugs (Stöhr and Dichgans, 1980) have been reported to cause ischemic lumbosacral plexopathy.

Because of the IIAs' proximity to the sacral plexus, any aneurysmal dilation may affect the latter. Therefore, IIA aneurysms or pseudoaneurysms may compress the plexus posteriorly. Pseudoaneurysms result from the accumulation of blood between an artery's tunica media and tunica adventitia, the vessel's two outer layers, as a result of vascular trauma (e.g., suture lines, catheterization, and vascular reconstructive surgeries). Incriminating risk factors for the development of pseudoaneurysms include infection, defective vascular anastomosis, and chronic atherosclerotic disease (Luzzio et al., 1999). IIA aneurysms and pseudoaneurysms represent unusual causes of lumbosacral plexopathy. In fact, isolated IIA dilations themselves are rare (Dix et al., 2005) and remain asymptomatic unless they rupture or compress adjacent structures. Furthermore, IIA aneurysms' repair can compromise the vascular supply to the sacral plexus, as bilateral ligation of the distal and proximal ends is required (Khanna et al., 2014). Above all, a high index of suspicion and low threshold for investigation of suspected aneurysms, particularly when symptomatic, and referring the patient to a vascular surgeon, should be maintained because of the risk of fatal rupture.

Retroperitoneal hematoma represents another infrequent cause of sacral plexopathy. They affect the lumbar plexus predominantly, as most of these hemorrhages occur within the psoas muscle, which contains this plexus' nerve roots. To a lesser degree, these hematomas will affect the entire lumbosacral plexus and the sacral plexus nerve roots. Several problems can cause retroperitoneal hematoma, including anticoagulation, ruptured renal aneurysm, ruptured aortic aneurysm, vascular injury (e.g., femoral vein dialysis and lumbosacral block procedures), as well as malignancy (Katz et al., 1997; Anastasiou et al., 2013; Al-Khulaiwi et al., 2000; Kaymak et al., 2004; Aveline and Bonnet, 2004). The mortality attributable to these retroperitoneal hemorrhages is significant, particularly when caused by injuries. The mortality rate was 20% in one report on 81 patients with retroperitoneal hematoma attributable to traumatic injuries (Selivanov et al., 1984). On the other hand, retroperitoneal hematoma—induced sacral plexopathies demonstrate good neurologic recovery (Kent et al., 1994).

Neoplasms

Tumor involvement of the sacral plexus occurs most commonly as a result of direct invasion of adjacent malignancies' part (Jaeckle et al., 1985). Less commonly, metastasis from other organs, lymphatic spread, and bone metastasis from the sacrum or pelvis, may occur. In addition, Capek et al. (Capek et al., 2015) suggested that "Tumor cells can use splanchnic nerves as conduits and spread from the end organ to the lumbosacral plexus." Similarly, Ebner et al. (Ebner et al., 1990) described a mechanism in which the tumor cells can track along the connective tissue around the nerve trunks and affect the involved nerves' function. This explains why many patients have a physical exam that is inconsistent with imaging findings.

The most frequent tumor affecting the sacral plexus is colorectal cancer (Jaeckle, 2004). Other tumors may include sarcomas, metastatic breast tumors, lymphomas, gynecologic carcinomas, and prostatic carcinomas, among others (Capek et al., 2015; Jaeckle et al., 1985). Moreover, neoplastic lumbosacral plexopathy may arise from benign tumors, such as uterine leiomyoma, neurofibromas, and schwannomas (Felice and Donaldson, 1995; Argyrakis et al., 1985; Freitas et al., 2018). In one study, the sacral plexus was involved in 51% of 85 cases of pelvic tumor, while the lumbar plexus was involved in 31%, and the entire lumbosacral plexus was affected in the remainder of the subjects. Symptoms normally present insidiously rather than acutely, and pain, typically aching and cramping, is the symptom encountered most frequently. Months later, patients develop leg weakness (86%), sensory disturbances (73%), diminished reflexes (64%), and leg edema (47%). Autonomic symptoms are rare; however, "hot and dry foot" represents an early sign of metastatic plexopathy in one-third of patients as a result of sympathetic plexus infiltration. In most cases, the prognosis is dismal, and the median patient survival is only approximately 5.5 months (Jaeckle et al., 1985; Chad and Bradley, 1987; Dalmau et al., 1989). Typically, the diagnosis is confirmed by MRI or CT. The former provides more sensitivity in detecting neoplastic plexopathy, and thus, is the preferred choice if available (Taylor et al., 1997).

Radiation Plexopathy

Radiation-induced sacral plexopathy presents usually as asymmetrical bilateral weakness in the lower extremities, loss of reflexes, and less commonly, sensory deficits. Unlike patients with neoplastic plexopathy, it causes only modest, if any, pain. In addition, bilateral involvement is more common with radiation plexopathy (Chad and Bradley, 1987; Thomas et al., 1985). The time between exposure to radiation and symptom onset varies widely and ranges from 1 to 31 years. Further, the amount of radiation does not determine this latency (Chad and Bradley, 1987). On the contrary, neurotoxicity is dose dependent, where doses above 100 rsads have been shown to cause pathological changes on the cellular level (Cavanagh, 1968). Gutmann (Gutmann, 1991) indicated that radiation may cause electrochemical disturbances along the nerve axons, and generate a characteristic pattern of discharges that is referred to as "myokymia," which can be detected via EMG; thus, electrodiagnostic studies can be used to distinguish radiation plexopathy from the recurrence of a tumor treated formerly. The management largely is symptomatic and should focus on pain control, particularly in patients with neuropathic pain.

Infectious and Inflammatory Etiologies

As with all other parts of the body, the sacral plexus and its branches can be sites of infections. Some infectious agents have a relative or absolute predilection for the nervous system, while others can affect many other organs as well as the peripheral nervous system. Systemic inflammatory conditions that affect various organs in the body also may cause acral plexopathy. In this situation, vasculitis is believed to be the basis for this plexopathy.

Infections can lead to sacral plexopathy, either by adjacent infected structures' direct involvement or through a "para-infectious" immune-mediated destruction mechanism. Tuberculosis, osteomyelitis, pyelonephritis, and appendicitis, among others, have been implicated in direct infections of the sacral plexus (Aichroth and Rowe-Jones, 1971). Organisms such as *Mycobacterium tuberculosis, Borrelia burgdorferi, Treponema pallidum,* HIV, Epstein-Barr virus, varicella-zoster virus, and HSV have been reported (Stoeckli et al., 2000; Sharma et al., 1993; Garcia-Moncó et al., 1993; Putti, 1927; Steiner et al., 1999; Archer, 2018). An abscess can form as the body attempts to eliminate these organisms through an inflammatory response. Abscesses within structures that rest in close contact with the lumbosacral plexus, most importantly the psoas major muscle, may compress the sacral plexus. Abscesses within the gluteal and pelvic regions typically are associated with gastrointestinal and urinary tract infections. The principal routes through which these infections gain access to the pelvis are the iliopsoas muscle and iliac vessels (Ergun and Lakadamyali, 2010). Patients with weakened immune systems (e.g., from HIV chemotherapy and severe trauma) are prone to develop more severe abscesses. Further, if the infection spreads to the sacral plexus, systemic symptoms may develop together with the manifestations of sacral plexopathy. Of note, a psoas major muscle abscess should be cosnidered in patients with a history of Crohn's disease who present with pain and progressive motor deficits in the lower extremities (Femminineo and LaBan, 1988). In general, surgical drainage is necessary to relieve the symptoms that result from the plexus' compression.

Inflammatory and autoimmune etiologies of sacral plexopathy are relatively rare; however, they can be clinically significant. Normally, they affect the plexus because of their tendency to cause vasculitis of the vessels that feed the nerve roots (vasa nervosum). Autoimmune disorders that may lead to lumbosacral plexopathy include systemic necrotizing angiopathies (Cohen et al., 1980) (Polyarteritis nodosa and Churg-Strauss syndrome), hypersensitivity vasculitis (Cream, 1976) (systemic lupus erythematosus, serum sickness, Henoch-Schonlein purpura, cryoglobulinemia), Wegener granulomatosis (Fauci and Wolff, 1973), and systemic sclerosis. Moore et al. (Moore et al., 1989) reported the first case of CREST (calcinosis, Raynaud's phenomenon, esophageal dysmotility, sclerodactyly, telangiectasias)-induced lumbosacral plexopathy. It has been speculated that vasculitis that occurs in systemic sclerosis is the plexopathy's primary mechanism. Although the nerves' watershed areas are the most susceptible to vasculitis-induced damage, the lumbosacral plexus roots are involved occasionally (Chad and Bradley, 1987). Zuniga et al. (Zuniga et al., 1991) reported on 10 patients with sarcoidosis and neurologic

manifestations, four of whom had atypical neuropathies, including unilateral lumbosacral plexopathy that appears to have an underlaying immune-mediated basis.

OTHER ETIOLOGIES
Diabetic Amyotrophy
Diabetic amyotrophy, also known as diabetic lumbosacral radiculoplexopathy (DLRP), is the most common cause of lumbosacral plexopathy. Diabetic amyotrophy is a nerve disorder that is a complication of diabetes mellitus. Although DRLP can occur in both type 1 and type 2 diabetes mellitus patients, it is found most commonly in type 2 diabetics. Despite its name, DLRP also can affect the sacral plexus' nerve roots and peripheral nerves. DLRP's principal mechanism has been the subject of considerable debate. Metabolic derangements that lead to impaired control of capillary blood flow secondary to loss of pericytes and thickening of the basement membrane were thought first to cause the nerve damage associated with the condition that ultimately results in hypoxic-ischemic insult. Nerve biopsies have shifted the view toward an immune mechanism that causes microvasculitis that eventually could lead to ischemia. Experimental treatments with immunosuppressive proteins have provided corroborative evidence of the immune mechanism theory. Moreover, nerve biopsy specimens typically show axonal degeneration, multifocal fiber loss, and neovascularization. These histological features most likely are attributable to microvasculitis with perivascular infiltrate that results in ischemic insult (Dyck et al., 1999).

Signs and symptoms of diabetic amyotrophy depend on the region of the plexus affected. Nevertheless, the first symptom typically is pain over the buttocks, thighs, and legs, as well as sensory changes. Frequently, the pain is unilateral and can occur suddenly followed by variable weakness in the lower limbs' proximal muscles. The sacral plexus scarcely is affected compared to the lumbar plexus. Therefore, most patients exhibit proximal symptoms on presentation. Although they begin often on one side, these symptoms also can progress to the contralateral side and become symmetrical. Denervation of the specific muscle regions the affected plexus innervates explains the weakness. The symptoms progress over the course of months; however, they are followed by complete resolution within months to years in nearly all patients. Infrequently, patients experience long-term or even persistent symptoms, such as foot drop and neuropathic pain (Dyck et al., 1999; Dyck and Windebank, 2002).

Patients with diabetes and proximal pain and weakness often are suspected to have diabetic amyotrophy. A more definitive diagnosis commonly is established with electrodiagnostic studies, including nerve conduction studies and electromyograms. Diabetic amyotrophy often is a diagnosis of exclusion in diabetic patients with lumbosacral plexopathy for whom no other cause of the condition can be determined. Proper management of diabetes can prevent diabetic amyotrophy from occurring repeatedly. However, once it occurs, its management largely is symptomatic. Although unproven, some studies have postulated that immunosuppressive therapy may result in clinical improvement (Pascoe et al., 1997; Krendel et al., 1995; Tamburin et al., 2014).

Idiopathic Lumbosacral Radiculoplexus Neuropathy

Idiopathic lumbosacral radiculoplexus neuropathy (LRPN) and diabetic amyotrophy share similar pathological, clinical, and prognostic features. However, idiopathic LRPN occurs in the absence of diabetes mellitus. The condition was identified only recently as a separate entity when Sander and Sharp (Sander and Sharp, 1981) and Evans et al. (Evans et al., 1981) first described it clinically. Typically, similar to diabetic amyotrophy, it begins suddenly with severe pain that affects one proximal lower limb, followed by weakness that progresses over weeks to months with gradual recovery (Dyck and Windebank, 2002).

Gynecologic Causes

The sacral plexus also may be affected as a result of compression by intrapelvic masses, such as retroverted uterus, leiomyoma, and adenomyosis, or ovarian and uterine tumors' infiltration (Ergun and Lakadamyali, 2010). In addition, endometriosis can infiltrate the sacral plexus and causes subsequent signs and symptoms of sacral plexopathy depending upon the region affected. These lesions' pathogenesis is uncertain and still debated. de Sousa et al. (de Sousa et al., 2015) suggested that perineural spread from the uterus is the main route by which endometriosis reaches the sacral plexus. Endometriosis may spread bilaterally; however, the right sacral plexus is involved more frequently, as the sigmoid colon seems to protect the left (Pham et al., 2010). Endometriosis is overlooked frequently as a potential cause of sacral plexopathy because it is extremely rare and because other more common causes (diabetic amyotrophy, compressive masses, and injuries) are considered primarily. Overall, the index of suspicion for sacral plexopathy attributable to gynecological etiologies should be high, particularly when no other causes of it are identified.

Amyloidosis within the sacral plexus has been described as well. In this case, imaging shows enlargement of the plexus' roots and branches (Soldatos et al., 2013). Sacral plexopathy also may be the result of adjacent inflammatory processes (Wong et al., 2005). In addition, genetic conditions, such as hereditary neuralgic amyotrophy, an autosomal dominant recurrent neuropathy, may result in sacral plexopathy. This condition is characterized by painful episodes of neuropathy with muscle weakness and atrophy, as well as sensory disturbances (Meuleman et al., 1999).

CONCLUSION

Knowledge of these pathologies is of utmost importance to clinicians and surgeons. Therefore, early diagnosis of sacral plexopathies improves the likelihood of relieving symptoms significantly, as well as avoiding any additional neurologic injury and unnecessary surgery.

REFERENCES

Aichroth, P., Rowe-Jones, D.C., 1971. Iliacus compartment compression syndrome. Br. J. Surg. 58 (11), 833—834.

Al-Khulaiwi, A., Razaak, F.A., El Shair, A., Bamehriz, F., 2000. Idiopathic retroperitoneal hematoma. Ann. Saudi Med. 20, 270—271.

Anastasiou, I., Katafigiotis, I., Pournaras, C., Fragkiadis, E., Leotsakos, I., Mitropoulos, D., Constantinides, C.A., 2013. A cough deteriorating gross hematuria: a clinical sign of a forthcoming life-threatening rupture of an intra-parenchymal aneurysm of renal artery (Wunderlich's Syndrome). Case Rep. Vasc. Med. 2013, 452317.

Archer, T.M., 2018. Varicella zoster lumbosacral plexopathy: a rare cause of lower limb weakness. BMJ. Case Rep. 2018.

Argyrakis, A., Teichmann, A., Kuhn, W., 1985. Solitary neurofibroma of the lumbosacral plexus. J. Neurol. Neurosurg. Psychiatry 48 (8), 844.

Aveline, C., Bonnet, F., 2004. Delayed retroperitoneal haematoma after failed lumbar plexus block. Br. J. Anaesth. 93 (4), 589—591.

Capek, S., Howe, B.M., Amrami, K.K., Spinner, R.J., 2015. Perineural spread of pelvic malignancies to the lumbosacral plexus and beyond: clinical and imaging patterns. Neurosurg. Focus 39 (3), E14.

Cavanagh, J.B., 1968. Prior x-irradiation and the cellular response to nerve crush: duration of effect. Exp. Neurol. 22 (2), 253—258.

Chad, D.A., Bradley, W.G., 1987. Lumbosacral plexopathy. Semin. Neurol. 7 (1), 97—107.

Cohen, R.D., Conn, D.L., Ilstrup, D.M., 1980. Clinical features, prognosis, and response to treatment in polyarteritis. Mayo. Clin. Proc. 55 (3), 146—155.

Colachis III, S.C., Pease, W.S., Johnson, E.W., 1994. A preventable cause of foot drop during childbirth. Am. J. Obstet. Gynecol. 171 (1), 270—272.

Cramer, G.D., Ro, C.S., 2017. The sacrum, sacroiliac joint, and coccyx. In: Clinical Anatomy of the Spine, Spinal Cord, and ANS-E-Book, p. 312.

Cream, J.J., 1976. Clinical and immunological aspects of cutaneous vasculitis. Q. J. Med. 45 (2), 255–276.

Dalmau, J., Graus, F., Marco, M., 1989. 'Hot and dry foot' as initial manifestation of neoplastic lumbosacral plexopathy. Neurology 39 (6), 871–872.

Day, M.H., 1964. The blood supply of the lumbar and sacral plexuses in the human foetus. J. Anat. 98, 104–116.

de Sousa, A.C.S., Capek, S., Howe, B.M., Jentoft, M.E., Amrami, K.K., Spinner, R.J., 2015. Magnetic resonance imaging evidence for perineural spread of endometriosis to the lumbosacral plexus: report of 2 cases. Neurosurg. Focus 39 (3), E15.

De Tommaso, O., Caporuscio, A., Tagariello, V., 2002. Neurological complications following central neuraxial blocks: are there predictive factors? Eur. J. Anaesthesiol. 19, 705–716.

Dhillon, S.S., Sarac, E., 2000. Lumbosacral plexopathy after dual kidney transplantation. Am. J. Kidney Dis. 36 (5), 1045–1048.

Dix, F.P., Titi, M., Al-Khaffaf, H., 2005. The isolated internal iliac artery aneurysm—a review. Eur. J. Vasc. Endovasc. Surg. 30 (2), 119–129.

Drake, R.L., Vogl, A.W., Mitchell, A.M., 2010. Pelvis and perineum. In: Schmitt, W., Gruliow, R., Adinolfi, A.M., et al. (Eds.), Gray's Anatomy for Students, second ed. Churchill Livingstone, Philadelphia, PA, pp. 404–502.

Dyck, P.J.B., Windebank, A.J., 2002. Diabetic and nondiabetic lumbosacral radiculoplexus neuropathies: new insights into pathophysiology and treatment. Muscle Nerve 25 (4), 477–491.

Dyck, P.J.B., Norell, J.E., Dyck, P.J., 1999. Microvasculitis and ischemia in diabetic lumbosacral radiculoplexus neuropathy. Neurology 53 (9), 2113.

Ebner, I., Anderl, H., Mikuz, G., Frommhold, H., 1990. Plexus neuropathy: tumor infiltration or radiation damage. Röfo 152 (6), 662–666.

Ergun, T., Lakadamyali, H., 2010. CT and MRI in the evaluation of extraspinal sciatica. Br. J. Radiol. 83 (993), 791–803.

Evans, B.A., Stevens, J.C., Dyck, P.J., 1981. Lumbosacral plexus neuropathy. Neurology 31 (10), 1327.

Fauci, A.S., Wolff, S.M., 1973. Wegener's granulomatosis: studies in eighteen patients and a review of the literature. Medicine 52 (6), 535–561.

Feasby, T.E., Burton, S.R., Hahn, A.F., 1992. Obstetrical lumbosacral plexus injury. Muscle Nerve 15 (8), 937–940.

Felice, K.J., Donaldson, J.O., 1995. Lumbosacral plexopathy due to benign uterine leiomyoma. Neurology 45 (10), 1943–1944.

Femminineo, A.F., LaBan, M.M., 1988. Paraparesis in a patient with Crohn disease resulting from septic arthritis of the hip and psoas abscess. Arch. Phys. Med. Rehabil. 69 (3 Pt. 1), 223–225.

Freitas, B., Figueiredo, R., Carrerette, F., Acioly, M.A., 2018. Retroperitoneoscopic resection of a lumbosacral plexus schwannoma: case report and literature review. J. Neurol. Surg. Cent. Eur. Neurosurg. 79 (3), 262–267.

Garcia-Moncó, J.C., Beldarrain, M.G., Estrade, L., 1993. Painful lumbosacral plexitis with increased ESR and Borrelia burgdorferi infection. Neurology 43 (6), 1269.

Gutmann, L., 1991. AAEM minimonograph# 37: facial and limb myokymia. Muscle Nerve 14 (11), 1043–1049.

Hefty, T.R., Nelson, K.A., Hatch, T.R., Barry, J.M., 1990. Acute lumbosacral plexopathy in diabetic women after renal transplantation. J. Urol. 143 (1), 107–109.

Jaeckle, K.A., Young, D.F., Foley, K.M., 1985. The natural history of lumbosacral plexopathy in cancer. Neurology 35 (1), 8.

Jaeckle, K.A., 2004. Neurological manifestations of neoplastic and radiation-induced plexopathies. Semin. Neurol. 24 (4), 385–393. PMID 15637650.

Katirji, B., Wilbourn, A.J., Scarberry, S.L., Preston, D.C., 2002. Intrapartum maternal lumbosacral plexopathy. Muscle Nerve 26 (3), 340–347.

Katz, R., Admon, D., Pode, D., 1997. Life-threatening retroperitoneal hematoma caused by anticoagulant therapy for myocardial infarction after SWL. J. Endourol. 11 (1), 23–25.

Kaymak, B., Özçakar, L., Çetin, A., Erol, Ö., Akoğlu, H., 2004. Bilateral lumbosacral plexopathy after femoral vein dialysis: synopsis of a case. Jt. Bone Spine 71 (4), 347–348.

Kent, K.C., Moscucci, M., Gallagher, S.G., DiMattia, S.T., Skillman, J.J., 1994. Neuropathy after cardiac catheterization: incidence, clinical patterns, and long-term outcome. J. Vasc. Surg. 19 (6), 1008–1014.

Khanna, S., Khanna, A.K., Mishra, S.P., Kumar Gupta, S., 2014. Pseudoaneurysm of internal iliac artery. Natl. J. Med. Res. 4 (2).

Kim, H., Kang, S.H., Kim, D.K., Seo, K.M., Kim, T.J., Hong, J., 2014. Bilateral ischemic lumbosacral plexopathy from chronic aortoiliac occlusion presenting with progressive paraplegia. J. Vasc. Surg. 59 (1), 241–243.

Krendel, D.A., Costigan, D.A., Hopkins, L.C., 1995. Successful treatment of neuropathies in patients with diabetes mellitus. Arch. Neurol. 52 (11), 1053–1061.

Kutsy, R.L., Robinson, L.R., Routt Jr., M.L., 2000. Lumbosacral plexopathy in pelvic trauma. Muscle Nerve 23 (11), 1757–1760.

Lang, E.M., Borges, J., Carlstedt, T., 2004. Surgical treatment of lumbosacral plexus injuries. J. Neurosurg. Spine 1, 64.

Lefebvre, V., Leduc, J.J., Choteau, P.H., 1995. Painless ischaemic lumbosacral plexopathy and aortic dissection. J. Neurol. Neurosurg. Psychiatry 58 (5), 641.

Luzzio, C.C., Waclawik, A.J., Gallagher, C.L., Knechtle, S.J., 1999. Iliac artery pseudoaneurysm following renal transplantation presenting as lumbosacral plexopathy. Transplantation 67 (7), 1077–1078.

Meuleman, J., Kuhlenbäumer, G., Schirmacher, A., Wehnert, M., De Jonghe, P., De Vriendt, E., Ringelstein, B., 1999. Genetic refinement of the hereditary neuralgic amyotrophy (HNA) locus at chromosome 17q25. Eur. J. Hum. Genet. 7 (8), 920.

Moore, M.E., Burke, J.M., Hartman, J.H., Korenzwitt, E., 1989. Lumbosacral plexopathy in a woman with CREST syndrome and vasculitis. Arthritis Rheum. 32 (5), 661–663.

Pascoe, M.K., Low, P.A., Windebank, A.J., Litchy, W.J., 1997. Subacute diabetic proximal neuropathy. Mayo Clin. Proc. 72 (12), 1123–1132.

Petchprapa, C.N., Rosenberg, Z.S., Sconfienza, L.M., Cavalcanti, C.F.A., La Rocca Vieira, R., Zember, J.S., 2010. MR imaging of entrapment neuropathies of the lower extremity: Part 1. The pelvis and hip. Radiographics 30 (4), 983–1000.

Pham, M., Sommer, C., Wessig, C., Monoranu, C.M., Pérez, J., Stoll, G., Bendszus, M., 2010. Magnetic resonance neurography for the diagnosis of extrapelvic sciatic endometriosis. Fertil. Steril. 94 (1). 351-e11.

Putti, V., 1927. New conceptions in the pathogenesis of sciatic pain. Lancet 2 (2), 53–60.

Qublan, H.S., Al-Sayegh, H., 2000. Intrapartum common peroneal nerve compression resulted in foot drop: a case report. J. Obstet. Gynaecol. Res. 26 (1), 13–15.

Sander, J.E., Sharp, F.R., 1981. Lumbosacral plexus neuritis. Neurology 31 (4 Pt. 2), 470–473.

Schmal, H., Hauschild, O., Culemann, U., Pohlemann, T., Stuby, F., Krischak, G., Südkamp, N.P., 2010. Identification of risk factors for neurological deficits in patients with pelvic fractures. Orthopedics 33 (8).

Selivanov, V., Chi, H.S., Alverdy, J.C., Morris, J.J., Sheldon, G.F., 1984. Mortality in retroperitoneal hematoma. J. Trauma 24 (12), 1022–1027.

Sharma, K.R., Sriram, S., Fries, T., Bevan, H.J., Bradley, W.G., 1993. Lumbosacral radiculoplexopathy as a manifestation of Epstein-Barr virus infection. Neurology 43 (12), 2550.

Soldatos, T., Andreisek, G., Thawait, G.K., Guggenberger, R., Williams, E.H., Carrino, J.A., Chhabra, A., 2013. High-resolution 3-T MR neurography of the lumbosacral plexus. Radiographics 33 (4), 967–987.

Steiner, I., Cohen, O., Leker, R.R., Rubinovitch, B., Handsher, R., Hassin-Baer, S., Sadeh, M., 1999. Subacute painful lumbosacral polyradiculoneuropathy in immunocompromised patients. J. Neurol. Sci. 162 (1), 91–93.

Stoeckli, T.C., Mackin, G.A., De Groote, M.A., 2000. Lumbosacral plexopathy in a patient with pulmonary tuberculosis. Clin. Infect. Dis. 30 (1), 226–227.

Stöhr, M., Dichgans, J., 1980. Ischaemic neuropathy of the lumbosacral plexus following intragluteal injection. J. Neurol. Neurosurg. Psychiatry 43 (6), 489–494.

Sugimoto, Y., Ito, Y., Tomioka, M., Tanaka, M., Hasegawa, Y., Nakago, K., Yagata, Y., 2010. Risk factors for lumbosacral plexus palsy related to pelvic fracture. Spine 35 (9), 963–966.

Tamburin, S., Magrinelli, F., Favaro, F., Briani, C., Zanette, G., 2014. Long-term response of neuropathic pain to intravenous immunoglobulin in relapsing diabetic lumbosacral radiculoplexus neuropathy. A case report. Pain Pract. 14 (2), E85–E90.

Taylor, B.V., Kimmel, D.W., Krecke, K.N., Cascino, T.L., 1997. Magnetic resonance imaging in cancer-related lumbosacral plexopathy. Mayo Clin. Proc. 72 (9), 823–829.

Thomas, J.E., Cascino, T.L., Earle, J.D., 1985. Differential diagnosis between radiation and tumor plexopathy of the pelvis. Neurology 35 (1), 1.

Tonetti, J., Cazal, C., Eid, A., Badulescu, A., Martinez, T., Vouaillat, H., Merloz, P., 2004. Neurological damage in pelvic injuries: a continuous prospective series of 50 pelvic injuries treated with an iliosacral lag screw. Rev. Chir. Orthop. Reparatrice. Appar. Mot. 90 (2), 122–131.

Wohlgemuth, W.A., Rottach, K.G., Stoehr, M., 1999. Intermittent claudication due to ischaemia of the lumbosacral plexus. J. Neurol. Neurosurg. Psychiatr. 67 (6), 793–795.

Wong, M., Vijayanathan, S., Kirkham, B., 2005. Sacroiliitis presenting as sciatica. Rheumatology 44 (10), 1323.

Zuniga, G., Ropper, A.H., Frank, J., 1991. Sarcoid peripheral neuropathy. Neurology 41 (10), 1558.

CHAPTER 22

Surgical Approaches to the Lumbosacral Plexus

AMGAD S. HANNA • PAUL PAGE

RETROPERITONEAL APPROACH TO THE ANTERIOR LUMBOSACRAL PLEXUS

Anatomy

The lumbosacral plexus is composed of anterior nerve roots from the twelfth thoracic to the fourth sacral vertebrae. The lumbar plexus can be described on the basis of its relationship to the psoas muscle as these nerves transition into the retroperitoneal space. The genitofemoral nerve is the only nerve to pass anterior to the psoas in this region. In cranial to caudal order, the iliohypogastric, ilioinguinal, lateral femoral cutaneous, and femoral nerves, respectively, traverse laterally. Medially, from cranial to caudal, the nerves include the obturator and accessory obturator nerves (the latter seen in approximately 10% of cases) and the lumbosacral trunk.

Regarding the sacral plexus, the ventral rami provide contributions from L4-S4 forming anterior to the piriformis muscle. The nerves of the sacral plexus can be divided into four groups according to their ultimate destination in the limb. Nerves exiting through the greater sciatic foramen traveling to the buttock include the superior and inferior gluteal nerves. The former traverses superiorly over the piriformis, while the latter exits below the piriformis. Nerves exiting through the greater sciatic foramen traveling to the lower extremity exit below the piriformis muscle and include the sciatic nerve and the posterior cutaneous nerve of the thigh. The third group of sacral nerves includes the pudendal nerve, which supplies the muscles of the perineum. It exits through greater sciatic foramen and re-enters the pelvis through the lesser sciatic foramen. A final group includes local innervation to the piriformis, superior and inferior gemellus, cutaneous nerves, and the parasympathetics splanchnic nerves.

Indications

Exposures of the lumbosacral plexus are much less common than exposures of the brachial plexus owing to its local anatomy and lower incidence of relevant pathologies. In general, trauma to the lumbosacral plexus is more rare than trauma to the brachial plexus. Pelvic neoplasms occasionally spread perineurally, and this can ultimately involve the lumbosacral nerve roots resulting in sciatica-like pain. A high degree of suspicion should be held for a patient with known pelvic neoplasms who develops sciatica-like pain. Iatrogenic injuries to this region are not uncommon and can occur during hip arthroplasty, direct interbody fusion, and a variety of pelvic surgeries. Given the large degree of exposure the retroperitoneal approach offers, it can easily be adapted to the specific need of the presenting pathology.

Technique (Fig. 22.1)

1. The patient is placed supine on the operating table or alternatively placed lateral on a bean bag.
2. Incision can be planned in the midline or parallel to the external oblique depending on the location of the pathology to be addressed. Dissection passes through Camper's fascia and then Scarpa's fascia.
3. Dissection then proceeds through the abdominal wall musculature, including the external oblique, internal oblique, and the transversus abdominis or alternatively through the rectus sheath.
4. Once the transversalis fascia is opened, the retroperitoneal fat is identified. Blunt dissection can then be used to expose the quadratus lumborum and iliacus. Further dissection allows the psoas major muscle to be identified medially.
5. Nerves lateral to the psoas muscle from superior to inferior include the iliohypogastric, ilioinguinal, lateral femoral cutaneous, and femoral. An additional layer of fascia overlying the posterior abdominal muscles must then be opened to identify the femoral nerve, which must be separated from the iliacus muscle.

Surgical Anatomy of the Sacral Plexus and Its Branches. https://doi.org/10.1016/B978-0-323-77602-8.00022-2

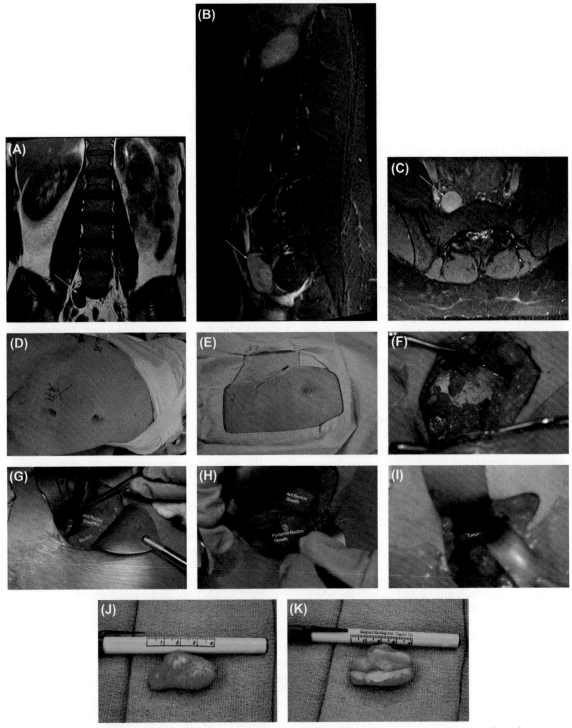

FIG. 22.1 A 32-year-old female presented with low back pain. MRI revealed an isointense lesion (arrow) on T1-weighted coronal **(A)**, hyperintense on sagittal T2-weighted **(B)**, and enhanced on axial with contrast **(C)**. A nerve sheath tumor was suspected. Surgical access was achieved by a vascular surgeon. An oblique right lower quadrant incision was performed **(D** and **E)**. The anterior rectus sheath was identified **(F)** and cut **(G)**. The posterior rectus sheath was then identified and opened **(H)**, allowing access to the retroperitoneal space and the tumor **(I)**. The tumor is shown after gross total resection **(J)** and in cross-section **(K)**. Pathology revealed schwannoma, WHO grade I.

6. Anterior to the psoas muscle, the genitofemoral nerve divides into its femoral and genital components. Medial to the psoas muscle, the obturator and the lumbosacral trunk are identified. However, their exposure requires mobilization of the iliac vessels.
7. The sacral plexus is located more deeply in the pelvis anterior to the piriformis muscle. For a complete exposure, the colon, rectum, and iliac vessels may require mobilization.

Complications

Given this dissection through the retroperitoneal space there is potential for injury to the vascular structures, including the iliac vessels, ureteric injury, and risk for bowel injury. Incisional hernias are rare but can occur with this approach, especially when the muscles are incised. Given the presence of these structures, an approach surgeon (usually a general, vascular, or trauma surgeon) is frequently recruited to limit those risks.

SCIATIC NERVE EXPOSURE
Anatomy

The sciatic nerve is formed by contributions from the L4 to S3 nerve roots after passing through the sacral plexus. Upon forming a single nerve, it traverses under the piriformis muscle and above the superior gemellus muscle, exiting the pelvis through the greater sciatic foramen. The sciatic nerve is composed of an anterior tibial component (L4-S3) and a posterior fibular nerve component (L4-S2). After exiting the foramen it passes through the buttock and then the posterior compartment of the thigh, superficial to the adductor magnus, to the popliteal fossa, where it divides into the tibial and common fibular nerves. The sciatic nerve itself supplies the biceps femoris, semimembranosus, semitendinosus, and the ischial portion of the adductor magnus.

Clinical Findings

Sciatic nerve injuries can result from a variety of trauma, autoimmune, musculoskeletal, and iatrogenic etiologies. Traumatic hip and hip fracture dislocations are frequent causes of such injuries at this level, occurring in approximately 10% of all cases of hip fractures (Cornwall and Radomisli, 2000). In such cases, the fibular component is most often injured, and there is 60%−70% nerve function recovery at least partially. In addition to trauma, sciatic nerve injury is a common complication following hip arthroplasty, especially when approached posteriorly. Overall sciatic nerve palsy occurs with hip arthroplasty in approximately 0.2%−2.5% of all cases and in up to 7.6% of cases following hip revision surgery (Stiehl and Stewart,

1998; Bistolfi et al., 2011). When the patient is evaluated for a potential sciatic nerve injury and for locating the lesion, it is important to note that the last branch of the fibular component in the posterior thigh supplies the biceps femoris, short head.

Exposures
Gluteal flap

1. Patient is positioned prone or lateral.
2. Incision is planned in a (reverse) question mark fashion starting at the lateral aspect of the hip, around the buttock, and vertically to the mid to upper thigh.
3. The superficial and deep fascia are incised.
4. The gluteus maximus insertion is identified and cut, ensuring a muscle cuff is left to suture to at the end of the procedure. After incision the gluteus maximus is lifted up and reflected medially.
5. The gluteus medius, gluteus minimus, and piriformis are subsequently identified. The fat pad below the piriformis is identified, and palpation then reveals the sciatic nerve as a cord-like structure.
6. The muscles deep to the sciatic nerve from cranial to caudal include the gemellus superior, obturator internus, gemellus inferior, quadratus femoris, and adductor magnus.
7. The pudendal nerve can be found medially and deep to the sciatic nerve.

Transgluteal (Fig. 22.2)

1. Oblique incision is made in the buttock along the fibers of the gluteus maximus.
2. Gluteus maximus is cut along its fibers.
3. The sciatic nerve is found in the fat pad deep to the muscle.

TIBIAL NERVE DECOMPRESSION
Anatomy

The tibial nerve is the medial terminal branch of the sciatic nerve originating at the lower third of the thigh or the cranial end of the popliteal fossa. After entering the popliteal fossa it continues in the midline and passes between the two heads of the gastrocnemius under the soleal arch. The tibial nerve supplies cutaneous innervation via the sural nerve, then travels in the medial aspect of the ankle. In the ankle it gives off a calcaneal branch prior to entering the tarsal tunnel and then divides into the medial and lateral plantar nerves. These nerves provide sensory innervation to the plantar surface of the foot as well as motor supply to the foot intrinsic muscles, while the medial calcaneal branches arise within the tarsal tunnel and innervate the skin over the heel.

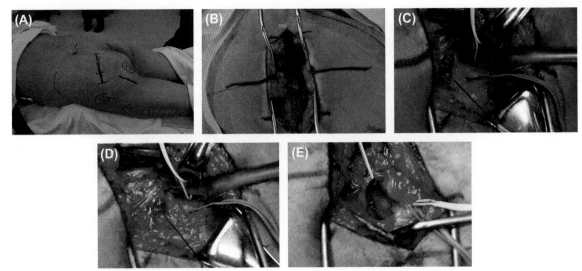

FIG. 22.2 **(A)**. Oblique incision made along gluteus maximus fibers. **(B)**. The gluteus maximus is identified and split along its fibers. **(C)**. Within the fat pad deep to the muscle, the sciatic nerve (blue loop) and posterior cutaneous nerve of the thigh (yellow loop) can be found. **(D)**. A black suture is placed along the piriformis inferior edge. **(E)**. Complete sciatic nerve decompression after resection of the piriformis muscle. *GT*, greater trochanter; *IT*, ischial tuberosity.

Motor innervation by the tibial nerve supplies muscles in the superficial and deep compartments of the leg. The superficial muscles in the posterior compartment innervated by the tibial nerve include the plantaris, soleus, and gastrocnemius. In the deep compartment the tibial nerve innervates the popliteus, flexor hallucis longus, flexor digitorum longus, and tibialis posterior.

Clinical Findings

The tibial nerve can be entrapped at the level of the soleal arch or the posterior tarsal tunnel. More distally, the tibial nerve can be a site of Morton's neuromas, which affect the digital branches of the medial plantar nerve between either the second and third or the third and fourth metatarsals. Clinically, tibial nerve compression can result in weakness of foot plantar flexion, pain radiating into the sole of the foot, and numbness in the plantar surface of the foot. Of note, tarsal tunnel syndrome can present as a part of the "heel pain triad" consisting of posterior tibial tendon deficiency, plantar fasciitis, and tarsal tunnel syndrome. This triad is believed to occur because the dynamic and static stabilizers of the medial arch are lost, resulting in traction neuropathy of the tibial nerve.

Exposures

Popliteal fossa exposure

1. Patient is placed in the prone position.
2. Incision is planned in the posterior midline to expose the lower thigh and upper leg. Care should be made to avoid crossing the knee crease if at all possible. If the knee crease is to be crossed, a Z-shaped incision can be considered.
3. Upon incision the superficial fascia is divided, followed by the deep fascia.
4. The fibular nerve can be found laterally, and the tibial nerve will be found in the midline.
5. Once the tibial nerve is identified it can then be followed distally to identify its branches to the gastrocnemius and contributions to the sural nerve. Further distally, the nerve passes under the two heads of the gastrocnemius. If compression is felt at this point, the 2 heads should be separated. The soleal arch should be opened. The plantaris and part of the soleus fascia could be resected for more complete decompression.

Tarsal tunnel

1. Patient is placed supine with leg externally rotated.
2. Procedure can be conducted under general anesthesia or local anesthetic with sedation.
3. Tourniquet can be used for bloodless dissection.
4. Incision is planned between the medial malleolus and the calcaneus in a curvilinear fashion.
5. Following incision, the superficial and deep fasciae are dissected to identify the flexor retinaculum.
6. The flexor retinaculum is opened with sharp dissection, allowing the tibial nerve and posterior tibial vessels to be visualized.

7. The first branch to be identified is usually the calcaneal branch, which arises from the posterior aspect of the tibial nerve coursing posteriorly and caudally.
8. As the tibial nerve runs distally, it divides into the medial and lateral plantar nerves traveling distally under the abductor hallucis.
9. The medial and lateral plantar nerves run in individual tunnels separated by a septum. Each nerve must be decompressed individually and the intervening septum resected to ensure adequate decompression.
10. Care should be taken during dissection to avoid injury to the saphenous nerve anteriorly and the calcaneal branch posteriorly.

Intermetatarsal

1. Patient is positioned supine.
2. Straight incision is planned between the second and third toes, or third or fourth, on the dorsum of the foot.
3. After incision, the intermetatarsal ligament is identified and transected. The digital nerve is then decompressed.
4. A swollen nerve in this location (so-called Morton's neuroma) is usually reactive and should be left alone to recover. However, a true neuroma should be resected and have a nerve graft placed, or resected and buried in a muscle.

FIBULAR NERVE DECOMPRESSION

Anatomy

The common fibular (peroneal) nerve is the lateral terminal branch of the sciatic nerve that conducts sensory information from the lateral aspect of the leg and dorm of the foot and provides motor innervation to the anterolateral leg. The common fibular nerve has three branches, namely, the superficial fibular nerve, the deep fibular nerve, and an articular branch.

The superficial fibular nerve provides motor innervation to the fibularis longus and fibularis brevis. This branch also provides sensory innervation to the lateral aspect of the lower leg and dorsal aspect of the foot. Contributions arise from the L4, L5, and S1 nerve roots. In contrast to the superficial fibular nerve, the deep fibular nerve provides motor innervation to the tibialis anterior, extensor digitorum longus, extensor hallucis longus, and fibularis tertius. The deep branch provides sensory innervation to the dorsum of the first web space. It courses under the extensor retinaculum through the anterior tarsal tunnel. The anterior tarsal tunnel contains the deep fibular nerve, tibialis anterior, extensor hallucis longus,

extensor digitorum longus, and anterior tibial artery. In contrast, the posterior tarsal tunnel contains the tibial nerve, posterior tibial artery, tibialis posterior tendon, flexor digitorum longus, and flexor hallucis longus.

Clinical Findings

Common fibular nerve compression can be consistent with clinical findings of motor deficits, sensory deficits, pain, or any combination of the above. Fibular neuropathy is common following trauma including knee dislocations or fractures; less direct causes include significant weight changes, increased activity overlying the knee joint, ganglion cyst formation, osteophyte formation, or other changes in medical history. Injury frequently results in a foot drop with intact foot inversion given the absence of involvement of the tibial nerve. A recent retrospective study of 217 patients presenting with paresis or complete paralysis of the foot dorsiflexors found that 68% had a nerve abnormality and 31% had weakness secondary to a common fibular nerve lesion (Van Langenhove et al., 1989). This neuropathy should not be confused with an L5 radiculopathy, which can also present with pain in this distribution and an associated foot drop with loss of inversion. A full clinical evaluation must be conducted to ensure the correct diagnosis.

Exposures
Around the fibular head (Fig. 22.3)

1. Patient should be placed lateral.
2. A curvilinear incision is made on the posterior border of the fibular head and lateral to the fibular neck. The fibular head should be easily identified by palpation at the level of the tibial tuberosity.
3. The superficial and deep fasciae are identified and opened. The common fibular nerve should be easily felt running laterally along the fibular neck.
4. The nerve sheath is opened and the common fibular nerve is decompressed posterior to the biceps femoris tendon, fibular head, and lateral to the fibular neck.
5. To ensure complete decompression the common fibular nerve should be followed proximally into the popliteal fat pad.
6. Distally, the nerve should be followed under the fibular fascia. The superficial layer of fascia should be identified first and cut followed by the deeper layer of fascia, which can be identified by retracting the muscle then cut.
7. Following this the superficial, deep, and articular branches of the fibular nerve should be easily identified with no evidence of compression.

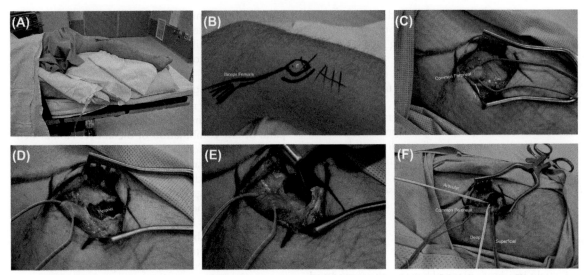

FIG. 22.3 The patient is positioned laterally on a beanbag **(A)**. The incision is made posterior to the fibular head (F) and lateral to the fibular neck **(B)**. Once the deep fascia is opened, the common fibular nerve can be identified (blue loop) **(C)**. The fascia superficial to the fibular muscles is opened **(D)**. The muscle is then retracted **(E)**, thus exposing the fascia underneath that needs to be released. After full decompression **(F)**, all the branches of the common fibular nerve can be identified.

Lower leg and ankle (superficial fibular nerve)

1. Patient is positioned supine.
2. Oblique incision is planned along the lateral aspect of the lower leg.
3. Terminal dorsal cutaneous branches are found piercing the deep fascia in the lower third of the leg in the subcutaneous fat; intermediate dorsal cutaneous branch laterally, medial dorsal cutaneous branch medially. For full decompression, the deep fascia should be opened widely.
4. Note: Ultrasound guidance may be helpful to identify small cutaneous nerves preoperatively or intraoperatively.

Anterior tarsal tunnel (deep fibular nerve)

1. Patient is positioned supine.
2. Incision planned for midline in the dorsum of the ankle.
3. Extensor retinaculum is opened.
4. The anterior tibial artery and vein are identified and should be preserved. The deep fibular nerve is found closely associated with these vessels.
5. Tibialis anterior and extensor hallucis longus will be identified medial to the deep fibular nerve. Extensor digitorum longus will be located lateral to the deep fibular nerve.

SURAL NERVE

Anatomy

The sural nerve is a purely sensory nerve formed by the union of the medial sural cutaneous nerve, a branch of the tibial nerve, with the lateral sural cutaneous nerve, a branch of the common fibular nerve. While the most common configuration involves contributions from both the tibial and fibular nerves, there are variations in which there are only fibular or only tibial contributions (Riedl and Frey, 2013). The medial and lateral sural cutaneous nerves unite in the distal third of the leg in as many as 84% of patients (Coert and Dellon, 1994). The primary function of the sural nerve is to provide cutaneous innervation to the skin of the lateral foot and ankle. This nerve lies in the plane between the lateral malleolus and Achilles tendon at the level of the ankle. The lesser saphenous vein is almost invariably adjacent to it (Strauch et al., 2005). During harvesting, care must be taken to ensure this vein is not mistakenly harvested given its close proximity.

Indications

Sural nerve harvesting has come to be used for a variety of indications. Most commonly, sural nerve biopsy is a common method for evaluating a variety of peripheral neuropathies. While a biopsy can be useful and necessary, it should serve as a supplementary test rather than a substitute for extensive clinical and laboratory investigations, including characterization of the disease inheritance, distribution, course, electromyographic findings, imaging findings, and availability of DNA testing (Said, 2002). In addition to nerve biopsy, the sural nerve is most commonly harvested in nerve reconstruction surgery for cable grafting owing to its ready accessibility and minimal neurological consequences following harvest.

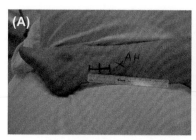 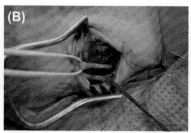 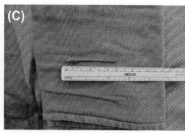

FIG. 22.4 **(A).** A 4 cm incision is made between the lateral malleolus and Achilles tendon. **(B).** The sural nerve (yellow loop), along with the short saphenous vein (red loop) are identified. **(C).** This usually allows about 6 cm of sural nerve to be harvested for biopsy.

Technique (Fig. 22.4)

1. For a standard sural nerve biopsy, the patient is positioned laterally under local anesthesia and monitored anesthesia care. In the setting of nerve grafting this harvest can easily be conducted in the supine position with leg elevated.
2. The incision is marked posterior to the lateral malleolus and anterior to the Achilles tendon. A 4-cm incision is sufficient to obtain up to a 6-cm nerve segment.
3. Following incision, dissection is carried through the subcutaneous space. A self-retaining retractor is placed, which allows the sural nerve and short saphenous vein to be visualized rapidly.
4. Dissection can then proceed circumferentially and vertically.
5. Upon proximal dissection the contributions from the tibial and fibular nerves can be encountered. Of note, these contributions occasionally fail to unite, and the sural nerve can appear as two separate nerves.
6. Upon sectioning the nerve for removal, the proximal section should be cut first to minimize discomfort to the patient.

Complications

Complications following harvesting include risk of wound infection, pain from neuroma formation, and loss of sensation on the lateral aspect of the dorsum of the foot and little toe.

REFERENCES

Bistolfi, A., Massazza, G., Deledda, D., et al., 2011. Operative management of sciatic nerve palsy due to impingement on the metal cage after total hip revision: case report. Case Rep. Med. 2011, 830296.

Coert, J.H., Dellon, A.L., 1994. Clinical implications of the surgical anatomy of the sural nerve. Plast. Reconstr. Surg. 94, 850–855.

Cornwall, R., Radomisli, T.E., 2000. Nerve injury in traumatic dislocation of the hip. Clin. Orthop. Relat. Res. 377, 84–91.

Riedl, O., Frey, M., 2013. Anatomy of the sural nerve: cadaver study and literature review. Plast. Reconstr. Surg. 131 (4), 802–810.

Said, G., 2002. Indications and usefulness of nerve biopsy. Arch. Neurol. 59 (10), 1532–1535.

Stiehl, J.B., Stewart, W.A., 1998. Late sciatic nerve entrapment following pelvic plate reconstruction in total hip arthroplasty. J. Arthroplasty 13 (5), 586–588.

Strauch, B., Goldberg, N., Herman, C.K., 2005. Sural nerve harvest: anatomy and technique. J. Reconstr. Microsurg. 21 (2), 133–136.

Van Langenhove, M., Pollefliet, A., Vanderstraeten, G., 1989. A retrospective electrodiagnostic evaluation of footdrop in 303 patients. Electromyogr. Clin. Neurophysiol. 29, 145–152.

Index

Note: Page numbers followed by "t" indicate tables and "f" indicate figures.

Printed and bound by CPI Group (UK) Ltd, Croydon, CR0 4YY

08/05/2025

01864763-0001